Ethical Dilemmas in Pediatrics

Cases and Commentaries

T0186151

Children in precarious health present particular problems for healthcare professionals because of their intimate relation to their family, and because of the family's need to provide major long-term support and to be actively involved in the decisions about their children's care. This collection of cases and commentaries in pediatrics highlights the difficult ethical dilemmas that can arise during high-tech hospital care of children in precarious circumstances. It serves as a teaching tool for clinical ethics, as an introduction for medical students and residents, and as a review for practicing physicians. Clinical cases are described in detail by the physicians involved, who focus on the ethical issues arising during treatment. Each case is then commented on in detail by a philosopher or other bioethicist. It thus serves as an introduction to contemporary clinical bioethics, but with a firm grounding in the practicalities of real-life pediatric care in the hospital setting.

Ethical Dilemmas in Pediatrics

Cases and Commentaries

Edited by

Lorry R. Frankel

Amnon Goldworth

Mary V. Rorty

and

William A. Silverman

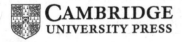

CAMBRIDGE
UNIVERSITY PRESS

CAMBRIDGE UNIVERSITY PRESS
Cambridge, New York, Melbourne, Madrid, Cape Town, Singapore, São Paulo, Delhi

Cambridge University Press
The Edinburgh Building, Cambridge CB2 8RU, UK

Published in the United States of America by Cambridge University Press, New York

www.cambridge.org
Information on this title: www.cambridge.org/9780521118613

First published 2005
This digitally printed version 2009

A catalogue record for this publication is available from the British Library

ISBN 978-0-521-84744-5 hardback
ISBN 978-0-521-11861-3 paperback

Contents

v

Contributors

Stephen Ashwal, M.D.
Department of Pediatrics, Division of Child
Neurology, Loma Linda University Adventist
Health Sciences Center, Loma Linda,
California 92350, USA

Roger Burne, M.B., B.S.
St. Bartholomew's Medical Centre, Cowley
Rd, Oxford OX4 1XB, UK

Ricardo Orlando Castillo, M.D.
Department of Pediatrics, Division of
Gastroenterology, Lucile Packard Children's
Hospital, Palo Alto, California 94304, USA

Clifford Chin, M.D.
Department of Pediatrics, Division of
Pediatric Cardiology, Lucile Packard
Children's Hospital, Palo Alto,
California 94304, USA

Ronald Cohen, M.D.
Division of Neonatal and Developmental
Medicine, Lucile Packard Children's
Hospital, Palo Alto, California 94304, USA

Joseph V. DiCarlo, M.D.
Department of Pediatrics, Division of
Critical Care Medicine, Lucile Packard
Children's Hospital, Palo Alto,
California 94304, USA

Douglas S. Diekema, M.D.
Department of Emergency Services,
Children's Hospital and Medical Center,
Seattle, Washington 98105, USA

Joel E. Frader, M.D.
General Academic Pediatrics, Feinberg
School of Medicine, 700 West Fullerton
Avenue, Chicago, Illinois 60614, USA

Lorry R. Frankel, M.D.
Department of Pediatrics, Division of
Critical Care Medicine, Lucile Packard
Children's Hospital, Palo Alto,
California 94304, USA

Manuel Garcia-Careaga, M.D.
Department of Pediatrics, Division of
Gastroenterology, Lucile Packard
Children's Hospital, Palo Alto,
California 94304, USA

Amnon Goldworth, Ph.D.
Senior Medical Ethicist in Residence, Lucile
Packard Children's Hospital, Palo Alto,
California 94304, USA

Linda Granowetter, M.D.
Columbia University Pediatric Oncology,
161 Fort Washington Avenue I-7, New York,
New York 10032, USA

Nancy S. Jecker, Ph.D.
Department of Medical History and Ethics,
School of Medicine, University of
Washington, Seattle, Washington 98195,
USA

Frances M. Kamm, Ph.D.
Kennedy School of Government,
Harvard University, 79 JFK Street,
Cambridge, Massachusetts 02138,
USA

John A. Kerner, Jr., M.D.
Department of Pediatrics, Division of
Gastroenterology, Lucile Packard
Children's Hospital, Palo Alto,
California 94304, USA

Eugene Kim, M.D.
Chief of Neonatology, Santa Clara Valley
Medical Center, 751 Bascom Avenue,
San Jose, California 95128, USA

Lawrence H. Mathers, M.D., Ph.D.
Department of Pediatrics, Division of
Critical Care Medicine, Lucile Packard
Children's Hospital, Palo Alto,
California 94304, USA

Richard B. Miller, Ph.D.
Poynter Center for the Study of
Ethics and American Institutions, Indiana
University, Bloomington, Indiana 47405,
USA

Robert Orr, M.D., C.M.
Director of Clinical Ethics, University of
Vermont College of Medicine, Burlington,
Vermont 05405, USA

Joy Penticuff, Ph.D., R.N., F.A.A.N.
School of Nursing, University of Texas at
Austin, Austin, Texas 78701, USA

Ronald M. Perkin, M.D.
Department of Pediatrics, Brody School of
Medicine, East Carolina University,
Greenville, North Carolina 27834, USA

Chester J. Randle, Jr., M.D.
Department of Pediatrics, Kaiser
Permanente, Oakland Medical Center,
280 West MacArthur Boulevard, Oakland,
California 94611, USA

Rosamond Rhodes, Ph.D.
Director of Bioethics Education, Mount
Sinai School of Medicine, One Gustav Levy
Place, New York, New York 10029, USA

Mary V. Rorty, Ph.D.
Stanford University Center for Biomedical
Ethics, 701 Welch Road, Suite 1105,
Palo Alto, California 94304, USA

William A. Silverman, M.D.
Professor of Pediatrics (retired), Columbia
University College of Physicians & Surgeons,
New York 10032, USA

Anita Silvers, Ph.D.
Department of Philosophy, San Francisco
State University, 1600 Holloway Avenue,
San Francisco, California 94132, USA

Simon N. Whitney, M.D., J.D.
Department of Family and Community
Medicine, Baylor College of Medicine,
3701 Kirby Drive, Suite 600, Houston,
Texas 77098, USA

Preface

The editors would like to offer their thanks to the authors of the chapters in this book for their thoughtful contributions. Inheritors of a long tradition of silent service, they have been willing to add their voices to an ongoing dialogue between providers of and observers of medical care in the late twentieth and early twenty-first centuries, for which we are grateful.

The children and the families for whom we have had the privilege of caring during their various illnesses are honored as well in these pages, though the details of the cases have been changed by the authors to prevent any identification of particular patients.

Although it is the physician's voice that is most often heard in this volume, we gratefully acknowledge that the work of the hospital involves many helping professions, including nurses, therapists, chaplains, social workers, and clinical ethicists.

The areas of pediatric medicine and of medical ethics have been impoverished by the loss of William A. Silverman, who died as this volume was in preparation.

The book has been greatly helped by the thoughtful comments of anonymous reviewers and the scrupulous and authoritative editorial work of Hugh Brazier, and is dedicated to our families, who support our work, and to the children.

Introduction

Medicine, dealing as it does with human beings when they are most vulnerable, is a combination of science, technology – and ethics. All human action has ethical implications, and this book is an exercise in making explicit the ethical implications of action by practicing physicians and other clinicians in the context of a particularly vulnerable population, the infants and children in pediatric medical practice. The book is aimed at several possible audiences, including the primary-care providers who care for children with a high mortality risk or the potential for significant debilitating morbidity, and the physicians in tertiary-care institutions, for whom the clinical scenarios described will sound very familiar. It can serve as a case collection for ethics education of ethics committee members, medical students, and residents. But it is hoped that it will be useful as well to those non-medical professionals who play a role in the ethical life of healthcare institutions, or to lay people who have reason to seek to learn more about the specialized and sometimes confusing world of high-tech care for seriously ill children and the thoughtful and well-intentioned healthcare professionals who wrestle with ethical issues in that world.

To maximize its usefulness to this variety of possible constituencies, the editors have chosen a case and commentary format, asking physicians (and in one case a nurse) to provide detailed clinical accounts of cases in their practice which presented perplexing ethical issues. We have then matched each case with a bioethicist, asking for an ethical commentary on the issue which seems most salient to the respondent, on the basis of the description given by the clinician. With each chapter the editors have included short discussions of ethical issues raised by or discussed in the case and commentary, including references for further reading in the medical and bioethics literature.

There is considerable variation in the way the cases are presented, reflecting different styles of case review. While the degree of attention to blood chemistry or particular pharmaceuticals in some cases may be bewildering to the non-clinician, it is attention to such empirical details that reveals the clinical picture to the physician;

and the ethical dimensions of a medical case are implicated by the clinical picture. Predictive clinical data provide the context in which value judgments are made about whether or not a medical intervention counts as a viable therapeutic option. Non-clinicians seeking to improve their familiarity with clinical culture will find the meticulous medical detail and attention to context of the clinical cases an illuminating change from the often schematic and spare examples typical of many introductory bioethics texts.

It is not surprising that many of the cases feature hard decisions around care at the end of life. Such cases are memorable, conflicted, and complex, and often incorporate tacit or explicit conflicts of obligation, of commitment, and of loyalty. Sometimes no good can be obtained without forgoing another good; sometimes the only choice is between equally bad options. The high emotions, the clinical unpredictability, and the heightened impact of decisions at the end of life can contribute to turning a clinical crisis into an ethical one. While this concentration on the frontiers of medical practice makes some ethical issues very salient, it remains true that the same range of issues arise in many more familiar cases drawn from primary-care practice, where the stakes may be as high and the consequences as tragic for patients and their families.

Pediatric medicine

Pediatric clinical ethics is to be distinguished from general clinical ethics for several reasons. Pediatric medicine must take account of a three-way relationship, involving physician, patient, and family (normally the parents) rather than the dyadic relation that is more typical in adult medicine. The adult patient can participate in the decision-making process. While husband or wife, mother or father may have an advisory role in determining treatment strategies, the adult patient has the final say in consenting to treatment. By contrast, in the pediatric setting the parents are usually the consenting parties. The pediatrician is thus more explicitly responsible to the parents than the oncologist or internist typically is to the family members of his or her adult patient.

Adult medicine also may deal with incapable patients – with individuals incapacitated by age, disease, or injury, as well as nominally adult patients who have for various reasons never attained capacity. For previously capable patients there is some possibility of considering what their treatment preferences might have been were they not incapacitated. Advance directives, previously expressed opinions, or remembered discussions give clues for surrogates attempting to exercise substitute judgment for now-incapable adults. The question of surrogate decision making for pediatric patients has different parameters. "Precedent autonomy" of the sort invoked by some writers in connection with treatment decisions for Alzheimer's patients (Dworkin 1993) is not available for very young infants, who have had no opportunity to form patterns of preference or to indicate their wishes. The only possibility is to invoke something like "precursor autonomy": to recognize that the presently incapable child is potentially a capable future person for whom the maximum of available options should be held open.

Such considerations, except for adolescent patients, are typically "best interests" judgments, not substitute decision making. One commentator has suggested that while respect for patient autonomy is the governing value in adult medicine, in pediatric medicine the duty of beneficence takes precedence over autonomy. Thus professionals may presume to protect or promote the patient's welfare with fewer limits on their authority than in the case of adult medicine (Miller 2003: 2).

All physicians seek to satisfy the best interests of the patient. When that patient is a minor, a helpless and vulnerable child, the importance of protecting those interests is particularly pressing. At the same time, the pediatric physician, more than many of his or her peers, must consider the situation, the interests, and the preferences of the family as part of the agenda. The child's interests cannot be viewed in isolation from the family, for it is the family that typically forms the major enduring and sustaining context for the child. The possibility of a conflict between the child's best interest and the family's best interest adds a dimension when ethical issues arise in the care of children. In cases where there is a clear conflict, such as parental abuse, negligence, or requests by parents for non-beneficial treatment, the professional duty to the child takes precedence, despite practical difficulties that arise in obtaining alternatives to the parents as advocates for the child. Pediatric medicine is an exercise in psychosocial, as well as technical medical, expertise.

Medical ethics, clinical ethics, bioethics

Healthcare organizations and the professionals employed or contracted with them have generally relied on professional or clinical ethics to provide guidance for difficult decisions. Physicians, nurses, and hospital administrators all operate under professional codes which are "Hippocratic" – that is, they acknowledge the primacy of the welfare of the patient as the governing value of their functions. The same is true of other health professionals. Professional ethics is fundamental to the dyadic relationship of the patient and the responsible physician, and enjoins honesty, confidentiality, attention to technical competence and good character, and advance of medical knowledge. Medical ethics is an important part of the education and professional socialization of medical professionals.

Clinical ethics, a patient-centered application of biomedical ethics, has developed for dispute resolution and mediation in clinical settings. A relative newcomer to the medical context, clinical ethics is premised on the assumption that people with a variety of professional (or personal) perspectives and roles may have an equal moral stake in the care of a particular patient, and need to have their voices heard in making treatment decisions in conflicted or ethically complex cases. This development has several roots. It is partially a result of a growing consumer activism that has extended into many areas, having as one result attention to patients' (and families') rights. It is responsive as well to shifts in healthcare delivery. Health care in the last few decades in the United States has increasingly been delivered through a team model in complex institutions. When numerous clinicians and hospital personnel are directly involved in patient care, cases can arise where inadequate communication, conflicts between caregivers, or differences between family members about appropriate treatments can create impediments to or interruptions in the implementation of plans of care for individual patients. It has thus become a condition of accreditation for US hospitals of more than 200 beds to establish an "ethics process," typically an ethics committee, to advise in the adjudication of such disputes. Discussions of these individual clinical cases may involve informed-consent issues, life-and-death decision making, pain and suffering, and the uses of power in clinical settings, as well as such issues as communication, disclosure, and truth telling. Clinical ethics focuses on making differing perspectives explicit and, where possible and appropriate, working toward agreement on the proper priority of shared values. It is typically a multidisciplinary practice, involving physicians and nurses, but also clinicians from allied health professions, social workers, chaplains, sometimes lawyers with health-related specialties, and individuals from such academic disciplines as philosophy, religion, or the social sciences who have familiarized themselves with clinical medical practice. People who identify themselves as clinical ethicists are involved in education, institutional policy deliberations, and ethics consultation in healthcare organizations, contributing to hospital ethics committees and engaging in discussion with clinical practitioners about ethical issues which arise in practice settings. Clinical ethics has been described as "a bridge between the clinical world of health care practice and the theoretical disciplines of bioethics and medical humanities in the academic world" (Fletcher *et al.* 1997: 7). Many of the chapters make reference to the presence and involvement of ethics committees in the cases discussed.

Bioethics as a social movement and academic practice has developed rapidly since the early 1970s. It is to some extent misleading to suggest that bioethics is a discipline. It is more properly described as a multidisciplinary research and practice, involving individuals with many different academic and professional backgrounds. Some sociologists, anthropologists, and historians, some philosophers, nurses, and theologians, some biologists, lawyers, and many physicians, draw upon and contribute to the burgeoning literature of bioethics. Nor is it solely theoretical. One scholar, contrasting bioethics with clinical ethics, characterizes bioethics as "greatly concerned with public policy issues" (Siegler 1979: 915), and in the USA as in many other countries one of the most visible forums for bioethical deliberation is in state- and federal-level bioethics commissions. The European Union and the United Nations have similar committees working on the international level.

When participating in policy or clinical discussions, participants with theological commitments may take those into consideration, just as lawyers may consider first the legal constraints or precedent cases. Philosophers who have turned their attention to bioethical issues, on either the policy or clinical levels, often have a temptingly rich body of philosophical ethical theorizing at their disposal. Those who prove most useful in those contexts, whatever their background, are able to draw from their areas of expertise elements which, when introduced into discussion, are able to broaden the range of issues under consideration, present perspectives that enlighten participants, and provide good reasons for one or another policy or course of action. In a pluralistic society the reasons that seem determinative for one participant or another, be they legal or theological, consequentialist or cultural, may be less persuasive to other affected parties. The purpose of a book on ethics and medical practice is not to provide definitive "right answers" that can silence dialogue, but to remind us that it is good reasons that provide both justification and motivation for action, and to encourage, and to illustrate, the search for reasons for treatment decisions.

Ethical approaches to clinical issues

There is a wide range of variation in the commentaries as well as in the cases, since the respondents come from different theoretical backgrounds and have a wide range of interests, reflecting the wide range of concerns in the changing field of bioethics. The commentators tend to be collaborators rather than critics, often tacitly entering into dialogue with the perplexities of the clinicians, or contributing their perspective with the freedom that can come from being an observer, rather than a participant. Philosophers predominate among the respondents, but clinical and legal training have also informed various commentaries.

Opening a dialogue between medicine and bioethics requires choosing a common vocabulary in which the issues can be discussed, and as the various respondents interact with the descriptions of the cases provided by the physicians, different commentators choose different vocabularies. One might think of the different uses of ethical vocabulary as "styles" of reasoning – principlism, casuistry, narrative. The common discourse of legal obligations features in some of the commentaries. Other commentators, and some of the physicians as well, utilize the vocabulary of the bioethics principles introduced in the first bioethics commission report in 1982 – beneficence and non-maleficence, autonomy and justice – to illuminate aspects of the cases which seem particularly deserving of ethical attention

(President's Commission 1982). The "methods" debate in bioethics is reflected in the different styles of commentary, with some commentators utilizing, others criticizing, application of ethical principles to specific clinical cases. Though each response is quite specific, the editors hope that the cumulative effect will broaden readers' appreciation of the range of ethical concerns clinical cases raise, and the variety of approaches available to deal with those concerns.

Ethical deliberation arises when agents ask "what should I do?" In some unproblematic situations the answer may be "whatever I can." In other situations agents may have cause to wonder whether something within their power is nevertheless a less preferable option, or find themselves wrestling with the consequences of doing their best. It is such cases that fill the following pages. In problematic situations, decision makers find themselves asking: What are the risks and benefits of each alternative? What are the rights of the individuals involved? How are the benefits and burdens of each possible course of action distributed (Foreman and Ladd 1991: 2–3)?

There is one consistent feature of the vocabulary, and of the concerns, of actors and commentators in the cases discussed: a recognition of the extent to which medical intervention, especially, if not uniquely, in pediatrics, is also an intervention into the varied, complex, and intimate arena of family relationships. The presumption, usually justified, is that parents have their children's best interests at heart, and are exercising affection and knowledge, as well as authority, over their children's lives. Anything that impacts the most vulnerable member affects the entire family, and this recognition permeates the book.

The complexity of the relation of children to their families in the light of third-party interventions, especially, although not only, medical interventions, has been the subject of considerable recent discussion. Contemporary liberal society has been characterized by a great emphasis on privacy and individual rights. Various critics, including feminists, communitarians, and disability-rights advocates, have complained that the liberal ideal insufficiently values intimate relations and devalues lives that include as central components various kinds of dependencies and interrelations. Several recent books have attempted to deal in detail with the relation of parental rights and family privacy to the general social and the specific medical obligations to protect the welfare of children, seeking to find a balance between acknowledgment of the importance of the family to the growing child, and the recognition that as a person-in-process the child may have some needs and interests other than those provided by the family (Nelson and Nelson 1995, Ross 1998, Miller 2003).

There is no doubt that the changing conditions of healthcare delivery in the United States, including the growth of managed care and the increasing emphasis on cost-containment and efficiency, is having an impact upon clinical medicine and clinical ethics. Often a subtext in our cases, questions of cost and third-party control of clinical decision making are explicitly raised by the last two contributions to this volume. As the impact of these changes is increasingly felt in clinical practice, there will be more need for explicitly addressing them, through institutional focus on ethics, through political processes, and through regulation and legislation (Spencer *et al.* 2000). Professional organizations, groups of concerned citizens, formal and informal ethics and policy processes, local, state, and federal governments, are increasingly focusing on the ethical and cultural, as well as fiscal, impact of clinical decision making. It is hoped that this volume can advance the integration of ethical and medical decision making in these changing times.

Structure of the book

The book is divided into four parts. Part I, "Therapeutic misalliances," includes three cases where for various reasons the root presupposition of medical care, a relationship of trust and collaboration between physician and patient or surrogate, is disrupted. The three cases call to our attention the extent to which alteration in the conditions of trust and communication within which medical care is expected to be delivered cascades into complications in both clinical and ethical decision making.

Part II, "Medical futility," addresses treatment decisions in circumstances where a variety of factors must be taken into consideration, but none of the options can provide the most hoped-for outcome. The interpenetration of facts and values complicates these cases where medical science alone cannot resolve all questions.

Part III, "Life by any means," presents three cases where only very complex, invasive, and high-risk interventions can postpone the death of pediatric patients, and in the case discussions and commentaries it becomes increasingly clear how much clinical decision making is influenced by the wider context – not only the institutional context, but the wider social environment, including the economic, technological, and cultural environment.

Part IV, "Institutional impediments to ethical action," focuses on the institutional context, calling attention to ways in which institutional arrangements – attention to continuity of care, or to mechanisms for appropriate consultation – can help or hinder ethically excellent medical care. The final contribution explicitly addresses the effects on traditional medical practice of contemporary alterations in the way healthcare delivery is financed.

References for the chapters are cited in the text, with complete references at the end of the book. Readings associated with each "Topical discussion" follow that section.

Part I

Therapeutic misalliances

The ideal relationship between physician and patient, or in the pediatric setting, between physician, patient, and parent, is a therapeutic alliance. In this alliance, both parties have a common understanding of the goals of treatment and the means by which to achieve them. The physician's perspective is that of the medical expert who best understands the appropriate means. The parent's perspective is that of an autonomous agent concerned with the well-being of his or her baby as this bears on the interests of the entire family.

The therapeutic alliance, once established, allows the physician to concentrate on meeting an adequate standard of care appropriate to the particular case without the need to justify his or her actions. In addition, it promotes parental trust and confidence in the physician. These important results are not possible when there is a lack of agreement between physician and parent concerning the ends and means of clinical care. Call this lack a therapeutic misalliance.

The three clinical cases that are discussed and commented upon in this section are examples of therapeutic misalliances. The first involves a mother's insistence upon the use of alternative medicine in the treatment of her seriously ill child. The second concerns confusions as to the goals of treatment and a concomitant breakdown in communication between the caregivers and the family. The third is about a mother's deceptive practices and miscommunications concerning her son's illness.

In Chapter 1, Chester Randle recounts the case of Melody, whose term baby girl, Ericka, had been seriously ill but was recovering. Melody believed that Ericka's immune system was weak and wanted her spiritual advisor to attend the child. Jonathan visited the child and prescribed an herbal tea that Ericka was to ingest and have applied to her chest. The attending physician believed he had an ethical and legal obligation to assure that all treatment of the child while she was under his care was safe and effective. After a meeting with the spiritual advisor it was agreed that the tea could be applied to Ericka's chest, but was not to be ingested.

In his commentary, theologian Richard Miller points out that Randle's belief, that allowing unconventional practices is morally permissible when these appear to be harmless, is inapplicable in this case because he did not have sufficient information to determine whether the tea was in fact harmless. Miller also suggests that Ericka's physicians did not address Melody's beliefs adequately as they pertained to the appropriate care of her child. Miller expands on the first issue by an analysis of the use of unconventional treatment, its therapeutic status and its admissibility, if non-therapeutic. His discussion of the second issue focuses on the lack of information about Melody's beliefs and practices and their possibly harmful effect on her past and future care of Erika.

Miller introduces a distinction between "transactional" and "transformational" approaches in the parent–physician relationship. The latter can reduce the likelihood of future illness and provide a means by which health-related habits are improved. He also notes that Melody's desire to use unconventional treatment for her baby reveals a significant difference between adult and pediatric medicine. Melody's autonomy permits her to use any treatment she wishes on herself. But autonomy plays no role in deciding on the treatment of her child, who does not have a liberty interest. This calls for a more expansive perspective in pediatric treatment than in adult treatment.

In Chapter 2, Ronald Cohen and Eugene Kim describe a fifteen-year-old unmarried mother who delivered a 23-week-gestation baby (Baby M) whom the neonatologists thought was not viable. This was explained to the mother and grandmother, who then consented to a plan of comfort care without mechanical ventilation. After she had survived for six hours, Baby M was re-examined, and with the concurrence of the family it was decided to intubate the baby and provide ventilation. She was transferred to a neonatal intensive care unit where she received complex treatment for nine months. Although conferences were held during that time in which the mother and grandmother were told of the infant's grave prognosis and high-risk status, they rejected these judgments. They had been told the baby was going to die and she was obviously alive. In addition, conflicting advice about appropriate treatment strategies was provided by a bioethics committee which was consulted; some members thought there should have been immediate and aggressive intervention at birth, and others thought no intervention should have occurred.

Respondent Simon Whitney, a physician who is also a lawyer, suggests that aggressive care of Baby M was inappropriate at any time. The fact that she survived, while good news, did not justify the treatment that kept her alive. In his commentary he discusses the issues of viability and legal doctrines that influence care decisions as they related to this case. He calls attention to the strained relations between the caregivers and the family, and notes that despite their protestations to the contrary the physicians made all the major decisions. Thus it was not the family that was inconsistent in their judgments, as suggested in the case history, but the physicians, who initially decided to do nothing but then decided to do everything.

He concludes by recommending a procedure that calls for two-way listening that would accurately and fully inform both the caregivers and the family of the material facts.

In Chapter 3, Manuel Garcia-Careaga and John Kerner introduce an 8-year-old boy who came to a pediatric gastroenterology clinic with reports of recurrent fevers, joint symptoms, chronic diarrhea, and abdominal pain. Over the course of a year the clinical picture included many visits to the GI clinic, fevers, and numerous hospitalizations. The physicians began to suspect that the mother, for complex psychological reasons, was inducing illnesses in her child. Self-induced illnesses as a means of getting attention are termed "Munchausen syndrome," and when as in this case the illnesses are in a second party, it becomes Munchausen syndrome by proxy (MSBP). The consequences of inducing illnesses in a child can be damaging, both psychologically and physically, and can lead to death.

But concrete proof of MSBP is difficult to obtain. When it is discovered, the moral obligation to protect the child from harm creates a heavy burden of responsibility on the caretakers, including the need to protect the child and help the offending parent, securing protective services and organizing adequate patient care. Overt efforts to uncover hard evidence of what one suspects can have the effect of frightening off the mother so that contact is lost with a child who is at risk. To avoid this calls for covert activities – video monitoring, searching the belongings of parents without their knowledge, as well as continuing lab tests to see if they give any clue to what is going on with the mother's interventions. The case report describes the consternation of the physicians as they began to eliminate all other causes of the child's symptoms, their growing suspicion, and finally a clear diagnosis.

The commentary by philosopher Frances Kamm consists of two parts. First she discusses the components of MSBP, conceptual issues with the use of the term "syndrome," child abuse, and the doctor's aims. Then she rigorously explores some of the ethical issues involved in the methods used to diagnose this unusual and counterintuitive pathology. She suggests that the major concern of the doctors is what is morally permissible for them to do in order to identify the child's illness. She questions whether secret monitoring can properly be described as a diagnostic tool, since it is done without the permission of the monitored individual and is not done to garner evidence for the purpose of criminal prosecution. She presents a series of possible arguments justifying secret monitoring, but finds that all of them have problems. Resolving them leads to revisions of the original arguments.

In her final analysis she notes that there are two kinds of procedures for determining whether a parent is responsible for a child's illness – those that prevent her from acting, and those that catch her in a wrongful act. She presents four procedures that fall under those two categories, and suggests an order of preferability.

1.1 Unconventional medicine in the pediatric intensive care unit

Chester J. Randle Jr.

The Lord hath created medicines out of the earth: and he that is wise will not abhor them.

Ecclesiasticus 38: 4

Introduction

Patients commonly use unconventional medical therapies such as chiropractic medicine, acupuncture, and herbalism to treat a variety of medical conditions. Many physicians have incorporated some unconventional therapies into their practice. Moreover, many third-party payers reimburse patients for a variety of unconventional therapies. It is less common to use unconventional therapy to treat a critically ill infant. In this case, a mother demanded that the medical staff use herbal therapy on her infant who was recovering from septic shock.

The case

Ericka was a vigorous 7 pound 12 ounce (3.5 kg) term baby girl. She stayed in the hospital two extra days after birth for evaluation of a low-grade temperature. At ten days of age, she developed a runny nose and a cough. Her mother, Melody, continued to breast-feed and gave her some of the special herbal tea she had used during the pregnancy. Two days later, Melody took her infant to the emergency department because she was lethargic, fed poorly, and breathed heavily.

In the emergency department, Ericka was in moderate respiratory distress. Her respiratory rate was 65 breaths per minute, her heart rate was 160, and her blood pressure was 65/40. Her color was pink, but her skin was slightly cool and her mucous membranes were dry. Bilateral crackles were heard over both lung fields.

Ethical Dilemmas in Pediatrics: Cases and Commentaries, ed. Lorry R. Frankel, Amnon Goldworth, Mary V. Rorty, and William A. Silverman. Published by Cambridge University Press. © Cambridge University Press 2005.

The rest of her exam was normal. The chest X-ray showed bilateral patchy infiltrates. She was admitted to the hospital for treatment of pneumonia and mild dehydration.

Within hours of admission to the pediatric unit her condition deteriorated. Her color was dusky and she was extremely obtunded. She was transferred to the pediatric intensive care unit for treatment of respiratory failure and septic shock. By now her respiratory rate was 80 breaths per minute, her heart rate was up to 200, and her blood pressure was 40 over barely palpable. She was intubated and given mechanical ventilatory support. Several fluid boluses of normal saline and 5% albumin failed to improve her circulation and blood pressure. Her vital signs did not improve until she received inotropic support, and she required 15 μg kg^{-1} min^{-1} of dopamine and 0.25 μg kg^{-1} min^{-1} of epinephrine to maintain normal blood pressures and good circulation. She received pancuronium as a neuromuscular blocking agent, and fentanyl and lorazepam infusions for analgesia and sedation. Ericka initially required high concentrations of oxygen, and high airway pressures to maintain adequate oxygenation and ventilation. The FiO$_2$ was 0.6, the peak inspiratory pressure was 35 cm H$_2$O and the positive end-expiratory pressure was 12 cm H$_2$O. As a result of her severe lung disease and the high airway pressures, she developed a right tension pneumothorax. Her condition stabilized after the air was evacuated with a chest tube. The gram stain of her purulent tracheal secretions showed many polymorphonuclear cells and both gram negative and positive organisms. Two days later, the bacterial cultures grew *Haemophilus influenzae*.

By the third hospital day, Ericka's condition began to improve. The dopamine drip, the epinephrine drip, and the neuromuscular blocking agents were discontinued. The intravenous feeds were slowly converted to enteral feeds of breast milk. By the seventh hospital day, Ericka's lungs expanded well with a peak inspiratory pressure of 28 cm H$_2$O and a positive end-expiratory pressure of 5 cm H$_2$O The physicians and nurses clearly saw that she was recovering. However, Ericka's mother Melody was skeptical. In spite of the reassuring words from the medical staff, she was afraid that her infant's immune system was extremely weak. She wanted to do something to make sure that she would regain all of her health and well-being. She wanted Jonathan to attend to Ericka.

Jonathan was a special man in Melody's life. He was her healer and spiritual advisor. Melody, raised a Methodist in Philadelphia, had adopted a New Age religion when she moved out west. She had a history of chronic headaches, and the drugs that the neurologists prescribed failed to control the pain without putting her in a confused daze. Her headaches were only controlled after she began seeing Jonathan, who prescribed daily meditations and an herbal tea. Her headaches disappeared and her mind remained sharp and focused.

In the early morning of the ninth hospital day, Melody brought Jonathan to the pediatric intensive care unit to see Ericka. After a period of deep meditation, he agreed with the medical staff that Ericka was getting better. However, he reported that, as Melody suspected, he sensed that the baby needed additional treatment to strengthen her immunity. He prescribed a special herbal brew that Ericka was to ingest and have applied to her chest two times a day for two days starting when the moon was full. According to the calendar, therapy was to begin in two days. Melody promptly gave the packet of ingredients to the nurse to use as prescribed.

Although sympathetic, the nurse could not hide her look of shock and disgust. Although she told Melody that she would notify the attending physician of her wishes, Melody read her response as, "Lady, we don't do that mumbo-jumbo stuff here!" Melody grew agitated and angry. Her voice escalated to a scream as she told the nurse that "her baby had better get her treatments" and that if she didn't, "You all would hear from her lawyer and the newspapers!"

The attending physician was astonished to hear about Melody's outbursts. Fearing a legal and public-relations disaster, he notified the chief of staff of the hospital, legal affairs, and hospital public relations. He then consulted one of the sociologists at the local university to gain more insight into Melody's religion. Unfortunately, there was little information about this group. This was one of many cults that had developed in the Southwest over the last 30 years. The New Age religious group had had a small commune that had disbanded in the early 1980s. Many of the doctrines adopted were from Eastern philosophy and valued natural cures and therapies. Herbal therapies, usually from indigenous plants and minerals, were commonly used by members in religious ceremonies and to treat a variety of ailments.

The following day, Melody returned to the hospital appearing much calmer. The attending physician reassured her that the medical and nursing staff were doing everything possible to make sure that her infant would make a full recovery, and explained that as the attending physician he was ethically and legally responsible for assuring that all treatments Ericka received were safe and effective. He could not guarantee that the ingredients in the herbal tea were safe for her baby, especially as she was recovering from a life-threatening illness. He asked that she not do anything until he had a chance to consult with Jonathan. Melody agreed to wait until the two could talk.

When Jonathan and the attending physician met, both agreed that Ericka was improving. Jonathan recognized the potential for conflict between the herbs he prescribed and the drugs she was receiving. The two agreed that placing the herbal tea on the infant's chest was not likely to cause harm and might still allow the infant to receive a form of therapy that the mother requested. Jonathan would defer prescribing ingestion of the tea until the infant was older and much healthier. The following day, the attending physician ordered that the mother or nurses would apply the herbal tea four times, as had been requested.

Melody was satisfied that her baby would receive all the therapy that would result in a cure. The reporters and lawyers never appeared. Ericka slowly improved and she was extubated on the fifteenth hospital day. She was discharged from the hospital four days later.

Discussion

In this case, a mother demanded that the medical staff use an unconventional therapy to treat her infant who was recovering from septic shock. Specifically, the staff were to give this infant a tea prepared from unknown ingredients that was prescribed by a lay herbalist. Although patients frequently use unconventional therapy to treat a variety of medical and psychological problems, such therapy is rarely used for critically ill children. The physician was forced to address the following issues. Is a physician obligated to provide unconventional therapy? Under what circumstances is it appropriate to incorporate unconventional therapy in the care of a sick child? How can a physician maintain a good working relationship with a family that has different cultural or philosophical beliefs about health and medical care?

In making therapeutic decisions, physicians should follow the ethical principles of beneficence (to use treatments based on the benefits they provide), nonmaleficence (to consider the potential of harm to patients), autonomy (to accept the possibility that different persons may judge benefits differently), and justice (to treat similar cases similarly). Because unconventional therapies usually fail to meet the first two medical principles, I believe that a physician is not obligated to provide unconventional therapy.

Physicians are obligated to provide therapy that is likely to improve the patient's outcome. Therapies such as intravenous fluids for hypovolemic shock, or insulin for diabetic ketoacidosis, are obvious examples of beneficial therapies. These therapies are based on sound scientific principles and supported by numerous clinical studies. In contrast, unconventional therapies rarely meet this standard of beneficence.

By definition, unconventional therapies are modalities that are promoted for general use in disease prevention, or are treatments that, based on careful review by scientists and/or clinicians, are not deemed to be of proven benefit nor recommended for current use. Furthermore, few unconventional therapies are taught widely at US medical schools or generally available in US hospitals. They include practices such as acupuncture, homeopathy, chiropracty, mind–body therapies, nutritional therapy, herbalism, and environmental medicine. Unconventional therapies are also termed alternative, complementary, or unorthodox medicine. Critics of unconventional therapies might use the terms unproven, ineffective, fraudulent, dubious, or questionable.

There is a large body of literature that provides examples of patients who were cured by unconventional therapies such as acupuncture, herbal therapies, and meditation (Micozzi 1996). However, too many of these reports are based on testimonials or poorly controlled clinical trials. Therefore, it may be impossible for a physician to appropriately evaluate the value of an unconventional therapy for their patients.

The case presented exemplifies the physician's dilemma. Melody had used herbal therapies for years. Her special herbal tea brought her relief from chronic headaches. In contrast, the conventional, "well studied" drugs had failed. However, the exact content of her herbal tea was unknown. Jonathan, the lay herbalist, prescribed another tea consisting of an unknown combination of herbs for Ericka to ingest and to have rubbed on her chest. Was this a beneficial or harmful therapy?

Herbal therapies may result in benefit, no effect, or harm. Clearly, there are many beneficial herbal therapies that have now become standard in conventional medicine. Aspirin, derived from willow bark (*Salix* species), and digitalis from foxglove (*Digitalis purpurea*) are well known examples. The herb *Coleus forskholii* is a powerful bronchodilator that has fewer side effects than the conventional bronchodilator fenoterol (Pillans 1995). However, other herbal therapies for asthma, such as a tea of eucalyptus, honey, lemon, and oregano, are benign, but have no clinical benefit as bronchodilators (Risser and Mazur 1995). Unfortunately, some herbal therapies for asthma are contaminated with poisons such as lead and arsenic.

The dangers of herbal therapies are due to toxicity, contamination, and adulteration (Huxtable 1992). For example the herb *Aristolochia fangchi* is nephrotoxic (Stefanovic and Polenakovic 1991). *Teucrium chamaedrys*, a plant used for weight loss, may cause hepatitis. Pyrrolizidine alkaloids, used as an expectorant, may also cause hepatitis. Moreover, infants are more susceptible to the toxic effects of this alkaloid (Roulet *et al.* 1988). Herbs containing aconite alkaloids are easily found in Chinese herb stores. Aconite alkaloids activate sodium channels and affect cardiac, neural, and muscle tissue. Side effects include hypotension, ventricular arrhythmias, paresthesias, and gastrointestinal symptoms. Some commercial herbal therapies contain drugs such as diuretics, corticosteroids, and nonsteroidal anti-inflammatory agents to enhance their potency. Moreover, it is frequently difficult to identify all components of herbal preparations.

In the case presented, Ericka was to ingest a tea to improve her immune system. From the herbalist's point of view experience told him that this was a beneficial therapy. From the physician's point of view, it was an unknown therapy that subjected the infant to a dangerous experiment. Thus, this unconventional therapy failed to meet the standard of non-maleficence.

Physicians have increasingly recognized and honored the principle of autonomy. In the spirit of taking control of their health care, patients actively participate in developing treatment plans, discuss cardiopulmonary resuscitation, and in some cases determine the time and mode of their death. In this atmosphere that encourages autonomy it is not suprising that some patients might look beyond conventional medicine for health care. Patients frequently use unconventional therapies for a multitude of diseases and ailments including headaches, cancer, arthritis, back pain, allergies, asthma, diarrhea, infections, renal failure, anxiety, depression, and acquired immunodeficiency syndrome. In one telephone survey, 34% of respondents reported using at least one unconventional therapy in the past year (Eisenberg *et al.* 1993). Eighty-three percent of the respondents who used unconventional therapy for a serious medical condition also sought treatment from a medical doctor. Unfortunately, less than 30% of the respondents who used unconventional therapy informed their medical doctor.

Although the use of unconventional therapies is common, it need not imply a rejection of conventional medicine. In a mail survey, 39% of the respondents who were highly satisfied with their conventional medicine also used alternative therapies (Austin 1998). These respondents felt that the philosophies of unconventional therapy were in keeping with their own values, including the need for a greater influence of the mind and spirit in curing illnesses and maintaining health. These respondents also had poor health status, and were more likely to have had a transformational experience that changed their world view in some significant way. Only 4% of the respondents relied primarily on unconventional therapies. This smaller group were more likely to distrust conventional medical practices, desire more control over health matters, and believe in the importance of one's inner life and experiences.

Some physicians have also incorporated unconventional therapies into their practice, because of their belief in the holistic approach to medical care, or to honor the traditions of folk medicine used by the patients and families in their practice. In one survey of physicians in the United Kingdom, 92% of trainee general practitioners wanted to receive more training in complementary medicine. Forty percent of general practices offered access to at least one unconventional therapy. In 21% of the practices, unconventional therapy was offered by a member of the primary-care team (Lewith and Watkins 1996). Third-party payers and some governmental agencies have also accepted the value of some unconventional therapy. For example, many insurance companies and managed care organizations cover acupuncture and chiropracty for common problems such as chronic back pain and headaches. The European Parliament Committee on the Environment, Public Health and Consumer Protection has advocated that national social services should reimburse the cost of unconventional therapy in line with conventional medicine (Lannoye 1994). Clearly, unconventional and conventional medicinces are intertwined.

In the case presented, Melody was a devoted follower of a New Age religion. Within this culture, she found a more vigorous life that was pain-free and increased her sense of well-being. It is little wonder that she wanted her infant to receive the same benefits. I agree with Pachter that physicians must work toward developing a culturally sensitive health care system (Pachter 1994), a system that is flexible, accessible, and respects the beliefs, attitudes, and cultural lifestyles of its patients. However, this flexible system does not imply that patients have unrestricted autonomy. Patients do not have a right to antibiotics just because they want them, or to chemotherapy because they are afraid they might have cancer. Similarly, parents and surrogates do not have a right to deny a child access to therapy that is medically indicated.

Distributive justice dictates that non-autonomous patients be given equal access to beneficial medical care. Using the best-interests standard, physicians are obligated to protect the health and welfare of children. No parent or surrogate is free to beat their child at will, use prayer alone to treat meningitis, or deny their child a life-saving blood transfusion because of religious prohibitions. In these cases, society expects the physician to intervene to ensure that the child is safe and receives appropriate medical care. How then does the physician incorporate unconventional therapy in the care of a sick child?

The physician should become aware of the medical beliefs and behaviors of the family and their community. The physician should learn more about reasons for use of unconventional therapy. With the help of the family, the physician can develop therapeutic plans that successfully negotiate between their beliefs and those of conventional medicine (Katon and Kleinman 1981). The physician identifies unconventional therapies that are potentially beneficial or benign, and then uses these therapies to complement conventional medical care.

In the case presented, the attending physician learned more about the background and practices of the New Age religion and met with Jonathan the healer. The attending physician and Jonathan were able to develop a therapeutic plan to provide herbal therapy that was unlikely to cause harm and was compatible with conventional medical care. As a result of these negotiations, Ericka received all the conventional medical care necessary, and Melody maintained a therapeutic relationship with her New Age religion and Jonathan the healer.

Conclusion

Many patients use unconventional therapies to treat a variety of medical conditions. Most patients using unconventional therapies also continue to receive, and are satisfied with, conventional medical care. A physician is not obligated to use unconventional therapies, as they are likely to lack proven benefit and may cause harm. However, when they believe the treatment to be safe, physicians may incorporate unconventional therapies into their practice to accommodate the different cultural or philosophical beliefs of their patients and families. The case presented demonstrates that a physician can maintain a good working relationship with a family that has different philosophical beliefs about health and medical care without sacrificing the ethical principles of beneficence, non-maleficence, autonomy, and justice. Thus, a therapeutic environment of mutual trust and respect is developed that increases the possibility of a positive clinical outcome.

1.2 Role responsibility in pediatrics: appeasing or transforming parental demands?

Richard B. Miller

Introduction

When thinking about cultural differences and the care of children, it is tempting to view a child's culture rather than the child herself as the appropriate recipient of diagnosis and treatment. That is because we have come to value cultural heritage as a defining feature of our identities. Of course, one's heritage has little meaning unless it is respected, perhaps affirmed, by others and by public culture at large. As Charles Taylor puts the point, today's concern for culture and respect is premised on the idea "that our identity is partly shaped by recognition or its absence, often by the misrecognition of others, and so a person or group . . . can suffer real damage, real distortion, if the people around them mirror back to them a confining or demeaning or contemptible picture of themselves." Our "sense of self" depends on internalizing the views that others have of us, and the lack of recognition "can inflict harm, can be a form of oppression," imprisoning us "in a false, distorted, and reduced mode of being" (Taylor 1992: 25).

That said, in healthcare settings, especially pediatric settings, respect for culture and identity might crowd out other important values. In an age that urges us to recognize and perhaps affirm particular cultural and personal backgrounds, there is the danger that respecting a patient's heritage might compromise care for that patient's bodily needs. In healthcare settings informed by identity politics, a child's true particularity, or particular claims to care, can get lost. Or so I want to argue here, focusing on a case that raises difficult questions about multiculturalism, medical treatment, and the limits of respect.

To help set the stage for this brief essay, let me state a baseline for pediatric medical ethics, and then refine that baseline a bit by identifying special challenges that are posed by cultural diversity. In my view, a pediatric paradigm is necessary

Ethical Dilemmas in Pediatrics: Cases and Commentaries, ed. Lorry R. Frankel, Amnon Goldworth, Mary V. Rorty, and William A. Silverman. Published by Cambridge University Press. © Cambridge University Press 2005.

for handling the moral world of children's medicine (Miller 2003). In adult settings, the care provider's responsibility is premised on the value of respecting a patient's autonomy. When treating adults, respect for the norm of autonomy has general priority over the norm of beneficence. What presents itself as beneficial treatment must be acceptable on the patient's own terms. Professionals must accept an adult patient's wishes to refuse treatment, even if those wishes are not in that patient's medical interests. In pediatric contexts, on the other hand, the norm of beneficence has general priority over respect for autonomy. With children, care providers may often act in ways that subordinate respect for autonomy, such as it is, to the value of patient benefit. Pediatric care providers thus have fewer limits on their authority. Children are generally not free to make decisions that put themselves at considerable risk; adults may discount a child's decision in order to protect that child's current or future welfare.

Making matters more complicated is the fact that the child is usually not a free-standing agent, but a member of a social unit in which parents enjoy the presumption of authority. One requirement of pediatric health care is for medical professionals to triangulate their care between the child, the parents, and the healthcare team. And because families come from different backgrounds and have different belief systems, connecting with families can be enormously difficult. This is especially true when it is not clear that a family's beliefs support the child's medical welfare. Given the demand to respect cultural differences, one question in the care of children is: How far must respect go? How much authority can parents rightfully claim?

In multicultural contexts, it is necessary to avoid two extremes in the care of children and respect for their families. One extreme is ethnocentrism – dismissing a family's views simply because they are unusual or different. The other extreme is what Taylor (1992) calls "respect on demand," the idea that people have the right to demand respect simply because they are unusual or different. Ethnocentrism is close-minded and callous; respect on demand asks us to be uncritical and patronizing.

I will explore these challenges as they frame disagreements between families and pediatric care providers in the case of Ericka. That case concerns whether, and on what terms, care providers should accommodate unconventional therapies and New Age religious practices. When pediatricians treat patients such as Ericka, they often consider whether to negotiate between the world of modern biomedicine and cultures outside the mainstream, either indigenous or transplanted from elsewhere. In such cases it might seem wise to coordinate conventional methods with nonmainstream practices, even at the expense of providing optimal care for patients. I want to discuss the merits of that idea in the course of commenting on Dr. Chester Randle's treatment of Ericka's case.

Treating Ericka when the moon turns full

In discussing the use of unconventional medicine in the treatment of infant Ericka, Dr. Randle poses two ethical questions and answers both affirmatively. The first is whether accommodating unconventional medical practices is morally acceptable when those practices seem potentially harmless to the patient. The second is whether Ericka's physicians adequately responded to Melody's beliefs within the limits of providing adequate care for her daughter. These questions are complicated by the fact that Melody's demands for unconventional treatment implicated religious and cultural values. Ericka's case reminds us that in pediatrics it is often necessary for healthcare providers to attend to family members' needs in the course of caring for a child. Pediatric medicine occurs within the context of a therapeutic alliance between healthcare providers and a child's family.

In this brief response, I will argue that Dr. Randle's answer to the first question is inadequate, for we are not given enough information to be confident that applying herbal tea to Ericka's chest will be harmless. I will also argue that Randle's answer to the second question is wrong, for the doctors failed to ascertain how Ericka acquired sepsis, and they made no attempt to educate Melody about how to avoid such crises in the future. As a result of these omissions, Ericka's physicians failed to respond adequately to the medical implications of their cultural differences with Melody.

Randle's manner of treating the first question blinds him to the deeper challenges of the second question. He tackles the first question by mechanically applying principles of biomedical ethics – beneficence, non-maleficence, autonomy, and justice – to Ericka's case. Approaching the second question requires us to ascertain the deeper meaning and practical implications of these principles for Ericka's ongoing health and well-being.

I will thus counsel greater caution about how Randle answers the first question and attempt to offer a different answer to the second question. My argument is that, when circumstances permit, the role responsibilities of pediatric care providers include challenging parental demands and educating parents about possible connections between their habits and their child's health. In this case, Ericka's physicians failed to exercise that educative responsibility, despite the fact that circumstances were favorable to discharging this duty. To see this point, we need to move beyond a mechanical application of the principles of biomedical ethics to ascertain their meaning and their (sometimes demanding) implications for physician responsibility. Let us consider each question in turn: the ethics of using unconventional treatment on Ericka, and the challenge of reckoning with Melody's religious and cultural values.

Unconventional treatment

Randle is correct to argue that Ericka's physicians were not obligated to have Ericka ingest tea that was prepared by Melody's healer, Jonathan, given the fact that Jonathan's remedy was of unknown effectiveness. This judgment is justified on terms that all treatments – conventional or unconventional – must be evaluated. Ericka's physicians exercised no cultural prejudice by barring Jonathan from having Ericka ingest a tea made from unknown ingredients. Treatment that is non-beneficial or potentially harmful is neither medically nor morally indicated. Ericka's physicians decided instead to allow Jonathan to apply his herbal tea to Ericka's chest. The grounds for this compromise are unclear. We are told that the physicians and Jonathan agreed that applying the herbal brew to Ericka's chest was not likely to cause harm and could "still allow the infant to receive a form of therapy that the mother requested." Immediately we should ask, what was the factual basis for this agreement? Were the contents of Jonathan's tea subjected to laboratory analysis? Was the tea potentially damaging to Ericka's skin, such that it might have caused dermatitis? More generally, how do we know that she was not put at risk by this treatment?

I raise these questions because herbal remedies and other forms of unconventional therapy are not subject to the same strict standards that are used to evaluate the pharmaceutical industry in the United States. The Dietary Supplement Health and Education Act of 1994 weakened the authority of the Food and Drug Administration (FDA) to regulate vitamins, herbal remedies, and dietary supplements by shifting the burden of proving their safety. Before 1994, the FDA could order a medically suspicious substance off the market until the manufacturer had proved it safe. As a result of the new act, the FDA must prove a product unsafe before ordering it off the market. Dangerous products may now be sold until someone is harmed by them and reports his or her case to medical professionals or governmental authorities. Risks to public health are not insignificant. In a recent test of herbal products from Asia, the California Department of Health Services found poisonous heavy metals such as lead, arsenic, or mercury in 83 of 260 samples (Grady 1998).

In fairness to Ericka's physicians, we should note that Jonathan's herbal remedy may have been subjected to laboratory analysis before the compromise was struck. Unfortunately, the case does not present data to assure us of this fact. Without these data, we cannot be certain that the caregivers have satisfied the duty of non-maleficence. In appeasing Melody, the physicians may have subjected Ericka to further risk and/or discomfort.

It appears that the compromise was struck less for Ericka's benefit than for the benefit of Melody and the house staff. By securing Jonathan's and Melody's agreement, physicians lessened the emotional tension between Melody and the nurses on the floor, and reduced the threat of legal action. But if that is the reason for the compromise, then the tea was applied to Ericka's skin in order to resolve problems other than those of her sepsis and respiratory distress. Without further information about why the tea is deemed beneficial when applied to Ericka, there is a danger that she is being used for others' benefit. To describe the compromise as one that allows the infant to receive a form of therapy that her mother requested is to ignore medical and moral concerns. On what basis can we confidently say that herbal treatment is indeed Ericka's therapy?

In raising this question, I do not mean to suggest that non-beneficial treatment of a child to benefit others is absolutely inadmissible. In one of the best discussions of a similar issue, non-therapeutic research on children, Thomas Murray argues that parents may volunteer their children for non-therapeutic research if the risks are small and the benefits to others are substantial. The latter outweigh the former; subjecting children to such risks resembles other kinds of actions that parents may reasonably take for communal goods. Murray considers an analogous case: may a family's church "borrow" their baby briefly to star as the infant Jesus in a Christmas pageant? In Murray's mind, that is a permissible action for a communal good, although it subjects the infant to possible risks and discomfort (Murray 1996). But in Ericka's case, the use of unconventional procedures is not deemed non-therapeutic and aimed toward the benefit of others. It is presented as therapy for her, and I have already called attention to reasons that should lead us to doubt such a description.

Cultural differences

Randle endorses what he calls a "culturally sensitive" healthcare system, adding that such a system must be constrained by considerations of patient benefit. He rightly urges flexibility, respect for different cultural practices, and accessibility all within the limits imposed by principles of biomedical ethics. In his view, Ericka's physicians operated within the broad contours of this vision, providing Ericka with the medical care she needed while forging a therapeutic relationship with Melody. Although it seems that Ericka's physicians were more culturally accommodating than physicians in the United States are sometimes reputed to be (see Fadiman 1997), Randle's judgment about how Ericka's physicians worked with Melody is too generous.

The most striking omissions concern Ericka's admission and the requirements for her future care. Both issues may involve Melody's cultural beliefs and practices, which could be harmful to her daughter. Consider Ericka's admission. No one seems to ask why Ericka developed sepsis and subsequent respiratory distress. Were these problems prompted by ingesting the herbal tea that her mother fed her? Might the tea be toxic to Ericka? (Hence another reason to subject the tea to laboratory tests.) Consider Ericka's return home. Will Melody feed the herbal brew to Ericka in the future? If so, what risks to Ericka are involved? Will Melody's cultural and religious beliefs put Ericka at risk in other ways? If so, shouldn't she be dissuaded from acting on beliefs that might affect her daughter adversely?

All of these questions bear upon and potentially challenge Melody's cultural and religious beliefs. Critically engaging Melody about her commitments and her treatment of Ericka are clear implications of the principles of beneficence and non-maleficence. Those principles bear not only on the immediate question of proper therapy in intensive care, but on the cause of Ericka's illness and the prevention of future illness. In failing to address such issues, Ericka's healthcare providers failed to exercise proper medical responsibilities; the therapeutic alliance they forged with her mother is medically and morally deficient.

In the words of William F. May, the relationship between Melody and the physicians is more "transactional" than "transformational" (May 1992: 38). A transactional approach involves an exchange of information and the guarantee that goods and services will be adequately provided. But such interactions do not require doctors to instruct patients or parents about how to decrease the likelihood of future illness or how to improve their health-related habits. May worries that a transactional approach privatizes professional responsibility by reducing it to a commodity to be bought and sold on the marketplace (see Sullivan 1995). A transformational approach requires physicians to get to the root of their patients' problems, and envisions professional life as part of the larger commonweal. A doctor confronted by an insomniac patient, for example, may be asked to provide the quick remedy of a sleeping pill. But in a transformational approach, a physician "may have to challenge the patient to transform the habits that led to the symptom of sleeplessness" (May 1992). The aim is not to satisfy patients' preferences or to strike compromises in order to reduce emotional tension and the danger of litigation, but to address patients' long-term problems with an eye to prevention and public health.

Method and substance

Earlier I stated that the problem with Randle's analysis lies with his method of evaluating Ericka's case. May's distinction between transactional and transformational dynamics enables us to see how that is so. Randle takes the principles of biomedical ethics and applies them in a "top-down" manner to Ericka's case and Melody's cultural and religious beliefs. The goal is to determine whether particular actions can be subsumed within a general principle, or to pick out features of a situation to see whether they abide by a more general value. Reflecting a transactional set of assumptions, Randle's analysis is limited to decisions within a narrow time frame, namely, the events in the intensive care unit. Although a top-down approach to practical reasoning and a transactional approach to medical care are not the same, they can enjoy an affinity in institutional settings that prize efficiency. Such an affinity crowds out considerations of causes or consequences – events prior or subsequent to Ericka's admission to the hospital.

A transformational approach requires a more longitudinal perspective, a larger frame of analysis. It thus generates greater expectations of the physicians responsible for Ericka, thereby enlarging the demands of beneficent and non-maleficent treatment beyond the immediate context of the hospital. These principles require physicians not only to provide care in the intensive care unit, but also to weigh the demands of future health and the prevention of illness. To be sure, such expectations are difficult to meet in intensive care; typically patients are in and out of such units in a few days. In many if not most cases, expectations of a transformational approach to patient and family care in intensive care units are unrealistic and unfair (Miller 1996a). But Ericka was in the unit for more than two weeks, enabling physicians to familiarize themselves with her situation and her mother's. That would normally allow them to make an informed assessment. Circumstances that would excuse physicians from adopting a transformational approach to patient care do not apply in Ericka's and Melody's case.

Randle might respond that my analysis pays insufficient attention to other principles of biomedical ethics, especially autonomy and justice. I appear to overlook autonomy insofar as I have failed adequately to respect values that are central to Melody's identity. Randle could point to the irony that a more robust understanding of beneficence in my argument seems not to include a robust respect for family autonomy and the distinct features of Ericka's background. That seems inconsistent, he might continue, for a more longitudinal perspective would seem to imply a more demanding account of all of the relevant principles in medical care. That is, a transformational approach would bid us to see Ericka's needs *and* her mother's commitments within a larger narrative. Scrutinizing Melody's beliefs in light of their possible medical implications seems not to grant her the kind of appreciation that is important to her ongoing self-respect. Moreover, considerations of identity, respect, and recognition are morally significant in multicultural societies, in which recognition of cultural difference is seen as a matter of social justice (see Taylor 1992). Accordingly, my analysis does not adequately respect Melody's autonomy, and her self-defining choices do not receive the justice they deserve.

Yet it is important to remember that Melody is not the primary patient in this case. Moral considerations that bear on her needs are derivative upon and subordinate to Ericka's needs. If, as this case suggests, Ericka's health is potentially compromised by respecting Melody's cultural and religious beliefs, the latter must give way to the former. Herein lies a key difference between pediatric and adult medicine. With adults, the duty of beneficence is constrained by considerations of autonomy and the liberty interests that autonomy enshrines (see Childress 1982). Physicians must treat a patient with the patient's consent or, when that patient is incompetent, with the consent of a patient proxy who first tries to represent the patient's background and choices. In adult medicine, patients have the liberty to make medically irrational decisions, and their proxies may represent medically irrational wishes. In pediatric care, however, autonomy is a lesser factor, and is sometimes irrelevant, for children are not assumed to be fully competent. Those who represent children's interests must represent their basic medical interests, not their liberty interests.

Thus we have two responses to the charge of insufficient attention to autonomy and justice as these bear on Ericka's family background: (1) those principles are relevant to Melody, who is not the primary patient; (2) Melody must represent her daughter's basic medical interests.

Principle and background

The use of unconventional treatment that is recommended by a parent's cultural and religious beliefs helps us understand some basic differences between adult and pediatric care. In pediatric medicine, beneficence is not constrained by autonomy in the same way that it is in adult medicine. Equally as important, considerations of beneficence cannot be confined to decisions that are made about treatment in the intensive care unit; a more capacious analysis is needed.

My disagreements with Dr. Randle's analysis are thus methodological and substantive, and these disagreements are linked. Methodologically, I have argued for situating ethical judgments within a larger context than Randle's analysis invites (see Miller 1996b). Enlarging the scope of that analysis, in turn, opens the door to substantive concerns about the requirements of responsible medical treatment, especially as they are implied by the principles of beneficence and non-maleficence in the treatment of children.

The fact that a transformationist approach to medical responsibility generates more robust moral expectations than we find in Randle's analysis points to an important idea in practical reasoning. How we interpret and apply moral principles relies in part on unarticulated, background assumptions (see Taylor 1995). In my argument, the principles of beneficence and non-maleficence have acquired an expanded set of implications for healthcare practitioners given what we can infer about transformational dynamics.[1] In this respect, the demands of biomedical ethics are amplified; their range of application is broadened owing to background assumptions regarding the proper responsibilities of healthcare providers. My differences with Randle are traceable to differences in those assumptions and their practical implications for role morality in pediatric intensive care.

ACKNOWLEDGMENTS

Portions of this essay were presented at the University of Northern Arizona and I am grateful for the comments and suggestions I received during that visit. I am grateful to Judith Granbois and Barbara Klinger for comments on an earlier draft. A fuller version can be found in Miller (2003).

---

[1] Amplifying the range of a principle's meaning or its concrete implications is one pattern of reasoning that is rarely noted in discussions of practical ethics. The reigning models of practical reasoning involve deductively applying a principle to a case, specifying, then weighing and balancing principles after they have been specified. For discussions, see Richardson (1990), Miller (1996a), Childress (1996). Although I do not have space to develop this point here, amplifying a principle is a pattern of practical reasoning that stands apart from the reigning models.

1.3 Topical discussion

Alternative or complementary medicine

This case presents possible problems associated with "unconventional medicine" in a particularly vivid form; the infant is seriously ill, the proposed treatment is completely unknown, and the frantic parent is obdurate.

The category of "alternative medicine" is commonly taken to include health practices that generally are not available from US physicians, are not offered in US hospitals, or are not widely taught in US medical schools. It covers a range of therapeutic modalities, some of which are currently being tested for efficacy by Western research methods, and some of which count as "conventional" in other countries. Some unconventional therapies are indigenous survivals of earlier schools of medicine, including homeopathy and chiropracty, while the waves of recent immigrants have introduced practices such as herbal medicine or acupuncture that are well established in other cultures. Schools of osteopathy and chiropracty medicine are accredited in the USA, and some homeopathic medicine is considered standard practice in Europe. Many medical schools and nursing schools now incorporate a unit on alternative medicine in their curriculum.

Underlying the concept of unconventional therapy is the question of whether medical judgments concerning disease and illness are objective or subjective. Are judgments based on Western science in a privileged position compared to judgments derived from non-Western sources? Or are all such judgments culturally determined? If the latter, then this requires changes in the medical curriculum and expanded efforts to determine which kinds of medical interventions, whatever their source, are most efficacious.

Whether medical judgments are objective or subjective, Randle seems well advised in calling for a healthcare system which is sensitive to the cultural

Ethical Dilemmas in Pediatrics: Cases and Commentaries, ed. Lorry R. Frankel, Amnon Goldworth, Mary V. Rorty, and William A. Silverman. Published by Cambridge University Press. © Cambridge University Press 2005.

differences of its patients. It is also worth considering what the implications of the "transformational" approach to medicine that Miller recommends are for patient (and family) privacy and freedom of choice. Does pediatric medicine, as contrasted with adult medicine, put different demands upon physicians?

Cultural sensitivity

Limits on parental authority in treatment decisions have been established by case law in the United States in some easily defined cases. Jehovah's Witness refusals of blood transfusions are honored for adults but may be overridden for minor children. Christian Scientists have been prosecuted for refusing to present ill children for standard medical treatment. Controversy still rages over parental refusal of public health measures such as vaccination against common and contagious childhood diseases. US society is rapidly becoming a multicultural one. In many communities well-established subcultures like Mormons or Amish are being joined by new immigrants from non-Western societies. Not only the expectations of health care of these new residents, but often the language in which they are able to express them, present additional problems to individual clinicians and their institutions. Although one need not be a member of a recognized religion or culture in order to hold strong convictions about matters of health or appropriate treatments, some such groups are readily identifiable, and a general, or at least local, familiarity with their beliefs on the part of the clinicians can make it easier to find common ground when children enter the health system.

Ethical principles

The physician author uses the language of the Belmont Report, invoking the ethical principles of beneficence, non-maleficence, justice, and autonomy, around which he organizes his discussion of what to do to resolve his perplexity. The four values often, as here, serve as much as a focus of mindfulness as a justification for action. The respondent invokes some of the same principles, but draws other implications from them. These principles are sometimes called "the Georgetown mantra" because of their virtual canonization in that institution's summer bioethics institutes and in successive editions of the influential textbook *Principles of Biomedical Ethics* by Thomas Beauchamp and James Childress. In the course of this book they will reappear in various forms. The pervasiveness of the vocabulary reflects the extent to which each of the "principles" expresses widely held moral commitments.

There is an ongoing discussion among bioethicists about the role moral theories play in moral judgment about particular cases. Few assume that solutions to complex cases can be resolved by simple application of a comprehensive theory such as utilitarianism or recourse to hierarchically ordered priniciples. Much of the popularity of the "principlist" approach to clinical ethics is its position on a meso-level of ethical abstraction. Seeking a ground common to and intelligible to holders of utilitarian, aretaic or deontological theories, it avoids a deductive or top-down approach to ethical decision making by emphasizing attention to the particular details of cases and recommending a tailoring of their prima facie principles to those contours. By consulting the ethical ideals and the brute details of the particular case, the bioethicist hopes to attain a "reflective equilibrium" in which participants find a common ground of reasons for adopting one position or another.

The "case" method

If "principlism" represents an ecumenicism of theory, casuistry as the term is used in bioethics represents a countervailing inferential intuitionism. As Jonsen and Toulmin argue in their influential book *The Abuse of Casuistry*, a shared perception of what is at stake in a particular case is more likely to lead to resolution than any agreement about self-evident rules or principles. In its purest form, ethical casuistry, like its legal counterpart, would rely on drawing analogies with precedent cases, which would then serve as models for resolution. Any more general "principles" would be merely thumb-rules, empirical generalizations over past experience. In practice, bioethical casuistry does not ignore ethical rules and principles any more than bioethical principlism ignores cases. Although the two approaches represent opposite epistemological commitments, the actual practice of ethical deliberation involves both. If principles without attention to cases are empty, cases in their brute particularity are unenlightening.

There is a growing literature on the role of cases, casuistry, and narrative in bioethics education and clinical ethics, Miller's own book, *Casuistry and Modern Ethics*, being a valuable contribution to that literature. Most medical education is case oriented, and pedagogically, case studies have been found to be useful in ethics education because of the importance of details in providing the basis for moral judgment. There are dangers in relying solely on cases for education, since no two cases are ever identical, and cases that are simplified for instructional purposes may make moral deliberation look misleadingly simple. Reading an account of a case, however scrupulously presented, is a poor substitute for ongoing dialogical interaction with a patient and family. Any participant in a case has a position, a point of view, from which the details are seen or heard. Before its demise, the journal *Second Opinion* of the Park Ridge Center for the Study of Health, Faith, and Ethics published lengthy and detailed case reports for ethics education in which a variety of stakeholders in a given case – physicians and family members, social workers, nurses and chaplains, involved community members and the patients themselves – contributed their own perspective.

What counts as a case report differs between a resident or medical student, a psychiatrist or a philosophy instructor, and throughout this book a variety of formats reveal the differences – and the difficulties – of case reporting, and the importance of what is included, and what is excluded, in a given example. Randle's report of Ericka's medical progress and his negotiations with her mother are lengthy and rich in clinical detail. However, it is what is not known that seizes the attention of respondent Miller. Miller stresses the importance for ethical deliberation of context and of a longitudinal history – what preceded the crisis, and what will follow discharge.

FURTHER READING

Beauchamp, T. L. and Childress, J. F. *Principles of Biomedical Ethics*, 4th edn (New York, NY: Oxford University Press, 1994).

The Belmont Report: Ethical Principles and Guidelines for the Protection of Human Subjects of Research (Washington, DC: Government Printing Office, 1979).

Berger J. T. Multi-cultural considerations and the American College of Physicians *Ethics Manual. Journal of Clinical Ethics* **12** (2001), 375–381.

DeVito, S. On the value-neutrality of the concepts of health and disease: into the breach again. *Journal of Medicine and Philosophy* 25 (2000), 539–567.

Eisenberg, D. M., Davis, R. B., Ettner, S. L., *et al.* Trends in alternative medicine use in the United States, 1990–1997: results of a follow-up national survey. *JAMA* **280** (1998), 1569–1575.

Ernst, E. Ethics of complementary medicine. *Journal of Medical Ethics* **22** (1996), 197–198.

Jonsen, A. and Toulmin, S. *The Abuse of Casuistry: a History of Moral Reasoning* (Berkeley, CA: University of California Press, 1988).

Miller, R. B. *Casuistry and Modern Ethics* (Chicago, IL: University of Chicago Press, 1996).

2.1 The extremely premature infant at the crossroads

Ronald Cohen and Eugene Kim

Case: Baby Girl M

Ms. M, an unmarried 15-year-old primigravida, presented at a community hospital accompanied by her mother. She reported a history of sporadic spotting for approximately four weeks, and a recent spontaneous rupture of membranes. Though she had not had prenatal care, she was confident that the pregnancy was at 23 weeks gestation as measured from dates. She was febrile and suspected to have chorioamnionitis, so she was started on intravenous antibiotics. Given the initial diagnosis of chorioamnionitis, neither tocolytics nor steroids were given. The maternal grandmother clearly expressed her desire that the baby should be supported aggressively if deemed viable at the time of birth. The neonatologist present at that time understood her wishes. The mother's desires were not appreciated, however.

The mother progressed to a spontaneous vaginal delivery approximately ten hours after the rupture of membranes. At delivery, the baby girl was obviously less mature than would be expected of a 24-week gestation. The one-minute Apgar score was 2. A partial placental abruption was noted. Her birth weight was 550 g. The neonatologist present at the delivery, who was different from the admitting neonatologist, felt that the patient probably was not viable, and chose not to aggressively intervene. This care plan was explained to the mother and grandmother, neither of whom expressed any disagreement with the plan, which was not to initiate mechanical ventilation and to provide comfort care only. The baby was kept warm in an incubator and given oxygen by hood. For more than five hours, she maintained a regular respiratory rate and heart beat, and her oxygen saturations were stable and greater than 90%.

At this point the neonatologist at the community hospital consulted with his partner, a neonatologist at the local regional medical center, to consider whether it

Ethical Dilemmas in Pediatrics: Cases and Commentaries, ed. Lorry R. Frankel, Amnon Goldworth, Mary V. Rorty, and William A. Silverman. Published by Cambridge University Press. © Cambridge University Press 2005.

would be appropriate medically or ethically to deviate from the initial decision not to provide aggressive support for this extremely immature patient. Furthermore, there was significant concern that several hours without IV fluids or ventilator support might have worsened the baby's prognosis. Given the course thus far, and the initial questionable prognosis, it was felt that further data would be helpful before any additional decisions were made.

A capillary blood gas at six hours of age showed a pH of 7.31 and a pCO_2 of 33 (within normal range). Her blood glucose screen at that time was greater than 45 mg dL^{-1}, an adequate level. These were felt to be reassuring results, certainly not indicative of any deleterious effect of the lack of aggressive support up to this time. Therefore, further discussion to review the situation with the mother and grandmother was initiated. They were told that the baby's prognosis was very poor, but that perhaps a trial of mechanical ventilator support was warranted. The grandmother stated that she had always wanted "everything" done for the baby. It was thus decided to intubate the patient and begin mechanical ventilation. Artificial surfactant was given, and Baby Girl M was transferred to the nearest level III regional center neonatal intensive care unit (NICU).

The mother became distant and passive in the care of the baby and in the decision-making process. The father was present at the birth and visited on a few occasions early in the patient's stay in the NICU. Thereafter he did not participate in Baby Girl M's care. The maternal grandmother always appeared to be the primary caretaker as well as decision maker.

Initially, and with the family's consent, the baby had a "no resuscitation" order. However, this status was later changed to full resuscitation when it became evident that her clinical condition had stabilized and her head ultrasound results were benign. Several multidisciplinary conferences were held with the family. From the start, the family was informed about the baby's grave prognosis and high-risk status. At one point, roughly halfway through the NICU course, the family informed the care team that everyone had told them that their child would die, and obviously that was wrong, therefore they did not believe all these pessimistic assessments that they were hearing from us.

When the patient was a month old and had already been transferred to another hospital, the ethics committee at the primary community hospital was consulted to discuss this child's initial care. There were two opposite opinions. One was that there should have been immediate and aggressive intervention at birth. The second was that the oxygen should not have been started and no intervention should have been made at all.

Family dynamics were a significant problem for the caregivers, as it eventually became evident that there was significant internal conflict. As indicated, the father of the baby seemed to be involved initially, and his opinion was sought and contributed to the formulation of the care plan. However, he soon disappeared. Meanwhile, the maternal grandfather was present frequently, participated actively in discussions about the care of the baby, was hostile to the caregivers on many occasions, and was often at odds with the rest of the family. At one point he claimed he was going to seek legal custody of the mother, and thus of the patient. Shortly thereafter, he too disappeared and played no further role in the care of the child. In retrospect, the confusion regarding the family's initial decision not to support the child aggressively probably reflected internal dissention within the family. The mother was an "emancipated minor" and thus had full legal custody of her daughter. However, she generally deferred to her mother. Unfortunately they were not always both present for discussions with the staff, and thus they initially gave mixed messages to the staff on many occasions.

Follow-up

Eventually the grandmother applied for, and was granted, foster-care custody of Baby Girl M. At 11 months postnatal age, and 7 months corrected age, her height was 60 cm, her weight 5.6 kg, and her head circumference 40.5 cm. All of these were below the 5th percentile for corrected age. She was alert, active, and smiling. Her behavior and temperament appeared appropriate for age. Her neurological examination showed no abnormal findings. However, she was functioning at a level of four months of age in all categories. It is not certain at this point whether this developmental delay is secondary to the prolonged and stormy NICU course and lack of stimulation, or reflects a permanent central nervous system injury.

At about a year and a half, she visited the NICU with her grandmother. Though obviously quite small for her age, she did not need oxygen and was walking normally and beginning to talk. Her grandmother was quite satisfied with her "quality of life."

2.2 The extremely premature infant at the crossroads: ethical and legal considerations

Simon N. Whitney

Introduction

The retrospectoscope is usually a pleasure to use. After someone else's case turns out badly, simply direct the retrospectoscope at the original clinical events and explain calmly how you would have made better decisions, resulting in a better outcome. In the case of Baby Girl M, it is plain that aggressive management from the moment of birth would have avoided the awkward six hours in which she received comfort care only, but that is not the whole story. In fact, it is my thankless duty to assert that aggressive care was inappropriate at any time, and that optimal management would have resulted, not in survival, but in her prompt and intended death. That did not happen, and I am pleased for Baby Girl M herself, who is doing well, but her good outcome does not vindicate her initial management. To understand how she should have been managed, we must begin with the issues raised by infants who are born at the margin of viability.

This essay reviews the determination of viability, moves on to the legal doctrines that influence care decisions, discusses the way these issues illuminate the case of Baby Girl M, and concludes with recommendations for a process designed to lead to better decisions.

Shades of viability

An infant's chance of survival gradually increases with gestational age, so the limit of viability is blurred rather than distinct. Fost and co-workers proposed that an infant is viable if it has the capacity "to survive for a designated period of time in a defined environment" (Fost *et al.* 1980). A slightly more concrete restatement might consider an infant to be viable if he or she has a chance of long-term survival if given maximal care. However, the decision to provide aggressive care does not

Ethical Dilemmas in Pediatrics: Cases and Commentaries, ed. Lorry R. Frankel, Amnon Goldworth, Mary V. Rorty, and William A. Silverman. Published by Cambridge University Press. © Cambridge University Press 2005.

turn on the chance of survival alone, for some very early infants face a high risk of major disabilities, and all will consume tremendous resources in their uncertain journey in the neonatal intensive care unit (NICU). Allen and co-workers found no survivors among infants delivered at 22 weeks gestation and 15 percent survival at 23 weeks (Allen *et al.* 1993), so in the mid-1990s, at the time of this case, an infant at 23 weeks gestation was potentially viable with optimal care. As medical management improves, the lower limit of viability will continue to be pushed back. This clinical progress does not alter the overall principles discussed here.

If no costs were incurred, it would be appropriate to try to resuscitate every infant that might conceivably survive, even if the chance of survival were one in a thousand. There are, however, costs: costs to the infants themselves when their life brings more suffering than joy, emotional costs to the family as very tiny infants struggle and usually die, and emotional costs to the professionals who care for them. For society there are the financial costs of paying for intensive care for these infants and then, for some that survive, the long-term cost of caring for children, and adults, with multiple disabilities.

Allen and colleagues found that only 2 percent of the infants born at 23 weeks survived *and* did not have severe abnormalities on cranial ultrasound. This rate rose to 24 percent at 24 weeks (Allen *et al.* 1993). A 1997 study found that a mother delivering at 24 weeks had a 26 percent chance of a child that survived and had a normal or borderline cognitive outcome (Piecuch *et al.* 1997). Even at 24 weeks, then, the chance of a baby surviving neurologically intact was one in four. In 1996 it was uncommon for infants of less than 24 weeks gestation to be given aggressive care. Baby Girl M was therefore not a typical premature infant, but the dilemmas her case poses are common.

Quality of life

Some people believe passionately that it is wrong to use the quality of life as a criterion in making decisions about extremely premature newborns; C. Everett Koop, former Surgeon General of the USA, has promoted this view eloquently. Of more importance to me, some parents with whom I work share this belief, often founded on a conviction that we can best respect the sacredness of life by preserving life at all costs, no matter what disabilities might result. As these parents struggle with difficult decisions, I struggle to help them on their moral home ground. I respect their perspective, but outside the exam room I do not find it useful when discussing matters that concern society as a whole. In this essay I therefore accept the deeply held belief of most people that it matters, for many reasons, whether a child grows up with full capacities or severely impaired.

The impaired infant's quality of life usually begins badly, for simply being in intensive care is a burden. In an academic NICU, this burden is recognized most clearly by the nurses, who restrain these infants as harried house staff or technicians perform procedures. Some may consider infant suffering to be transitory, something that will never be remembered and is in any case inevitable if the infant's life is to be saved. This answer is too easy, and while there has been progress in providing sedation and pain medication to infants in recent years, their suffering deserves far more attention. Our neglect may be due in part to the fact that we measure pain only very indirectly, through catecholamine release and changes in vital signs and behavior. New neuroimaging techniques, new computer analysis of EEG waveforms, and other advances in technology persuade me that one day we will be able to measure pain far more directly than we do now. That will open the door to studying the effects of chronic pain in the neonate, both in the moment and in terms of later development. When that day comes I believe we will look back on today's practices with regret.

Decisional authority

The law vests parents with the right and duty to make medical decisions for their newborn so long as their decisions are in the child's best interests. It is often said that parents have this authority because infants themselves cannot make the decisions, but surely this is not the entire reason. The parents know their own values and their own resources, which are part of the child's endowment and shape his or her prospects (Shaw 1977). The decision to aggressively treat a very premature infant commits the parents and society to prolonged, often lifetime, care that can be of tremendous intensity and cost. This should not be done reflexively.

Commentators sometimes say that every baby deserves love. It is one thing to say that every baby deserves love, and quite another to provide it. Clinicians who care for children with chronic health problems are well aware of the difficulty these children can create for other children in the family and for the relationship of the parents to each other. A family that plans to have a child, and is prepared to manage the emotional and financial burdens of raising that child, may be entirely unprepared for the multiple demands of an infant that requires intense care for months or years. All too often, emotional, marital, and financial disaster result. Of course, there is another possibility: a few children benefit from the generous emotional and social resources of loving, stable families. These situations remind us of the potential for love and growth in families with even very impaired children.

Neonatologists have a wide range of personal views on whether it is better to sustain life at all costs or to make decisions based on the infant's anticipated quality of life. Therefore, they often disagree on which infants should be treated aggressively, but almost all agree that some should receive aggressive care, some should be allowed to die, and some are in a middle zone. In this middle zone physician and parental discretion make individual determinations of the best course. Beginning in 1982, the federal government has intermittently asserted its authority to second-guess these decisions. The laws in place may reduce egregious misconduct, but they also make ordinary decision making more difficult. Fortunately, a careful examination of the legal milieu shows that this threat is more theoretical than real.

The role of the law

Hospital attorneys commonly invoke legal doctrine as binding; their response can be quite dogmatic if a physician proposes a course of treatment that could be construed as violating the law or posing a hazard of malpractice liability. Nevertheless, the law should play third fiddle in medical decision making, with ethical and medical considerations (in that order) normally dominating legal concerns. When there are no ethical factors at play, what is medically right should always be determined first, and this will almost always be what is legally appropriate. When there is conflict between medical and legal obligations, that conflict should be confronted directly and an explicit decision made about how to resolve it.

There are three areas of the law that pertain to the care of Baby Girl M: state criminal law, federal and state civil law, and malpractice law.

Criminal

Occasionally a sick or injured child is given no medical care or inappropriate alternative care, and those responsible are charged with child abuse or homicide under state criminal laws. A few scholars have argued, by extension, that the selective non-treatment of infants of marginal viability violates the criminal law (Robertson 1975, Robertson and Fost 1976). This argument resides in a theoretical never-never land, for no United States physician has ever been found guilty of a criminal offense for the considered non-treatment of an impaired newborn (Fost 1995), nor is such a case likely to happen. This is because the safeguards built into the criminal law reduce to the vanishing point the chance of such an outcome.

If parents and physicians decide not to provide aggressive care to a severely handicapped or very premature infant, they can be convicted of a criminal offense only if every one of an unlikely series of events occurs. This is because, whatever a scholar believes *should* be criminal, no person can be found guilty of a crime except through due process. California procedure is typical: first, a bystander (nurse, for instance, or social worker) must feel the decision not to treat an impaired infant is wrong and notify the prosecutor. The prosecutor, in turn, must agree that a crime has been committed and file a complaint; then (in the case of any felony charge) a judge must hear evidence, agree that a crime has been committed and that there is reasonable evidence to hold the defendant(s) for trial, or a grand jury must hear evidence and return an indictment; the trial judge must allow the case to proceed through trial; and the trial jury must convict. These actions turn on legal language that is not directed specifically at the management of a marginally viable infant, so there is room for different interpretations. Each of these individuals must believe that this infant should have been treated and that not treating the infant violated the law; the prosecutor, judge, and jury must also believe that setting this precedent will do more good than harm. Thus, when parents and physician act reasonably, the chance of criminal conviction is nil.

Civil

The civil law presents different considerations. Here a judge or official may have the sole power to decide that a newborn should be treated, and this has happened from time to time (Weir 1984). Although most of the cases and controversies have involved defective newborns, the principles apply equally to very premature infants.

The federal government first intruded itself into this previously private area in 1982. After public controversy over a Down-syndrome newborn that died when her parents refused corrective surgery for her esophageal atresia, the Department of Health and Human Services (DHHS) sent a letter to hospitals stating that handicapped newborns must be treated and that it was a violation of their civil rights not to do so. This policy attempted to wipe out the middle zone in which a decision to treat aggressively is made on an individual basis. To DHHS, every baby that was not terminal, however badly impaired, had to receive maximal care. This position was solidified when an interim final rule was promulgated by DHHS in 1983. Statutory authority for this was claimed from the 1973 Rehabilitation Act (29 USCA sec 794(a)), which provides, "No otherwise qualified individual with a disability . . . shall, solely by reason of his or her disability, be excluded from participation in, be denied the benefits of, or be subjected to discrimination under any program or activity receiving Federal financial assistance."

This initiative meshed well with President Reagan's pro-life philosophy, but many pediatricians viewed it as imposing a prefabricated solution on a wide variety of complex clinical situations. As a result of the regulations, NICU administrators lived under the threat of investigation by a Baby Doe squad if an anonymous tipster complained that a defective infant was not receiving maximal care. After a series of tactical skirmishes, the Supreme Court found that the regulations exceeded DHHS's authority (*Bowen* v. *American Hospital Association*, 476 US Supreme Court 610 (1986)).

The Baby Doe regulations are defunct, but other federal statutes (now often generically called "Baby Doe") have been or could be used to intervene in the nontreatment of a defective newborn. Chief among them are the 1984 amendments to the Child Abuse Prevention and Treatment Act (CAPTA). Under CAPTA as amended, state agencies that choose to participate in the program (all but three do) must develop procedures for reporting alleged or suspected "medical neglect," defined as the withholding or withdrawal of a life-sustaining medical treatment that is "medically indicated." CAPTA provides that withholding medical treatment does not constitute medical neglect when, "in the treating physician's . . . reasonable medical judgment," one of these narrow conditions apply:

(a) the infant is chronically and irreversibly comatose; (b) the provision of such treatment would merely prolong dying, not be effective in ameliorating or correcting all of the infant's life-threatening conditions, or otherwise be futile in terms of the survival of the infant; or (c) the provision of such treatment would be virtually futile in terms of the survival of the infant and the treatment itself under such circumstances would be inhumane. (Child Abuse Prevention and Treatment Act (CAPTA) sec. 5106g(6))

CAPTA is intended to ban all judgments made on the basis of quality of life or the chance of survival (Merrick 1995). Some commentators feel that the use of the phrase "virtually futile" allows some room to maneuver, but this is overoptimistic. Futility has proven a difficult concept to pin down, but most definitions of futile care specify a low probability of success – say, one in 10 or one in 100. If we define "success" in treating an extremely premature infant as survival, considered without regard to the chance of neurological disability, the observed survival rate of 15 percent in infants at 23 weeks gestation means that aggressive care of these infants is not futile. CAPTA, then, would require that we treat Baby Girl M.

Although CAPTA's intention is to force aggressive treatment for many infants that are now allowed to die, that does not mean that we must or should bow to its command. CAPTA only requires states to develop mechanisms to respond to allegations of the medical neglect of infants. It does not require the states to take any additional action, nor does it address the actions of physicians and hospitals. Any intervention in the care of impaired infants prompted by this law would have to be undertaken by a state child protective service acting under the aegis of state law. Not surprisingly, child protective services, which usually carry overwhelming caseloads of urgent problems, have shown little interest in second-guessing a physician in the NICU. I have been unable to find a single instance of a child protective service taking action when treatment has been withheld from a defective newborn in the type of circumstance under consideration here. There are no court cases, no precedents to help hammer out the contours of the physician's duty. Simply silence. Nonetheless, some neonatologists, acting out of fear, reluctantly treat infants that they feel should be permitted to die (Kopelman et al. 1988).

A second law, the Emergency Medical Treatment and Active Labor Act (EMTALA), has been applied to the non-treatment of handicapped newborns. This law was enacted for the worthwhile purpose of preventing patient dumping, as when a hospital turns away an indigent patient who comes to the emergency room in active labor. In 1993 a federal district judge applied EMTALA to the case of an anencephalic infant, Baby K. This infant was given aggressive care at her mother's request and survived to go home, but then underwent a series of respiratory arrests and could be kept alive only with intermittent mechanical ventilation. The physicians objected that Baby K, who had no brain, was certain to die soon and in any case was incapable of any human interaction and that re-intubating her was purposeless. A federal judge disagreed, ruling that EMTALA required the hospital to provide continued treatment. The Fourth Circuit Court of Appeals agreed, holding that no exception could be carved out for an anencephalic patient simply because of her quality of life (*In re Baby K*, 832 F. Supp. 1022 (E. D. Va. 1993), aff'd 16 F. 3d 590 (4th Cir. 1994), cert. denied, 115 Supreme Court 91 (1994)).

The courts may be a poor forum in which to resolve treatment decisions, in part because these decisions often must be made in hours or minutes. In the case of Baby K, we have a federal appellate court that took three months to reach a decision. Surely this is time enough to review the records, consult with experts, re-read the legislative history, and deliberate the issues. Despite this, the court's decision in Baby K seems terribly wrong to many physicians. This may be a predictable result, however, when physicians ask the courts to set practice standards (Annas 1994).

This dubious precedent, and these laws, should not change the care of Baby Girl M. A nurse is unlikely to complain that Baby Girl M was not being given aggressive treatment; nurses are with these infants continuously and know, perhaps better than the physicians, the suffering that heroic treatment imposes. Even if there were a complaint, and it were upheld, the physicians are unlikely to be in any legal jeopardy. CAPTA frightens physicians but no actual enforcement appears to have followed. Similarly, EMTALA was used to compel physicians to treat Baby K, but the physicians involved were not censured. I am unaware of any physician being penalized under either of these statutes for withholding or withdrawing treatment of a handicapped newborn. Physicians make many tough decisions; sometimes a precondition to the right decision is to disregard a remote legal risk.

Malpractice

The most serious legal hazard for the physicians who cared for Baby Girl M is a medical malpractice lawsuit. To gauge the likelihood of suit being brought, and of its success, we must suspend this legal discussion and review the case history.

Baby Girl M at the crossroads

We are not told if the physicians in this case followed their own standard practice; I suspect that they did. Unfortunately, standard practice is occasionally inadequate to the challenge presented by a very premature infant. I state this not to criticize the physicians involved but to urge a change in the routine care of pre-viable infants.

Neonatologists, like most physicians, provide two levels of care: aggressive care and comfort care. Aggressive care employs every stratagem to increase the likelihood of healthy survival. Comfort care is undertaken in the face of insurmountable obstacles: an inoperable tumor, for instance, or congenital absence of the kidneys. There is no uniform agreement on what comfort care involves, and it could include withholding all medical interventions, but more typically one sees the provision of warmth, oxygen, IV fluids, and medications for pain and dyspnea. In comfort care, medicine's power is turned toward easing the physical symptoms of dying and making the experience of death peaceful for the patient and the family. This requires a plan.

The decision not to provide aggressive support for this 23-week infant fell within the realm of good practice, but the comfort care she received shows a lack of forethought. Unlike an infant with a lethal congenital anomaly, Baby Girl M had the potential for life. Comfort care supported her long enough to thrust her into an uncertain voyage in the NICU. In retrospect we know that she survived and is doing reasonably well, but the odds against this were long, the price was high, and the level of residual disability remains unknown. These decisions must be made on the basis of what is likely to happen, not the best that might happen (Sinclair and Torrance 1995). If a decision is made not to treat a marginally viable infant, what should be done next?

Management of such an infant should have three goals: to permit death, to prevent suffering, and to help the family take this child into their hearts. Intelligent choices foster family understanding and involvement and promote normal grieving (Pearson 1997); the interpersonal dimensions of this process ripen best outside the high-tech setting of the NICU. First, of course, the diagnosis must be certain; for a premature infant, that occurs when the attending physician confirms that this infant should not receive aggressive care, after considering its gestational age, its condition, the facilities available, and the wishes of the family. If the infant is not deemed viable, her care should be changed immediately and unequivocally to true comfort care.

An infant like this should be wrapped in a blanket and given to her family to hold. She should not be dried, warmed, or stimulated in the delivery room, nor should she be placed in a warm incubator, given oxygen, or monitored. Death will come easily, and a sedative can be administered if she shows signs of distress. The family's questions should be anticipated, and the social worker and hospital chaplain often have much to contribute. The family will be very grateful if there is a camera available so that mother, father, and grandparents can be photographed holding the infant. It may be more descriptive to call this family care rather than comfort care, for this child will be held, not by a nurse, but in the arms of her own family, and to the extent that this child will experience human affection, it will be in these moments. Ask a NICU nurse what her birth plan would be if she were to deliver an infant that is probably not yet viable. She will probably say she would do anything to keep her infant out of the NICU, and would prefer to deliver among her loved ones and hold her baby in her arms as death comes. I have great respect for the wisdom of nurses.

Some may feel that this approach moves toward death too briskly. It can be hard to admit that death is sometimes a goal that one should steer directly toward, but sometimes that is the best medical choice. Here I am not discussing actively causing death, say by lethal injection. The neonatologists did not need to cause death, they simply needed to permit it. However, they did not permit death, so it did not occur. Their intention was not to give Baby Girl M a trial of deprivation of care, but that is what happened. The case report describes the ethics committee as having "two opposite opinions" about how this infant should have been managed at birth; it would be equally true to say that the ethics committee was unanimous that a plan should have been formed early on and that plan adhered to, although members of the committee might have chosen different specific plans. This is not to say that a plan must be cast in stone at the moment of birth, or that it cannot be changed in response to unexpected events. A baby who is given family care could survive longer than expected and force a reassessment of the situation. But that did not happen here: this baby was resuscitated, monitored, and given oxygen in a warm incubator, dramatically increasing the chance of this kind of awkward situation developing. We are not told why the neonatologist chose this course of action; perhaps there was concern that doing less would violate CAPTA. Theoretically this is understandable, but the chance of this resulting in legal problems is almost infinitesimal – certainly less than the chance of other legal trouble from events as they unfolded.

Because this baby was given mid-level care, the ground was laid for another mistake when the baby looked better than expected at five hours. Reading between the lines, the clinician probably panicked when Baby Girl M did not deteriorate as expected. At this point two neonatologists considered the peculiar question of whether a change in plan would be "appropriate, medically or ethically." This is an odd comment, as a medically appropriate action is almost invariably ethically appropriate as well. Ethics is not free-dwelling; it is grounded in a context, which is here the medical care of this infant. Good medicine and good ethics walk together; bad medicine is bad ethics by definition. The real question seems to have been whether a change would be appropriate medically *or legally*; in other words, at this point, are we more likely to get sued if this child lives or dies? Because the law travels its own road, observing ethics and medicine at some distance and paying them no homage, this is an understandable question.

The neonatologists were now in a tough situation, and obtaining objective data – the blood gas and glucose – was a smart move. Their decision to change course, however, shows the same tentativeness as in the earlier provision of comfort care. The neonatologist comments that "perhaps a trial of mechanical ventilatory support was warranted" and full support was instituted. What kind of trial was this, and how was it explained to the family? The trial of an intervention should last for a specified period of time with the child's condition to be evaluated again at the end. As far as one can tell from the case history, the trial was ongoing on the day Baby Girl M was discharged. It would be better to tell the family, for instance, that a trial of full support is proposed, with the infant re-evaluated in 12 hours, with support to be continued if she showed good blood gases and there were no other signs of trouble.

What is Baby Girl M's outcome so far? She needs no oxygen, she's walking and talking; this is good. On the other hand, she also has a developmental delay, one that may result in significant problems in the future. This brings us back to the issue of malpractice. In order for a malpractice suit to be filed, two elements must be present: a bad result and an unhappy family. When things do not go right, one looks anxiously to the family to see if they are satisfied with what has happened or if they seem angry. Good communication has prevented many an otherwise plausible claim. In this case, the grandmother brought M back for a visit and is pleased with her, which is good for all concerned.

This brings us back to the family. The neonatologists appear to feel that this family is dysfunctional, difficult, and perhaps simply not very bright. Granted, some families are easier to work with than others, but so far we have heard only the clinicians' story. What about the family's perspective?

We know, as a beginning, that this family – teenage mother, disappearing father, and dominant maternal grandmother – is not atypical. As the President's Commission noted,

Women who have LBW [low birth weight] infants are more likely than other mothers to be poor, nonwhite, single, poorly educated, or under 18 or over 35. Inadequate prenatal health care is also strongly associated with low birth weight and infant mortality. (President's Commission 1983: 201)

Of course the neonatologists would prefer to deal with a Standard Family (distraught mother, pained but rational father, kids at home with the nanny, grandparents out of state), but this is the family they got.

For Baby Girl M, as for many babies in this plight, the parents are not the primary decision makers. Baby Girl M's mother is 15 and is portrayed as passive. Baby Girl M's father and grandfather are both involved early on, but soon disappear. The one person who emerges from this as a strong person is the grandmother. She is the glue that holds this family together, that coaxes her daughter along, outwaits or exiles her husband, is there for the baby, and brings the child back at 18 months. This woman is Baby Girl M's greatest asset.

A medical case history provides meager evidence from which to judge the interactions of family and physicians, but what we have suggests that the physicians made all the major decisions. This is occasionally appropriate, for some families are too shaken or too indecisive to make choices. But the clinicians do not say that; rather, they implausibly assert that the family did make decisions. At the end of the case history, they comment, "In retrospect, the confusion regarding the family's initial decision not to support the child aggressively probably reflected internal dissension within the family."

What "initial decision"? As often happens in the NICU (Anspach 1993), the physicians made the decisions, the family assented. When the neonatologist first explained that Baby Girl M did not appear to be viable and proposed that no aggressive intervention be undertaken, this care plan was "explained to the mother and grandmother, neither of whom expressed any disagreement with a plan for comfort care only." This family did not actively decide, it acquiesced. The family understood that this baby would not live and accepted it.

Imagine the family's surprise when the neonatologist reappeared and told them that although the prognosis was "very poor," a trial of mechanical ventilation might be appropriate. Again, the physician decided and the grandmother acquiesced. The family consented to a DNR (do not resuscitate) order early on – here there is no pretense that it was their decision – and later to a withdrawal of that order.

The case history complains that the family was inconsistent, but consider the events from the family's point of view. At first the physicians say "Let's do nothing," then "Let's do something," and then "Let's do everything," while still saying "This baby will probably do badly anyway." In terms of cardiopulmonary resuscitation (CPR), early on the physicians say "Let's not do CPR if she stops breathing"; later they say "Now things are different, let's do CPR if she stops breathing." There were reasons for these changes, but it still seems small to accuse the *family* of inconsistency.

Malpractice considerations

I do not like talking about malpractice in this setting. Malpractice law is a creature of the courts; it tells us nothing about the medical and moral duties of physicians. Yet when a situation suggests a high likelihood of malpractice allegations, it is a rare physician who can serenely carry forward without at least thinking of covering his legal backside.

At one point, confronted with a severely compromised infant, doing everything was a safe harbor. This is no longer true, and liability can follow if the physician intervenes and a baby that would otherwise have died survives impaired. In the first important case of this kind, a Texas family brought suit against the hospital where their extremely premature infant was resuscitated against the family's wishes. At trial, the hospital argued that the baby was believed to be viable at birth and the hospital was therefore obligated to treat her. The child, who has cerebral palsy and is legally blind, is almost totally incapacitated. The jury returned a verdict for the family, awarding them $46.9 million in medical expenses and interest and $13.5 million in punitive damages (Annas 2004). This verdict was overturned on appeal. However, the resuscitation of an extremely premature infant against the wishes of the parents clearly holds significant liability for physician and hospital alike. This line of attack would probably not work for Baby Girl M's case, though, assuming that there is adequate documentation of the family's acceptance of aggressive care when that recommendation was discussed with them.

Just as it can be hazardous for a physician to do too much, liability can also result if an infant is given only minimal care and then survives with neurological or other impairments. What if the family later asserts that her condition was worsened by the six hours of comfort care? This situation is reminiscent of a discredited custom that was once common:

In an earlier era, the practice was indeed different. Infants who were extremely premature were given a "trial of life"; that is, they were left alone and were reassessed at a later time. Those who were still alive were then resuscitated and supported. Unfortunately, for many of these infants, significant *post-natal* hypoxic-ischemic injury had already transpired. (Donn 1996)

The keys to preventing a malpractice suit are to make good decisions, deliver good care, maintain good communication, and document what has been done and why. The physicians who cared for Baby Girl M failed on at least two accounts (good decisions and good communication). Their actions probably stemmed, at least in part, from concern over a perceived legal obligation to treat even this very premature infant aggressively, a concern that may have increased their malpractice risk. How vulnerable are they?

It is impossible to determine the extent of the injury resulting from this period of neglect, but this uncertainty might provide ground for a settlement to avoid the risk of going to a jury. Nonetheless, the studies obtained from Baby Girl M at six hours do not demonstrate obvious deterioration, the care provided appears impeccable from that point forward, the hospital bills are apparently not a problem, and the grandmother is satisfied with the child's quality of life. These are encouraging signs that a lawsuit is unlikely to result.

Toward better decisions

Baby Girl M's physicians did their best to make reasonable decisions; a more systematic approach, however, would reduce the frequency of this kind of troublesome case. These recommendations are intended to be consistent, even if they do not please everyone:

(1) Society should accept responsibility for rationally distributing (i.e., rationing) the resources that are committed to health care, resources that are currently irrationally allocated. We know that hundreds of thousands of dollars were spent on Baby Girl M, but we do not know if her mother had access to birth-control services. For some it will matter whether or not she lived in an area in which abortions are available, and it should matter to us all that despite spotting for four weeks, she did not receive prenatal care, care that might have prevented her premature delivery.

(2) Until action on a societal scale occurs, the appropriate professional societies should promulgate recommendations for the management of the very premature infant that could be adapted as needed for use at the local level. These guidelines, which should include a provision for discretion when appropriate, would provide medical, ethical, and legal support to clinicians who follow them.

(3) In the absence of action by professional societies, individual neonatologists and neonatologist groups should establish their own guidelines rather than relying on ad hoc decisions, simply because guidelines promote better decision making. These guidelines can only be a first step; it would be far better to take formal account of economic and social costs as well as clinical outcomes, something individual clinicians are not trained to do.

(4) Infants in the gray zone, those who are neither viable nor not viable, should be managed with aggressive care, family care, or a trial of aggressive management, according to the wishes of their parents. This requires an active effort to learn about the parents and to inform them about the life of very premature infants. Whenever possible, this two-way learning should take place before the infant is born. If it cannot be, the infant should be given basic supportive care for an hour or two while the family reaches a decision. Many people might have useful input into this process if time permits – a minister, the obstetrician or other clinicians, the nurses, parents of similar children. The parents need information both about premature infants in general and about their own child. This kind of program makes good medical sense. It reduces confusion within the professional team and ensures a more consistent approach to these very sick infants. It also makes clear communication with the family much easier. For all of these reasons, it also reduces the likelihood of a malpractice suit.

(5) When maximal care is suggested by the clinician, or demanded by the parents, for infants that would be considered pre-viable by expert neonatologists, the following should be obligatory:

    (a) the parents should be informed that although there is a chance of the infant surviving, trying to salvage such early babies is not community practice and there is a substantial risk of neurological impairment and unpredictable costs; and

    (b) if the parents consent, the outcome of such attempts should be meticulously tracked, preferably as part of a formal research protocol. This should be continued into childhood and beyond so that we can learn more about their short- and long-term prospects.

Conclusion

The impulse of clinicians to provide some minimum level of medical intervention reflects the understandable desire to do something even when death is anticipated. In a few circumstances, such as the extremely premature infant, even the minimal intervention of comfort care may be enough to cause problems. For the pre-viable infant, planned family care is better than haphazard comfort care. It is better for a family to hold their infant during its brief life than to watch it die in an incubator.

When an infant is not viable, the family should be compassionately informed of the situation and their assent to family care sought. When the baby may be viable but it is unclear if aggressive care will do more harm than good, the family should be helped to make their own decision as much as possible. Federal initiatives to impose a standard solution harm all the participants in this intimate drama; the greatest victims are usually the parents. Normally they have the legal right, and obligation, to make decisions on behalf of their infant. No one but the parents knows their inner responses when suddenly faced with responsibility for a desperately ill child; no one else knows if they feel capable of rising to this challenge, or terrified and overwhelmed. Of course, most parents know nothing about the treatment and prognosis of premature babies, and it is the responsibility of the physicians to instruct them in these matters insofar as it is possible. But the parents' ignorance does not, cannot, justify the physicians simply following their own instincts or moral or religious preferences. The experienced physician also understands that promoting parental decision making leads to better decisions and improves family satisfaction; these in turn reduce the chance of a lawsuit.

The selection of which gravely impaired infants should be given aggressive care is controversial, with commentators (and practitioners) arrayed along a spectrum that may be oversimplified as extending from the religious right to the utilitarian left. What I have presented here is my own perspective, and I feel it reflects reasonable medical practice and ethical thought. Some will disagree, even in matters that I consider open and shut, and I respect their convictions. No moral position eliminates those difficult cases when a baby is in the medical and moral middle zone of ambiguity, it simply shifts the zones to left or right. However, having a position, almost any position, provides a foundation for action.

Some people feel that the extremely premature infant is different from the infant with a severe congenital malformation, for instance absent kidneys or hypoplastic lungs. The premature infant, they say, is entirely healthy and normal, simply born too soon, and not disabled, at least not yet. This view misses a critical point – that until the moment of birth, an infant's most important organ is the mother. A premature infant who must survive without this organ can be as disabled as a term infant born with no kidneys, and it is appropriate to treat both as impaired.

Because legal theory differs from the law as it actually functions, it is a mistake to unthinkingly do what someone says the law "requires." The best medical decision is almost always the right legal decision. The law is imperfect, but it is no fool, and generally when medical and legal imperatives appear to conflict, the situation requires more thought. The physician who says in court, "This was the best medical course of action," may not prevail, but there is rarely a better justification. The legal hazards that crowd the minds of hospital administrators should not prevent us from making clear decisions with the families of these infants.

ACKNOWLEDGMENTS

I am grateful for the editorial assistance of Anna Kieken, Ph.D., and the helpful comments of Judy Levison, M.D., Maude Pervere, J.D., David E. Woodrum, M.D., and an anonymous peer reviewer.

2.3 Topical discussion

The paradoxical neonate

The treatment of the extremely low-birth-weight baby, as in this case, is as challenging ethically as it is medically. A fragile baby able to fit in the palm of a hand can have remarkable reparative and adaptive potential, but short-term (and long-term) morbidity is unknowable. The parameter of "viability" is itself a moving target: it shifts downward with new technologies or treatment modalities, and varies among institutions as well as among infants. The difference of one week of gestational development can, as in this case, alter expectations for the medical course of a newborn.

For infants born at a gestational age of 26 or more weeks, or weighing more than 800 g, treatment is the standard of care. There is some consensus that for an infant of less than 23 weeks or 500 g at birth, the presumption should be against resuscitation. This recommendation, based on empirical results in such cases, is like the writing on ancient mariner's maps warning "here be dragons." It is all very well to be told not to go there – but, as in this case, you may find yourself there anyway.

Acting for the best in the face of uncertainty

Despite the availability of statistical compilations of complications of prematurity, the long-term results of any short-term intervention can be unpredictable for any given infant. For the extremely low-birth-weight baby, there is, in addition, a vulnerability that is based on the fact that the neonate is uniquely individual and resistant to classification. Thus, the short-term, as well as long-term, results of interventions can be unpredictable. The ethical course of action might be very clear

Ethical Dilemmas in Pediatrics: Cases and Commentaries, ed. Lorry R. Frankel, Amnon Goldworth, Mary V. Rorty, and William A. Silverman. Published by Cambridge University Press. © Cambridge University Press 2005.

if only the medical prognosis were certain; and conversely, early decisions about the ethically appropriate course of action have implications for the medical outcomes. This case report is the neonatologist's equivalent of a ship's log after a treacherous sea journey. Its anomaly is not the uncertainty of prognosis, or the changes in care plan to accommodate changes in the infant's status, but the degree of access the case gives us to those changes, and the frankness with which these shifts are charted.

Relation of law and ethics

The relation of law and ethics is far from simple. Although researchers and practitioners are constrained in their practice arenas by the laws and regulations that apply to it, they also stand under a professional obligation to critically scrutinize extant or proposed laws and offer arguments for their imposition or reform. Clinical ethics and health law evolve together in a dynamic and interactive relationship. Within the parameters of what is not forbidden by law at any given historical point may lie behaviors considered ethically problematic. Changes in either general social expectations or professional standards of care may precede the associated legal cases that then codify them. Conscientious professionals may find themselves driven by professional (or personal) ethical considerations to challenge current practices. Ethics committees serve a different role in healthcare institutions than do the legal officers or risk managers of those institutions, and can be a useful resource for discussion of cases where law and ethics seem to conflict.

The "Baby Doe" laws discussed at length in Whitney's response serve as a useful example of the relation of law and ethics. Prompted by publicity of problematic cases, the laws were promulgated on the federal level in order to prevent discrimination against individuals with handicaps. Quickly overturned on procedural grounds, the regulations were also problematic because of the extent to which they restricted parental and professional judgment. The development of "infant care review committees" on the institutional level was encouraged, in an attempt to keep decisions about the care of individual infants in the hands of experienced professionals and the affected parents, and out of the courts. Such local committees were one of the precursors of the contemporary clinical ethics committee.

Communication and documentation

Insofar as this case is a "misalliance," it is because of the communication problems that beset it from its onset. Any hospital ethicist will report that the majority of the "ethical dilemmas" that lead to consultations are in fact problems resulting from failures of communication – within the care team, within the family, or between the team and family. Many failures of communication are not personal failings of individual caregivers, but have systemic causes, stemming from the complexity of the modern healthcare system. It may be easy for a primary physician in an individual community practice to establish excellent relations of communication and trust with patients. But the inpatient in a tertiary care institution may be under the care of several physicians, sometimes even treated by several teams. Explicit responsibility for communication and coordination is essential, and in some cases it has proved useful to have one team member designated as the sole communicator to the family, or one family member designated as responsible for communication and coordination with the caregivers and within the family.

In the case of Baby Girl M the neonatologist present at the birth was not the same as the one present for the initial admission, and the infant was shortly transferred from the initial community hospital to a second, larger hospital. Unless establishing and maintaining clear communication lines within the team and with the family is given a high priority, complications of the sort described can ensue. Although not a factor in this case, culture or language barriers between patients and families and their caregivers can render communication even more difficult, requiring more attention.

FURTHER READING

Ariagno, R. L. and Greely, H. T. Government regulations in the United States, and Baby Doe and beyond. In *Ethics and Perinatology*, ed. A. Goldworth, W. Silverman, D. K. Stevenson, and E. W. D. Young (New York, NY: Oxford University Press, 1995), pp. 279–306.

Fischer, A. F. and Stevenson, D. K. The consequences of uncertainty: an empirical approach to medical decision making in neonatal intensive care. *JAMA* **258** (1987), 1929–1931.

Rhoden, N. K. Treating Baby Doe: the ethics of uncertainty. *Hastings Center Report* **16** (4) (1986), 34–42.

Saigal, S. Stoskopf, B. L., Feeny, D., *et al.* Differences in preferences for neonatal outcomes among health professionals, parents and adolescents. *JAMA* **281** (1999), 1991–1997.

Stevenson, D. K. and Goldworth, A. Ethical dilemmas in the delivery room. *Seminars in Perinatology* **22** (1998), 198–206.

3.1 Munchausen syndrome by proxy

Manuel Garcia-Careaga and John A. Kerner Jr.

Introduction

Munchausen syndrome by proxy (MSBP), first described by Professor Roy Meadow in 1977, is a form of child abuse where there is persistent fabrication of symptoms of illness on behalf of an unsuspecting or helpless victim that causes the victim to be regarded as ill by others (Meadow 1977). Methods of fabrication include: (1) fictitious history (false reporting of symptoms), (2) simulation, (3) induction, (4) withholding medications in a chronically ill child (e.g., in a child with asthma). The perpetrator may use more than one of the above methods. Criteria have been established (Table 3.1). MSBP can occur in individuals with a "true physical disorder" in which case the symptoms are exaggerated to the point that the child is subjected to multiple unnecessary treatments and/or investigations (Rosenberg 1987).

In a survey of all pediatricians in England and Ireland, the two-year combined annual incidence of MSBP was at least 0.5 per 100 000 children and at least 2.8 per 100 000 for children under one year of age (McClure et al. 1996). As of 1997, there were close to 300 articles published on MSBP in professional journals worldwide, with authors representing disciplines such as medicine, law, nursing, psychology, psychiatry, and social work. In more than 300 cases described by Meadow (1977), the perpetrator was the child's biological mother in ~90% of the cases (another female caregiver, baby-sitter, or nurse in ~5%, and the child's father in ~5%). Common clinical presentations of MSBP include false history of seizures, factitious bleeding, alleged allergies, vomiting, diarrhea, fever, apnea, and rashes.

Some of these child victims of MSBP die at the hands of their mothers. Mortality rates reported in the literature are said to be 9–10% (Rosenberg 1987). The majority of victims suffer physical and psychological damage, either directly from

Ethical Dilemmas in Pediatrics: Cases and Commentaries, ed. Lorry R. Frankel, Amnon Goldworth, Mary V. Rorty, and William A. Silverman. Published by Cambridge University Press. © Cambridge University Press 2005.

Table 3.1 Criteria used in the diagnosis of MSBP

The caregiver fabricates signs and symptoms in a child so that the child is considered to be ill by others

The caregiver (usually persistently) presents the child to medical professionals for assessment and/or treatment of the fabricated signs or symptoms

The caregiver denies knowing what is making the child ill

When the caregiver and the child are separated, the child improves or experiences complete disappearance of the symptoms

Source: Rosenberg 1987.

Table 3.2 Warning signals

(1) Recurrent illness where a cause can not be found

(2) Discrepancy between the history and the physical findings: the illness makes no clinical sense

(3) Symptoms fail to respond to treatments that "should work"; offered treatments are repeatedly not tolerated

(4) The child is labeled as having a rare disease: astute and experienced physicians remark that they have "never seen a case like this before"

(5) If "witnesses" other than the perpetrator are questioned closely, they are unable to conclusively support the picture presented by the perpetrator

(6) There is a cessation of symptoms when the victim is separated from the parent

(7) The perpetrator appears to be a model parent

(8) Despite the supposed severity of the child's illness, the perpetrator appears less concerned than are the consulted health professionals

(9) The parent is well-versed in medical terminology and the latest treatments

(10) The parent has a history of Munchausen syndrome or may have symptoms similar to those of the child

(11) A history of similar health problems in the victim's sibling(s)

(12) A parent who welcomes medical tests

(13) Stories that change over time

outright harm or indirectly from painful procedures, unnecessary medications, or hospitalizations ordered by unwitting physicians. As physicians, we have to be alert and have a high index of suspicion when certain "red flags" start to appear (Table 3.2). This form of abuse differs from others in a number of ways: the perpetrator is almost always female and usually presents as a model parent; there is little or no indication of family discord; and the abusive behavior is clearly premeditated, not impulsive or in reaction to a child's behavior (Bryk and Siegel 1997).

Since the mother not infrequently appears to be a caring and concerned parent, many physicians frequently do not include MSBP in their differential diagnosis of an unexplained illness, leading to under-recognition and undertreatment of this syndrome by healthcare professionals. Early recognition of MSBP may prevent physicians, nurses, social workers, and legal professionals from becoming unwitting collaborators with the parent (Zitelli *et al.* 1987). In Rosenberg's review, the mean time from onset of signs and symptoms of illness to the diagnosis of MSBP was 14.9 months, although "the diagnosis was made easily and quickly" once MSBP entered the differential (Rosenberg 1987).

MSBP is particularly sinister because physicians – especially those who treat small children – depend on accurate histories from parents. We need to learn that parents will sometimes fabricate symptoms or deliberately cause a disease (Lerer 1990). Our medical training has led us to listen to and trust the medical histories that parents provide. We have not been trained to be distrustful of parents or to investigate when our diagnostic work-up is unrevealing. The natural instinct of a physician is to continue searching for a disease, to comfort and support the patient and the family, and to offer solutions or palliation for the afflicted member. Unfortunately, it is this basic principle of medicine that makes the physician vulnerable to manipulation by the parent and sets him up to be a collaborator, potentially exposing the child to undue medical tests and procedures which could carry considerable risks both physically and emotionally. In essence, we become victims of deceit, and we add to the victimization process by continuing to subject these patients to unnecessary diagnostic evaluation.

Munchausen syndrome by proxy carries medical, ethical, and legal ramifications. In the great majority of instances of this condition, a "smoking gun" – concrete proof of a crime (e.g., direct observation of a parent suffocating a child, injecting feces into a central line, or giving the child a laxative to induce "diarrhea") – is not found, making the diagnosis difficult. Once the diagnosis is seriously considered, the first priority should be to protect the child from harm. When the suspicions are strong, the physician carries a tremendous burden of responsibility. It is at this point that an organized multidisciplinary team is of utmost importance to assist in securing the safety of the patient, helping the offending parent, contacting the protective agencies, and organizing adequate follow-up of the patient. Such teams should include pediatric psychologists, psychiatrists, social workers, and risk-management specialists who are familiar with hospital policy and procedures regarding child maltreatment, as well as with the special circumstances involved in assessing, diagnosing, and reporting MSBP. At our children's hospital, our physicians can now consult the SCAN committee (SCAN = suspected child abuse and neglect), which was launched to oversee child-abuse issues.

We physicians may confront difficulties in coming to terms with our own suspicions, and in that process a patient can lose his or her life, or we can unwittingly perpetuate the cycle of abuse. In many instances physicians are ill-equipped to deal with the complexity of MSBP, and for that reason adequate action may be dangerously delayed. The ability of these parents to convince both laypeople and professional persons of their innocence cannot be overemphasized (Zitelli *et al.* 1987). Many judges and attorneys still lack familiarity with MSBP and may require extensive education in this complex area.

Our case report starts with deceit, progresses to suspicion, and ends with a diagnosis. In many instances ethical questions will emerge; the answers to such questions are frequently not black or white. MSBP attacks the foundation of the parent–patient–physician relationship, the sacred axis of medicine.

Case report

An eight-year-old white male was referred to the pediatric gastroenterology clinic with reports by the mother of recurrent fevers, joint symptoms, chronic diarrhea, and abdominal pain of two years' duration. Prior to the onset of those symptoms two years ago, he was thriving and doing well, according to the mother's report. His mother reported fevers as high as 104° Fahrenheit (40 °C) repeating every ten days. The reported articular pain was found primarily in the large joints and did not involve any swelling or redness. These joint symptoms could occur with and without temperature elevation. There was no history of skin rashes, oral sores, or vomiting. The abdominal pain was described as diffuse and was relieved by defecation. Stools were described as diarrheic, not bloody and not foul-smelling, but just prior to the clinic visit blood was reportedly seen in the stools. The mother was also concerned about weight loss in the patient.

Past medical history

The medical history was positive for chickenpox, multiple food allergies, and hay fever, with no history of allergies to medications. The medical records received from the child's primary pediatrician revealed very frequent visits for diarrhea, fever, sore throat, runny nose, vomiting, viral syndrome, postnasal drip, and headaches. The patient had received multiple courses of antibiotics, decongestants, and antipyretics. The presence of fever was rarely corroborated in the physician's office. The physical exams on most occasions were normal; others were conclusive for a pharyngitis, flu, sinusitis, or bronchitis. The child's tonsils and adenoids had been removed, but the fevers and diarrhea persisted. He was initially referred to the division of pediatric infectious diseases, which performed a complete evaluation to determine the cause of his recurrent fevers and diarrhea. An extensive laboratory investigation disclosed no abnormalities.

Family history

The family history was remarkable for peptic ulcer disease, gallbladder and heart disease, allergies in an older sibling, and a maternal history of an ovarian tumor, for which she was receiving chemotherapy.

Social history

The history was notable for a number of social stresses. The nuclear family consisted of three members: the mother, an older sibling, and the patient. The mother stated that she had been separated from her husband for six months and was going through a divorce and custody battle over the children. The mother had taken the patient out of school for three months in an attempt to decrease his exposure to infectious illnesses. During this time of home study he continued to have fevers.

Physical exam

The exam revealed a thin young boy. He was alert, active, and in no distress at the time of the exam. His weight was 20.7 kg and his height 123.4 cm. Physical exam was essentially negative, except for tenderness over the complete abdomen, most notably over the right lower quadrant and upper part of the abdomen. There was no abdominal distension or organomegaly, or rebound tenderness. The rectal exam showed a normal sphincter tone, with trace guaiac-positive stools.

Assessment and plan

The differential diagnosis initially included inflammatory bowel disease, peptic disease, and food allergies, but none of these conditions could be confirmed. The child was seen one month later. The mother reported that he had diarrhea and abdominal pain. His appetite remained good, as did his level of activity. The physical exam was again essentially negative, except for mild discomfort on deep palpation of his right lower abdominal quadrant.

A social-service consult was obtained. Among the most salient features from this evaluation was that the parents' separation had been because of another woman. The couple had been experiencing marital problems for years. The parents were in a bitter custody battle. The mother had a 17-year-old son who had been suicidal in the past in reaction to family tensions. The mother also reported that she had had ten miscarriages before successfully delivering the patient. Both mother and child were receiving counseling. The impression of our social worker was that the mother's mental health appeared severely compromised. In addition, she was extremely involved with the patient. Because of the joint pain and elevated ESR (erythrocyte sedimentation rate), the patient was referred to the pediatric rheumatology clinic, and once again no abnormalities were found. The clinical course over the next year included numerous visits to the gastrointestinal (GI) clinic for evaluation of diarrhea and fevers, and recurrent hospitalizations for the same. In essence there were no changes in his physical examination with the exception of mild weight gains. Repeat laboratory tests and stool studies were essentially negative.

The social worker consulted with the therapists for both the mother and the child. The mother's therapist reported that the mother's anxiety was high and that she had a histrionic presentation. The therapists expressed confusion over the mother's medical condition. The mother led them to believe that she had stage 4 endometriosis which was cancerous but in recovery.

The GI nurse voiced her concerns about the medical history and felt that there was something "not right" with the mother. She stated that the boy looked too well, given the severity of the history. The attending physician started to become suspicious but did not believe that he had sufficient evidence of deceit. Eventually, the gastroenterologist met with both parents in the presence of the nurse and social worker to present them with a plan to hospitalize the patient. Since all test results were negative, they felt that the best way to diagnose this child was to evaluate him as an inpatient, in order to view his symptoms the moment they occurred. In view of the strong social stresses, the child psychiatrists could also be involved in an effort to deliver a comprehensive evaluation. This hospitalization did not yield a diagnosis since the child's symptoms resolved.

Follow-up

Two months later he returned to the GI clinic. The mother reported seeing him fatigued the night before, along with fever of 103 °F (39 °C). The boy was readmitted to the general pediatric ward. The mother reported that she had changed his diet over the last couple of months. She was also concerned about joint pains in his shoulders, knees, and wrists, and concerned that after spending the weekends with his father his diarrhea recurred.

This time the physical examination revealed his weight unchanged, height of 125 cm, fever to 38.7 °C, a greenish exudate in the posterior pharynx with a posterior cervical lymphadenopathy on the left side. The node was tender to palpation. There was no hepatosplenomegaly or palpable masses. The remainder of the examination and laboratory tests were essentially negative. The patient was admitted to the hospital and initially started on augmentin, but flagyl was added when reports of stool cultures (revealing several minor intestinal parasites) were returned. No other abnormalities were revealed in the laboratory tests. Repeat lab tests two days after the admission showed an ESR of 48. Because the father had a cat at home, further studies which included cat-scratch and *Toxoplasma* antibody panels were performed, and found to be negative.

Again the psychiatry service was consulted. The mother reported being treated with amitriptyline for depression. The psychiatry service recommended that the child be transferred to their unit. This would allow the psychiatrists to perform a better evaluation in a controlled environment. On the second hospital day, the patient was interviewed alone by the psychiatrist. The patient related that he had not had any diarrhea for the last two months and that he had been hospitalized because of the fevers. He said he was going to be in third grade and that he missed school. It upset him to have to wake up at 9:00 a.m. on Sunday to visit his father. He was allergic to cat fur, and his father had a cat. During the interview he was cooperative. His affect was appropriate, and his gait and speech were also normal. The impression of the psychiatrist was that of psychological factors affecting his physical condition. The differential diagnosis included Munchausen syndrome by proxy, somatization disorder, conversion disorder, and vulnerable child syndrome.

The mother was always by the bedside. The father visited on the first day, and the nurses noted that both son and father played video games for most of the shift. No abnormal interactions were seen until the last day of the hospitalization, at which time the nurse noted that mother seemed to be hovering over the patient during his meal.

After his discharge from the hospital, the patient returned to GI clinic, and seven months into the evaluation the patient returned to the GI clinic with a history of diarrhea lasting 17 days. The physical examination and various laboratories from blood, stools, and urine were negative. A few days later the patient was readmitted for persistence of the diarrhea. The mother reported that the patient was having 8–15 episodes of diarrhea per day, without blood or mucus but with crampy abdominal pain. The child had been afebrile. The physical exam demonstrated a slight weight increase, normal vital signs, and a negative exam. The plan was to restart a regular diet, lactose-free (as was being kept by the mother), with strict intake and output monitoring. A stool flow sheet was to be kept with recorded volume, pH, reducing substances, and testing for blood. Additional laboratory orders included a urine toxicology screen, and urine and stools were ordered to be tested for phenolphthalein (a laxative) due to the physician's growing suspicion of factitious or induced illness.

After the first day of hospitalization, the patient reported feeling well. The mother reported ten bouts of diarrhea from 5:00 p.m. to 10:00 p.m., but only three were recorded in the stool flow sheet. During the following two days he did not pass any stools. One of the ova and parasite tests again showed the presence of minor pathogens. He was prescribed iodoquinol (an antiprotozoal agent) for 20 days. Laboratory results from the hospitalization were again normal. Over the entire hospitalization, the patient did not complain of any abdominal pain.

Shortly after the hospitalization, he returned to the GI clinic. The mother reported that after being discharged he did well until the day of the clinic visit when he had four episodes of loose stools. The stools were described as yellow to completely clear. He also had abdominal cramping that only stopped when he had a bowel movement; there was no fever or vomiting. He was still taking iodoquinol. The exam did not suggest any pathology, with a completely benign abdominal exam. In the clinic he produced a colorless bowel movement, very mucosy.

Continuing confusion

Prior to this last appointment, the gastroenterologist discussed the patient's complicated course with the primary pediatrician. The pediatrician was asked if there was any concern on his behalf that the mother may be inducing the illness in this patient. He replied that it was possible. Both felt puzzled about the history of the fevers. The only documented fever was associated with his lymphadenitis. After that instance, and up to this appointment, there had never been another elevated temperature corroborated.

In his eighth month of follow-up, he was seen in GI clinic with a history of loose stools for the last eight days. However, the mother stated that the diarrhea had resolved one day prior to the appointment, and his fever had also resolved. His appetite was good, as was his level of activity. Again his exam was negative, except for a weight gain of 2 kg in 31 days to 23.2 kg. In view of the persistence of the symptoms, the GI attending solicited a second opinion. The patient was seen at an outside institution and the consultant commented on possible infectious etiologies and inflammatory conditions. He thought that at the moment of the consultation the patient was recovering from his illness. He recommended that a repeat endoscopy should be performed if the symptoms persisted, in order to re-evaluate for inflammatory bowel disease.

The patient returned to the GI clinic in the eleventh month of his illness. Reportedly, he had continued to have intermittent episodes of fever and diarrhea. Prior to this appointment, he was seen by the pediatrician, and found to be febrile with a temperature to 39 °C, and to have pharyngitis, probably not bacterial in origin. For three days he had had a fever as high as 104° Fahrenheit (40 °C). The fever broke one day prior to this visit, but the diarrhea resumed. The mother had been giving him Lomotil (atropine and diphenoxylate) tablets but without much success. During the appointment the patient had two loose bowel movements, which were negative for blood and reducing substances. The physical exam was negative. A blood count and ESR were normal. The patient had lost 400 g in the last three months. The symptoms were increasing in intensity, according to the history. Additional tests were negative. It was decided to re-endoscope the patient to rule out the possibility of a colonic inflammatory process. No definitive abnormalities were found.

After discharge, the mother called several times because the child had persistent vomiting and abdominal pain. She initially did not want to come to the hospital but wanted advice as to how to treat him at home. The patient was brought to the emergency room by the mother at 10:25 p.m. The nurse who did the initial assessment was told by the mother that for over three hours the patient vomited 15 times and had a fever of 38.5 °C. In the past medical history questionnaire, the mother stated that the patient had inflammatory bowel disease. On examination, the patient was afebrile and with no findings suggestive of an abdominal process. He was well hydrated. Abdominal X-rays were normal. The child was discharged home and followed the next day in the pediatric GI clinic where he was found to be essentially normal and sent home. He returned two days later to the GI clinic for persistent vomiting. His exam and weight were essentially unchanged. Repeat laboratory tests and stool studies were normal. Since the patient looked well and had tolerated his breakfast, he was discharged following lunch.

Unfortunately, the child began having large water-loss stools (400 and 250 cm^3). The attending was mystified, placed the discharge on hold and ordered a test for phenolphthalein on the patient's stool. Both stools were negative for blood and reducing substances. The attending physician expressed a desire to keep the patient in the hospital, but the mother insisted that since he was tolerating fluids by mouth, she could continue taking care of him at home. The attending agreed to the discharge with the request that he be called if the situation persisted or worsened.

Suspicion grows

Over the next 48 hours, a chain of events unfolded which led to the diagnosis of this child's medical problem. The day after the discharge, the attending received multiple calls from the mother reporting that the diarrhea continued but that the patient continued to be active, alert, and voiding. In the last call she sounded overwhelmed and tearful. The mother told the physician that the patient had had a total stool output of 1.8 L. He decided that the patient needed to be re-hospitalized, but the mother refused and assured him that his hydration was under control and that he was not looking dehydrated and he was active as usual. She would call the physician the following morning.

At 4:30 a.m. on the second day after discharge, the physician received a call from the mother who informed him that the patient was having bad diarrhea and she now wanted to hospitalize him. She told him that she had called the admitting office at the hospital and verified that there was one bed available. There was another call from the emergency department alerting the attending of the patient's situation and informing him that the mother had requested direct admission to the hospital from the ED. The patient was admitted at 9:00 a.m. His weight was 20.9 kg (his weight three days prior to the hospitalization was 23 kg). The physical exam was essentially negative with the exception of dryness of his oral mucosa and orthostatic changes in his blood pressure and heart rate, accompanied by dizziness. Obviously he was dehydrated with shock. Intravenous hydration was started. The mother was tearful and distressed about her financial situation, since she was close to bankruptcy and worried about hospital costs. She stated that she was going to have surgery herself the next day. The father arrived during the afternoon. The child was initially angry, but then readily engaged with the father in a board game. Within 24 hours of admission the child was eating pasta and potato chips and denied having any further bouts of diarrhea.

The attending physician was informed by the laboratory that stool was positive for phenolphthalein. He called the social worker, the psychiatry service, risk management, and the central pharmacy. In light of the positive phenolphthalein in the stool, he feared for the safety of this boy and filed a suspected child abuse report. The psychiatrists, social worker, and risk management specialist concurred with the decision.

The child-protection services (CPS) worker met with both parents, the social worker, psychiatrists, and the primary GI attending. The mother was not upset; she listened attentively and acted coldly. She said that she sometimes sent her son to the medicine cabinet alone for Imodium (loperamide), and the laxatives were next to it on the shelf. She did not think the older brother could have given the patient the laxative. She also volunteered that sometimes when she cleaned the toilet at home, the water would turn red. She then said that she may have inadvertently given him a laxative. Following this encounter, the diarrhea completely resolved. The patient's weight three days into the hospitalization was 22.1 kg, an increase of 1.2 kg since admission. Laboratory tests revealed a guaiac-positive stool on the day of admission. Thereafter, the hemoccults of the stools were all negative. The patient had a superb recovery from the physical standpoint. He ate a regular meal with no side effects and engaged in the ward's daily activity.

A key criterion for the diagnosis of Munchausen syndrome by proxy was met. The patient was able to eat a whole variety of foods without any untoward side effects and the symptoms of recurrent diarrhea, abdominal pain, joint symptoms, and fever vanished. The patient was placed in foster care. The District Attorney's office followed him closely, and the symptoms did not recur.

Trust is forever tarnished in cases like this. This child underwent multiple hospitalizations, numerous laboratory tests, colonoscopies, and endoscopies, as well as multiple separations from his home environment. A physician must always keep an open mind when analyzing a patient's illnesses, but one can not escape the haunting sense of distrust that stemmed from this experience. The physician's fear of being deceived again, and the personal risks, may result in delay in diagnosis and repeated unnecessary testing in an effort to rule out an organic etiology.

Legal and ethical issues

(1) If MSBP is suspected, should we perform covert video monitoring in the hospital room? (Southall *et al.* 1997, Wilde and Pedron 1993)

There is considerable controversy about covert monitoring, with legal entanglements as a possible consequence of such monitoring. We did not have covert video technology in our hospital when this case occurred, but without a doubt this type of surveillance should be readily available when the diagnosis of Munchausen syndrome by proxy is suspected. Prior to its use, we believe that cases like this should be discussed with the physicians involved, psychiatrists, risk-management staff, and the ethics committee.

(2) In an effort to corroborate our suspicions, should we search the belongings of parents and patients without their knowledge?

This should only be considered when there is a documented finding or a strong suspicion that some drug or medication is the cause of the patient's symptoms. This may require that the whole team agree to the search. Can this search extend to the parents' home? If there is a documented finding that points towards medications or chemicals as the causative agent of the patient's symptoms, there should be a call to the District Attorney's office. A search warrant may prove highly valuable in finding the offending agent in the household.

(3) Can we limit parents' direct contact with the patient by limiting their visitation or rooming-in rights?

Such action is a step that we did not consider. Merely entertaining the possibility of MSBP may not legally justify limiting the parents' contact with the patient, especially if it is a baby or a young patient that is directly or emotionally dependent on the mother's presence. The case is different when there are strong suspicions that there is imminent risk to the patient's life. If parental presence needs to be limited, an attempt to convince the parents of the importance of observing the patient's behavior in their absence should be attempted. The problem most commonly seen is that of parents objecting to the medical recommendation. If this happens, the next option is to put a 24-hour nurse or sitter in the room to supervise the parents and child, which in turn will make the parents suspicious of your intentions. This is likely to arouse the parents' suspicions concerning the intentions of the hospital.

(4) Once the doctor suspects the possibility of MSBP but has no proof, should he or she be allowed to continue doing laboratory tests and procedures in an effort to find a clue to the diagnosis that is quite improbable in light of previous studies? (Ludwig 1995)

The role of the physician is to heal and provide support, and one of our worst fears is to miss a diagnosis. Missing an organic disease may degrade the patient's health and result in serious medicolegal consequences. We believe that once there is a reasonable investigation of the patient's presenting symptoms and the results are negative, then consultation with our peers should be obtained. The psychiatry service, social worker, and the risk-management office should be immediately involved. Further invasive testing should come to a halt if the consensus supports the suspicions.

(5) Once MSBP is suspected, should the physician step aside and let the psychiatrist and social workers confirm the diagnosis before calling the child-protection agency?

The physician should not step aside, but he or she should continue to facilitate the work of other services. A sudden disappearance of the primary physician will probably end with the patient leaving the hospital against medical advice.

(6) Should the parent be informed that we have done tests to verify if the illness has been induced?

The parents should not be informed about specific tests done to find out whether the disease is being induced, since doing so may carry the risk of losing the patient.

(7) Should third-party payers (e.g., insurance or Medicaid) cover the cost of hospitalization to allow physicians to evaluate these extremely difficult cases?

With ever-increasing healthcare costs and restrictions imposed on hospitalization, hospitalizing a patient with the admitting diagnosis of "rule out Munchausen syndrome by proxy" will more than likely be denied. Such hospitalizations are multiple and at times prolonged and frustrating. Physicians are always left with the responsibility and burden of having to proceed with doing what is best for the patient knowing that there may be no reimbursement for medical services collected by the hospital or for the involved physicians and ancillary professional services. A very difficult problem results. The government and the private payers should take responsibility for covering these expenses. Munchausen syndrome by proxy should be recognized as a psychiatric phenomenon that may lead to the demise of the patient or to serious emotional and/or physical sequelae. The legal establishment needs to be clear that MSBP constitutes child abuse. Prompt and effective intervention is necessary once MSBP is suspected.

Conclusion

The management of MSBP is troublesome, time-consuming, and often not financially rewarding for the health care and other practitioners involved. There may be adverse publicity and even legal or personal risk directed against individuals (e.g., the physician reporting the case to CPS) and institutions. Thus, there are many reasons why it may be advantageous to avoid identifying cases and thus avoid the long process of management. This concern, that there may be vested interests against the identification of cases, raises a further ethical issue. (Mitchell 1995)

3.2 Some conceptual and ethical issues in Munchausen syndrome by proxy

Frances M. Kamm

Introduction

Munchausen syndrome by proxy (MSBP) involves someone who is responsible for a patient (often the mother) lying about and possibly even producing his or her symptoms while persistently presenting the patient (most commonly a child) for medical assessment.[1] Doctors are most interested in getting advice on morally permissible means of collecting evidence that MSBP is occurring, as a way to stop harm to the patient. However, there are also other issues of a conceptual nature raised by MSBP such as its relation to child abuse, the distinction between deceiving and harming, and between diagnosis and prevention of harm. In this chapter I will first discuss conceptual issues and then move on to the more clearly ethical concerns related to diagnosis and prevention of harm.

Conceptual issues

The use of the term "syndrome"

Suppose a small percentage of doctors deliberately gave their patients laxatives inappropriately and wrote notes in the patient's record, on which other physicians and nurses in a hospital rely, attesting to the patient's being diarrhetic. Would it be most appropriate to refer to the doctors' behavior as a "syndrome" and think that confirming its occurrence was most appropriately referred to as "diagnosing" the patient's problem? Surely this would be inappropriate language to use, because

---

[1] Since this article was originally submitted for publication there has been increasing skepticism about whether many cases presumably thought to involve MSBP actually did so. There has also been concern that hostility to women may sometimes have prompted the MSBP diagnosis. I shall simply assume for the sake of argument that MSBP actually occurs at least sometimes.

Ethical Dilemmas in Pediatrics: Cases and Commentaries, ed. Lorry R. Frankel, Amnon Goldworth, Mary V. Rorty, and William A. Silverman. Published by Cambridge University Press. © Cambridge University Press 2005.

it medicalizes what is essentially criminal behavior. Similarly, finding out if A was poisoned by B is not best described as diagnosing the cause of A's ill health. Crime may be bad for people's health, but trying to find out which particular person committed the crime as a result of which A's health is jeopardized is not best described, I think, as a diagnosis of A's ill health. Yet, when a parent[2] does essentially what the doctor in my imaginary case has done, it is referred to as a syndrome and finding evidence confirming her action is described as diagnosing the child's medical problem. Here is a quote (to which I shall return to make several different points) from an article on MSBP:

> In general, once MSBP is a part of the differential diagnosis, hidden camera or other monitoring may be viewed as a diagnostic tool like any other. Monitoring is not performed to collect evidence of criminal activity against the parents, but to make an appropriate diagnostic finding and to protect the child. The evidence may subsequently be used in child protective proceedings. (Wilde and Pedron 1993)

Perhaps both the doctors in my imaginary case and the parent in MSBP are being discovered to have psychiatric problems and so should themselves be thought of as patients. But it is odd to think that this turns discovery of their problem into a diagnosis of a syndrome from which their victim is suffering. (In this connection, it is interesting that Drs. Garcia-Careaga and Kerner say nothing about what motivates mothers in MSBP; understanding why they act might help us not only in treating them but in proving that they are victimizing the child.)

Why might one medicalize a criminal act so that confirming its occurrence is thought of as diagnosing the cause of its outcome? Perhaps because, as the quote above suggests, we think we could more easily justify ordinarily impermissible means of collecting evidence of criminal acts if we can label these means "diagnostic tests." This is one way the conceptual point about ways of describing an act can bear on the ethical issues to which I shall turn later.

Components of MSBP

Commonly, cases of MSBP involve (1) a parent deceiving a doctor about (i) symptoms had by a child, and/or about (ii) the causes of these symptoms. It is worth distinguishing (i) and (ii), because if the parent actually makes the child diarrhetic, she is not lying if she says he is diarrhetic. The cases also involve (2) something harmful happening to the child either because (i) the parent does something potentially harmful to the child (e.g., giving it laxatives), or (ii) because she does something that leads the doctor to do something at least potentially harmful to the child

---

[2] For stylistic reasons, this chapter generally uses "mother" and "she" in referring to the parent, although fathers and male caretakers have also been associated with MSBP.

(i.e., excessive tests). When a parent adds blood to an infant's diaper so that doctors will do tests, but does not cause the infant to bleed, we have (2)(ii) and not (2)(i).

Factor (2)(ii) is interesting in highlighting the role that doctors can play in themselves harming patients, since they are made the instruments of the parent's attempt to harm the child. In turn, the parent becomes the powerful, manipulating figure. This also makes MSBP interesting because it is usually doctors who have deceived patients, especially in the days before informed consent and full disclosure of diagnostic findings became standard practice. Doctors' shock at the violation of their trust in the parent of the patient is great in MSBP. This may not be because they are shocked at lies per se, having themselves lied to patients, but because they think that health and diagnosis, of all things, are goods that should not be interfered with. It would be useful to know if the desire to switch power roles in the medical scenario plays a part in the parent's motivation, especially since it is reported that a large number of the Munchausen parents have lower-level medical roles in work-life.

Note also that a child could have real symptoms and the parent deliberately omits to report some of these to the doctor. If the parent truthfully reports some symptoms, this can prompt the doctor to do tests and yet they may fail to reveal the real illness because of the missing information. In this case, no lies are told and yet the deliberate withholding of information with the intention of misleading should lead us to classify the behavior as MSBP. Hence, factor (1) should include a parent's intentional omission of information in order to mislead as well as a lie.

MSBP and child abuse

Often, in ordinary cases of child abuse, the abuser harms the child (so (2)(i) is present) and then lies about it or otherwise deceives only if, contrary to his or her wishes, someone finds out about the harm already done. Sometimes, the abuser takes a child to a doctor so that the harm can be discovered in order to have it treated and lies about its cause. Both these scenarios differ from MSBP, where one aim that motivates the activity that is harmful to the child is to deceive doctors while continuing to harm the child, and to involve doctors in harming the child.

It is also (theoretically) possible that the deceiving and harming criteria for MSBP are met, and yet we would be reluctant to call the case one of child abuse because the aim is not to make the child worse off overall, either as a means (to a goal like obtaining power over doctors) or as an end in itself. (This is consistent with there being an aim to cause *some* harm.) For example, suppose a homeless mother believes correctly that her child will be better off overall in a hospital than living on the streets, even if unnecessary tests risking harm are done. Deception and doing some harm may be the only way to get hospital admission. Of course, a child could be harmed in the ordinary way (e.g., beaten up) for this same reason, as well.

Hence certain types of justification for harm and deception will defeat an ascription of MSBP.

Doctors' aims

We can distinguish three aims doctors may have in relation to their patient: (a) diagnose why the child is ill, (b) prevent further harm to the child, (c) treat the child. These are distinct. For example, we might need to diagnose why the child was ill, even if the parent is no longer in a position to do further harm. In MSBP, (c) often collapses into (b), because there may be no need for treatment of past harm done (e.g., bruises induced during tests) once future harm is prevented by a treatment which involves separating parent and child.

Ethical issues

General considerations

As I have noted, doctors are most concerned with what it is morally permissible to do in order to discover the cause of the child's illness. (I shall use "discover" instead of "diagnose" so as not to over-medicalize.) This question should be distinguished from whether the permissible acts are effectual. For example, what is morally permissible may be ineffectual because it scares the mother into taking the child elsewhere. So we could refuse to do something not because it would be intrinsically unethical but because it would be ineffectual or even counterproductive.

Let us first consider the question of permissibility. Consider again the quote cited above (Wilde and Pedron 1993). It says that secret monitoring is like any diagnostic technique. This may be true in the sense that many diagnostic techniques invade privacy, but just because this is so, it would be prima facie unethical to use them without consent of the person on whom they are to be used (or his or her authorized proxy). But secret monitoring in the cases under consideration seems to be done without consent of the person monitored. This is the ethical issue. Notice that warning signs posted to the effect that secret monitoring will take place do not ensure that someone has consented to their use simply by entering the premises. And signed contracts that do not make explicit the specific kind of monitoring that may take place also do not satisfy the requirements of informed consent (Connelly 2003). There is also the conceptual problem of a concealing description. Just as "diagnosis" did not seem the best word to use when speaking of uncovering an act that victimized someone, so "diagnostic technique" conceals the moral impact of what is done in secret monitoring. Analogously, if a doctor's lying to a patient prompts the latter to do something that reveals the cause of his illness, the lie is a diagnostic technique, but this description conceals morally relevant properties of that technique.

The quote also suggests that the monitoring may be permissible merely because doctors are not aiming at collecting evidence for a criminal prosecution of the parent. But ordinary diagnostic techniques are also not used in order to collect criminal evidence and yet using them without appropriate consent can be unethical. In addition, it is noted that "the evidence may subsequently be included in child protective proceedings." Even if this is not intended by doctors, a foreseen consequence of one's acts could be morally relevant in deciding what to do. Possibly, the evidence might also be used in criminal prosecution of the parent, unless the evidence were barred for that purpose because of the way in which it was obtained (for it might be legally permissible to collect evidence in a certain way for some purposes and not for others). An ethical (not legal) question is what we should do if we know that the evidence would not be barred from use in criminal prosecution.

As an aid in considering this situation further, hypothesize a situation in which a patient lies to a doctor about her own condition, though she does not fabricate an illness. Suppose having an abortion is a criminal act and a doctor is required to report any person she knows to have had an abortion. The patient has a gynecological problem but conceals its origin in an abortion, though knowledge of the origin of the problem would be helpful in treatment. If the doctor searches out secret records without the patient's permission and finds that the patient had an abortion, this will aid her in diagnosis and treatment. But once she has the knowledge of an abortion, she is required to turn over the patient for trial. The patient can thus be made overall worse-off as a result of getting superior medical treatment than if inferior treatment had taken place. Should the doctor not consider the ultimate result and also the illicit means she uses, and refrain from getting a perfect diagnosis?

So far, we have seen that acting without patient consent to uncover truth about the cause of an illness is not necessarily permissible merely because one does not aim at criminal prosecution. But, of course, one important difference between the case in which a patient lies about him- or herself and MSBP is that in the latter the deceiver is harming *someone else*, and if collection of evidence can prevent that harm to another – harm which the liar either induces and/or helps cause – it may possibly be justified, even if it involves non-consensual monitoring and ultimately leads to prosecution. Whether this is so must now be considered.

A possible argument

Let us consider some arguments that aim to justify secret monitoring and secret bag searches, when preventing harm to others is at issue. One argument takes note of the fact that doctors are increasingly permitted to detect and report on patients who pose a threat to others. For example, one may draw blood and, without telling a patient, search for a particular disease and report the results to others who are at risk because of the patient. Suppose a doctor is taught to conceive of the patient's family, for example his mother, as also his patient. Why not monitor this patient (the mother) to prevent harm she may do to others?[3] Call this the parent-as-patient argument.

There are problems with this argument. First, taking a blood test is not done without the patient's consent, even if searching for an item in his or her blood and reporting this information is done without permission. Absence of permission also differs from absence of information, because a patient may be told what the doctor will do even if the patient's permission is not requested. But secret monitoring is begun not only without the person's permission, but also without his or her knowledge. Second, while a doctor may have to take account of the child's family in treating the child, that alone does not mean the parent is also a patient in the sense of having sought treatment or agreed to some diagnostic procedure. The parent is primarily the child's agent until proven otherwise.

Two other arguments

It is interesting to compare MSBP with a case in which the parent harms the child but not deliberately and there is no deception, for example, in the case of *folie à deux*. In this case, we can think of the parent as what philosophers call a morally innocent threat. Suppose secret monitoring were the only way to uncover the effect of a mother on a child in such a case. Since there is no attempt by the mother to harm or deceive, we could assume that given her current motives and intentions, she would want the discovery technique to be used and would consent to it, were it not that her knowledge of the monitoring would interfere with its effectiveness. The fact that we could presume her *hypothetical consent* in the absence of actual consent, based on her current motives and intentions, makes it easier to proceed with secret monitoring in this case, I believe. However, since there is an intention to harm and to deceive in MSBP (a morally guilty state of mind), we cannot assume the same hypothetical consent based on current motives and intentions in MSBP in order to help justify secret monitoring.[4]

Nevertheless, it might be suggested, hypothetical consent could play a role in a possible justification of monitoring in MSBP. *First point*: If we knew for certain that the mother was lying and trying to harm the child, she would have forfeited her moral right not to be lied to or even harmed in the process of stopping harm to the child. *Second point*: If we have only a suspicion of her guilt, it is possible that we should proceed as we would if we were certain. An argument for doing so is that if she is morally innocent, she probably would want the interests of her child

---

[3] This argument was made to me by Dr. Kurt Hirschorn, the head of the Ethics Committee of Mt. Sinai Hospital, New York City.

[4] I do not wish to foreclose the possibility that the reason the parent has the guilty state of mind is that she is psychiatrically ill, and this may be an excusing condition that makes it wrong to declare her legally guilty.

to be protected even by secret monitoring of herself. This is a hypothetical-consent justification based on *possibly* current motives and intentions. It is an analogue of the justification given above for monitoring, where the woman is harming her child without intending to do so. For example, if monitoring secretly a morally innocent mother, who also caused no harm, was (somehow) the only way to stop a third person from harming her child, she would probably want it to be done.

Putting the two points together, it might be thought that we can get a four-step argument: (1) If she is morally guilty, she has no right not to be monitored to prevent harm she will cause. (2) If she is morally innocent, she would want to be monitored to prevent harm. (3) She is either morally guilty or innocent. (4) Hence, it is permissible to secretly monitor her. Call this the hypothetical-consent argument (for the permissibility of secret monitoring).[5]

There are several problems with this argument. First, if there is any reason to secretly monitor a morally innocent parent, it must be to gather information to prevent harm. But (by hypothesis), the only way in which the harm is coming about in MSBP is if the parent is not morally innocent, because there is no chance that she is a threat without knowing that she is one. Hence, she is either guilty or there is no avoidable harm that monitoring a morally innocent person will prevent. This means step (2) is confused.

I think this problem can be remedied as follows. If a mother were morally innocent, she would want us to be so vigilant about the welfare of her child that we would even try to find out if she were guilty. Further, we need not even assume she hypothetically approves of being monitored. We need only assume that she hypothetically approves of our having an attitude (vigilance), one of whose necessary side effects is that we suspect even her. An analogy may help here. Suppose a chief of police wants all his officers to guard a VIP by checking the ID of everyone who comes in the building. When the chief himself tries to enter the building, his officers demand even *his* ID. He may be angry with this, but he can see that it is a consequence of their fulfilling his orders.

In sum, we should change the hypothetical-consent argument for monitoring in MSBP so that we no longer hypothesize that the parent is both morally innocent and that monitoring is necessary to stop harm. Instead, we hypothesize that the morally innocent mother would wish us to be vigilant and a side effect of this is our suspecting her of being guilty. In particular, we can revise the argument slightly, to produce hypothetical-consent argument II: (1) If she is guilty, she has no right not to be monitored to prevent the harm she will cause. (2) If she is morally innocent, she would want us to be vigilant and this makes us secretly monitor her. (3) She is

---

[5] An alternative strategy is to focus on our expectation that an innocent parent would endorse our behavior after the fact when it is revealed.

either morally guilty or innocent. (4) Hence, it is permissible to secretly monitor her.

There is still a problem with the first premise of this argument. If someone is guilty, he has forfeited certain rights. But at the time we collect evidence to prove someone guilty, we do not know that he is guilty and so we do not know that he has forfeited rights. Hence, it was wrong of us to act on the assumption that he had forfeited rights. Put another way, even if someone is found to be guilty, that does not mean that we could not have done anything wrong when we collected the evidence of his guilt before his guilt was proven. In the collection of evidence, even those who will turn out to be guilty are to be treated no worse than those who will turn out to be innocent.[6]

But step (2) in the argument claims that it would be permissible to secretly monitor someone who is, in fact, innocent. Hence, it seems we can construct a new, shorter hypothetical-consent argument III: (1) Treat those we do not yet know are guilty no worse than the innocent. (2) If a parent is innocent, she would want us to be vigilant even if this leads us to secretly monitor her. (3) Hence, it is permissible to secretly monitor the parent. Notice that treating those who turn out to be guilty no worse than the innocent may result in more problems for them, if the evidence leads to a criminal prosecution. But this does not invalidate the argument. When the fact of guilt alters the effect of otherwise permissible procedures, the additional bad effects are not a reasonable complaint against those procedures.

I do not think this is an airtight argument. First, even a parent who was innocent of MSBP still might not be the sort of parent who cared more about her child's welfare than about not being secretly monitored. She might not want us to be so vigilant that we suspect even her. She might be insulted that we would suspect her and also wish not to be embarrassed if monitoring reveals her doing other things she should not be doing but the prevention of which would not justify monitoring. She may also be correct to insist that we had to have strong grounds to think harm was going to be done to her child before we were justified in monitoring her. Furthermore, she might believe that privacy is necessary in order for her to interact with the child in ways beneficial to that child (Connelly 2003).

The hypothetical-consent argument seems to depend upon it being reasonable to attribute a certain state of mind to a parent innocent of MSBP, namely that she cares more about her child than about aspects of her own dignity. That depends upon this not being an unreasonable standard to which to hold a parent.[7] It also seems to depend on the view that a parent's beneficial interaction with a child does not require an assurance of privacy.

---

[6] Derek Parfit emphasized this point to me.
[7] Much more would have to be said about why we should hold parents to the standard of such good parents.

There is a further problem with this argument, however. It may also justify searching a parent's bag in secret, for would not a morally innocent good parent want us to be so vigilant that we even do this? Yet, intuitively, there seems to be a big moral difference between secret monitoring and secret bag searches. If this is so, then the argument is too strong. Finally, we should consider that the hypothetical-consent argument III is in a way too weak and so may be unnecessary. Many people besides the parent can come into the child's room and so be subject to secret monitoring. It is true that we may not intend this monitoring; observing them is a side effect of targeting the parent. But we could imagine that we had no idea who was making a child sick and truly aimed to observe everyone. These people, if morally innocent, cannot be assumed to be so concerned with the child that they would want us to maintain a degree of vigilance that leads us to monitor them secretly without their explicit prior consent. If we could nevertheless justify intentionally monitoring everyone simply because avoiding harm to the child justifies this intrusion, regardless of what these people would want given their concerns, we do not need step (2) in the hypothetical-consent argument III in order to justify secretly monitoring the parent.

Another argument

An alternative argument, unlike the parent-as-patient and the various hypothetical-consent arguments, would not focus on the parent in particular. One such argument claims that privacy is not expected in a hospital room; it is understood to be part of a public place and no more immune from secret surveillance than hospital corridors. Furthermore, bag checks of which one is aware as a condition for admission to a patient's room are no more impermissible than as a condition for admission to the hospital first. Let us call this the expected-public-zone argument.

I do not think it is correct. First, if visitors did not expect that privacy was achievable in a hospital room, why would they bother to close the door or draw a curtain? Why would they whisper (under the impression that then they would not be heard)? Even in an emergency room or hospital corridor where one least expects privacy one may not expect explicit violations of privacy. That is, one may expect people to observe patients and family, but not by secret video or audio machines. Second, undergoing a bag check when one retains the option of simply not entering if one refuses is different from a secret bag check that is, therefore, beyond one's control. Ordinarily, people expect surveillance in a public space only if a sign gives warning of it, as is done in banks.

Still, it might be said that a hospital has a right to monitor its property and hence people have no (or an easily overridden) right to privacy in a hospital, even if people do not expect to be monitored. Residents on a hospital's property are like guests, but unlike those in a hotel, they are guests whose welfare is of special concern to the hospital. (They are also guests who would presumably consent to losing much of their own privacy for the sake of their own well-being.) The hospital seeks to protect its residents from "visitors." This account helps explain why, while the hospital may monitor its property without being given permission by visitors, it may not search visitors' bags without their permission. The bag is the visitor's property, not the hospital's. Hospitals may have a right to monitor; but suppose it was generally known that they did not take advantage of that right. Then it would be reasonable for people not to expect to be monitored, although they would not be entitled to expect not to be monitored.

According to this argument, which I shall call the public-zone argument (by contrast to the expected-public-zone argument), the primary moral problem in justifying secret monitoring is not showing that people's right to privacy may permissibly be overridden in a hospital. That has just been done. The moral problem is that in order for monitoring to be effective (i.e., for it to stop harm), it must be kept a secret. If we defeat the public's expectation of privacy by announcing the fact that the hospital will exercise its right to monitor without permission, monitoring will not be effective. Acting without someone's consent is different than acting without his or her knowledge. The ability to effectively monitor in order to rule out a diagnosis of MSBP and prevent harm depends upon parents believing they are not being monitored. Hence the moral problem according to the public-zone argument turns out to be having to either lie or not be open about acting on a right to monitor. The next step in the public-zone argument, therefore, would be to show that we have a right to lie or not be open in this way. Such a right may depend on how urgent it is to resolve the diagnosis and what alternative means there are to this end. A possible solution is to post notices or to use admission agreements that include paragraphs saying "The hospital reserves the right to monitor in the interests of its patients without giving further notice when there is good reason and alternatives are not available." This makes it rational to believe one might not be monitored when doing something wrong, and hence it does not eliminate the effectiveness of monitoring.

Balancing

Suppose some argument justifies secret monitoring. This still does not mean that we do not wrong the person we monitor in the course of doing what is permissible. There may be "wrong-making characteristics" still present in what we do, even though they are overridden by "right-making characteristics" that speak in favor of the act. For example, it may be overall right (not wrong) to lie to an innocent person to save a life, and while the result is tainted the victim should not resist what we do. Sometimes, however, we may even "wrong someone" in the course of doing what is justifiable. This involves more than a negative moral residue, because it implies that a person might even legitimately resist our doing to him or her what we are justifiably doing.

What wrong we do to the morally innocent or those we are obliged to treat as morally innocent depends on what wrong-making characteristics deception and invasion of privacy have. Even if a person is guilty and has forfeited his right not to be lied to or misled, there could be reasons aside from violating his right that make our lying or misleading morally offensive. For example, it may simply be inappropriate to someone's nature as a rational being – even criminals can have this nature – not to be dealt with honestly. These wrong-making considerations can speak in favor of using other means besides deception and invasion of privacy, if they are as (or nearly as) effective in stopping harm to the child.[8]

Now let us consider the issue of the effectiveness of various discovery procedures and the balance we can achieve between effectiveness and moral considerations.

There seem to be essentially two types of procedures for finding out whether the parent is involved in causing the child's illness: (1) those that stop her from doing harmful things, whereupon the child improves, and (2) those that catch her while she is doing harmful things. The second may give a more definitive proof of wrongful acts, since some ways of stopping her acts (e.g., barring her presence) leave it open that it is merely her psychological interaction with the child that causes the problem. Hence, the second type of procedure would also be more useful in yielding evidence (if it were admissible) for a criminal proceeding or child-custody case. However, since the medical establishment's aim is not criminal prosecution or child custody per se, this cannot provide a reason for choosing (2) over (1).

Consider four specific procedures that fall under these two types: (A) the parent is barred from child's room; (B) a nurse is obviously present at all times; (C) secret monitoring; (D) secret alarming of the child's IV line or other equipment so that tampering will be detected if it occurs. (The last option is not one that was described in the literature I have read.) Procedures (A) and (B) are type 1; (C) and (D) are type 2. We could evaluate each of these procedures with respect to (i) their effectiveness and (ii) moral considerations as they bear on (a) innocent people and (b) those people we must treat as innocent until proven guilty. (It is possible that if something is objectionable from the perspective of the innocent, that should count against it more than if it is objectionable from the perspective of those proven to be guilty.)

---

[8] Notice that there is a distinction between wronging and harming; a lie can be a wronging of someone even if it does not harm him. Paternalistic action is by definition action that promotes someone's interest, and yet can be a wronging of a person.

Procedure (D) seems best from all points of view, since only if one is doing what one should not does any monitoring or interference by others take place. The question is whether it is feasible and effective. Now consider (A) and (C). The innocent would probably find being barred from the child's room more objectionable than being monitored. Secret monitoring is also more effective if barring a guilty parent may lead her to remove the child from the hospital. Hence, it would seem there is more to be said for secret monitoring than for barring. But we should keep in mind that even if the innocent would hypothetically prefer monitoring to barring, monitoring which involves deception seems intrinsically morally more objectionable than simply not allowing someone in a room. That is, monitoring is more disrespectful of the person, even if it causes less suffering to an innocent parent and her child. (This helps bring out the difference between wronging someone and harming him.) If it were possible to prevent a parent from removing a child from the hospital, or to alert other hospitals in the vicinity if there is an attempt to transfer, this would increase the effectiveness of barring. Finally, consider (B). Having a nurse in the room seems as effective as barring in catching the guilty and imposes less of a burden on the innocent.

On the basis of all this, a possible ranking of the four procedures in order of overall preferability is D, B, A, and C, but monitoring would move up on the list if A and B would lead to the child being removed.

Finally, we might consider telling the truth about our suspicions. Suppose we openly suggest (non-secret) monitoring or alarming. The innocent might be tempted to reject it because they are insulted. But would they risk the health of their child by removing it from the hospital, especially if all hospitals had the same policy? I doubt it. If someone refuses non-secret monitoring and removes the child, I think we have at least enough grounds for further investigation by child-abuse authorities, as well as grounds for temporarily restraining the parent from removing the child from the hospital.[9]

Summary

Having first characterized MSBP, I have considered several possible approaches to justifying at least secret monitoring of a parent. One approach relies on what a good parent would hypothetically be willing to agree to undergo. A second approach focuses on the right of a hospital to monitor its premises but faces the moral problem of the need to conceal whether it is acting on its right. Finally,

---

[9] Wilde and Pedron (1993) seem to think it is a more serious step to keep a parent from a child than to monitor her secretly. This may be true in terms of burden on an innocent mother and child, but barring lacks some moral problems that secret monitoring has.

I have evaluated, on effectiveness and moral grounds, several specific means that might be used to deter and stop wrongful behavior.

ACKNOWLEDGMENTS

I thank Derek Parfit, Roger Crisp, Rosemond Rhodes, Arthur Applbaum, the editors of this volume, and the audience at the Oxford–Mt. Sinai Colloquium on Medical Ethics, New York, April 1999, for helpful comments.

3.3 Topical discussion

Munchausen syndrome by proxy (MSBP)

Munchausen syndrome, poetically named in 1951 after German fables of the fictitious Baron Munchausen, denotes factitious or imaginary illnesses intentionally feigned in order to gain access to medical care. The label of Munchausen syndrome by proxy entered the literature in 1977. Confusion about whether it is a diagnosis of the perpetrator or the victim has been recently resolved by distinguishing between "pediatric condition falsification" (PCF), a diagnosis of the victim, some cases of which have other causes, and "factitious disorder by proxy" (FDP), a diagnostic category for the caretaker, referring to fabricating or inducing illnesses in another person in order to assume the sick role by proxy. MSBP is then characterized as the disorder that includes a diagnosis in both the child and the caretaker.

One reason for wishing to abandon the terminology of MSBP is the recognition that a caretaker may be led to fabricate or induce illness in another by a number of different psychiatric disorders, not only through projected Munchausen syndrome. As there is no single psychological profile and the label makes assumptions about the parent's mental state and motivation, the label is gradually falling out of use in clinical contexts, although still common in the popular press and imagination. Further, it appears to be a diagnosis of a parent rather than of the true patient, the child.

Factitious disorder by proxy is a form of child abuse, and may result in criminal prosecution of the perpetrator or in the removal of the child from the home. It is extremely difficult to diagnose, and misdiagnosis can be disastrous, not only for affected families, especially if criminal charges result, but also, as some recent legal cases in both Britain and the USA have shown, for the individuals and agencies involved. If a parent claims to have been wrongly accused of child abuse, the resulting

Ethical Dilemmas in Pediatrics: Cases and Commentaries, ed. Lorry R. Frankel, Amnon Goldworth, Mary V. Rorty, and William A. Silverman. Published by Cambridge University Press. © Cambridge University Press 2005.

publicity, professional complaints, and possible countersuits create a hostile climate. Thus exactly those professionals who are most obligated, by professional ethics as well as by law, to report possible child abuse, may face a strong conflict of interest in doing so.

Apnea, seizures, infections, fever, vomiting, diarrhea, asthma, and skin lesions are among the illnesses that have been associated with this syndrome, and in cases of serious abuse such as poisoning or suffocation, the high risk of further abuse is extremely dangerous to the child. Evidence suggests that recidivism in FDP caretakers is very high, and the death rate for children can be as high as 6%.

Trust: confidentiality and disclosure

This case reveals the practical implications of some of the most central issues in clinical ethics and the physician–patient relation: trust, privacy, and confidentiality. The physician–patient relationship frequently requires breaching normal social conventions of privacy, laying bare, for therapeutic ends, details of patient behavior usually considered private. In exchange for access to details that will aid diagnosis or treatment, physicians or other clinicians are expected to keep that information confidential. This conventional, if often implicit, exchange is the basis for the trust essential for a positive physician–patient relationship.

In the unconventional-medicine case that opened this section, impediments to parental trust led to ethical complications in treating a newborn. In this case, suspected duplicity on the part of the mother in reporting her child's symptoms, and physical evidence that she may have been causing them, led to a breakdown of trust on the part of the caregivers.

Covert surveillance: privacy versus care

The need to care for the pediatric patient led the reporting physician to consider alternative methods of determining the actual cause of the presenting symptoms Not every hospital is equipped for covert video surveillance of the sort suggested by Garcia-Careaga and Kerner, and considered in Kamm's response, but it has frequently been suggested as a method of differential diagnosis before confronting the caregiver. One reason given for considering it is the disruption in physician–parent trust that would be caused by an unjustified accusation, since videotaped evidence can exculpate, as well as incriminate, caregivers suspected of inducing illnesses, and the need for firm evidence if a charge of this seriousness is to be leveled. Though the parent is not the patient in pediatric cases, the importance of maintaining a strong relationship of trust with the patient's surrogate and most consistent support system weighs heavily with caregivers, and is being balanced in such cases with the pressing need to determine the cause of the symptoms, since clinicians' prime responsibility remains the welfare of their patient, the child.

To what extent are the expectations of privacy normal to the intimate family circle appropriate when, as here, one member of the family is in the institutional context of a hospital? Would the mother be justified if she considered her privacy invaded by the presence of a nurse or a camera? What procedures or safeguards are appropriate to protect the interests of the child's family?

Family reunification

All states have statutes that require physicians to report specific medical conditions. A failure to do so can result in the revocation of a medical license. One of the specific medical conditions that must be reported is an indication of child abuse. This often results in the abusing parent losing at least temporary custody of the child. In the case of MSBP, the resulting separation between mother and child results in the disappearance of the symptoms experienced by the child. It can also result in court-mandated psychiatric treatment for the mother. Berg and Jones believe that in certain cases such treatment can lead to successful family reunification. Several reasons offered for the importance of psychiatric treatment with this as the goal are: (1) all children have a right to be brought up in their birth family; and (2) improving the mother's psychological state may improve the quality of life of current and future siblings. Thus, an improvement in and protection of the physical and emotional health of the family is in the best interests of the abused child.

FURTHER READING

Allison, D. B. and Roberts, M. S. *Disordered Mother or Disordered Diagnosis? Munchausen By Proxy Syndrome* (Hillsdale, NJ: Analytic Press, 1998).

Annas, G. J., Glantz, L. H., and Katz, B. F. *The Rights of Doctors, Nurses, and Allied Health Professionals: a Health Law Primer* (New York, NY: Ballinger, 1981).

Ayoub, C., Alexander, R., Beck, D., *et al.* Position paper: definitional issues in Munchausen by proxy. *Child Maltreatment* 7 (2002), 105–111.

Barber, M. A. and Davis, P. M. Fits, faints or fatal fantasy? Fabricated seizures and child abuse. *Archives of Disease in Childhood* 86 (2002), 230–233.

Berg, B. and Jones, S. P. H. Outcome of psychiatric intervention in factitious illness by proxy (Munchausen syndrome by proxy). *Archives of Disease in Childhood* 81 (1999), 465–472.

Craft, A. W. and Hall, D. M. B. Munchausen syndrome by proxy and sudden infant death. *BMJ* 328 (2004), 1309–1312.

Hall, D. E., Eubanks, L., Meyyazhagan, S., Kenney, R. D., and Johnson, S. C. Evaluation of covert video surveillance in the diagnosis of MSBP: Lessons from 41 cases. *Pediatrics* **105** (2000), 1305–1312.

Morrison, C. A. Cameras in hospital rooms: the Fourth Amendment to the Constitution and Munchausen syndrome by proxy. *Critical Care Nursing Quarterly* **22** (1999), 65–68.

Pasqualone, G. A. and Fitzgerald, S. M. Munchausen by proxy syndrome: the forensic challenge of recognition, diagnosis and reporting. *Critical Care Nursing Quarterly* **22** (1999), 52–64.

Schreier, H. Munchausen by proxy defined. *Pediatrics* **10** (2002), 985–998.

Smith-Alnimer, M. and Papas-Kavalis, H. Child abuse by a different name: how to recognize Munchausen syndrome by proxy. *American Journal of Nursing* **103** (6) (2003), 56F–56J.

Part II

Medical futility

"Futility" is one of the most controversial issues facing contemporary health care – both in theory and in application. The three cases in this section illustrate the difficulty faced in theory and practice.

The term itself can be confusing. The futility of a particular treatment may be evident in either quantitative or qualitative terms. That is, futility may refer to an improbability or unlikelihood of an event happening, an expression that is quasi-numeric, or to the quality of the event that treatment would produce. In the absence of specific objective criteria consistently applied across different diagnoses and settings, subjective judgments about what is appropriate in a specific case can and do clash. A treatment judged "futile" from one perspective is liable to be termed "desirable" or "necessary" by another participant or affected party: "You may think it is futile, but it does not seem futile to me." Such conflicting reactions to a situation may reflect different formulations of the goals of treatment. One party may consider an intervention "futile" which only postpones death; another may find an extended time to resolve emotional or family issues priceless. The reliability of factual information cannot settle conflicts arising from these different value positions.

Even in cases where considerable outcomes research has generated probabilistic data about the likelihood of positive results for life-sustaining treatments such as cardiopulmonary resuscitation or mechanical ventilation under some medical conditions, the chance, however minimal, of postponing death can be of great psychological value to grieving parents. For the physicians involved in cases where there are conflicts, professional responsibility to provide medically appropriate care and payer emphasis on efficiency and cost-containment conflict with their legal, ethical, and professional deference to the best interests of their patients and their surrogates.

There has been a movement to avoid the term "futile," replacing it with terms like "medically inadvisable" in many of the forums in which these issues are being addressed. At the same time medical futility policies are being formulated in many hospitals, professional organizations, and bioethics forums. The dilemma represented by the conflation and interpenetration of fact and values in futility judgments will not be finally resolvable without a wider political and social consensus about the goals of our healthcare system.

In Chapter 4, Lawrence Mathers offers a nuanced description of the terrain that must be traveled when physicians have only bad news to deliver to frantic parents. A three-year-old suffered severe anoxia in connection with a swimming-pool accident, and within two days was determined to be neurologically devastated. Bad news of this magnitude precipitates professional obligations to propose withdrawal of support, but Dr. Mathers is clear that such withdrawals cannot be undertaken unilaterally. He sketches a series of negotiations in which the family, initially resistant to discontinuing care, eventually accepted the fact of death. The focus of his discussion then moves to the options available to the medical team for maintaining or withdrawing support, and the importance and difficulty of communicating with the family to determine a mutually agreed-upon plan of care.

In his response, Simon Whitney takes advantage of the ambiguities in Mathers' account to emphasize the primacy of the parents as decision makers. Professionals and family may agree about the desirable course of action in tragic cases. Timely, comprehensive, and unambiguous communication may make such agreement more likely. When they disagree, however, the question arises of what steps need to be taken, and who is in a position to make decisions about how to proceed. Whitney emphasizes the legal authority of the family.

The difficulty of withdrawing life-sustaining treatments in the absence of agreement between family and caregivers is already complicated by the professional responsibility physicians have to provide only indicated or appropriate treatments. Various mechanisms of contemporary healthcare financing are increasingly holding physicians responsible for resource allocation as well. This conflict of responsibilities can only serve to increase the moral perplexity in tragic cases.

In Chapter 5, Perkin, Orr, and Ashwahl sketch out the difficulties facing medical professionals confronting subjective disagreement about whether a specific proposed treatment is "futile." This case involves the care of a child with severe central nervous system impairment from a prior cardiac arrest. The child was in a chronic care facility, but suffered recurrent pneumonias, requiring frequent readmission to the hospital for mechanical ventilation. The question arises of whether it is desirable to initiate long-term ventilation in the chronic care facility. Although professional standards, empirical evidence of similar cases, and general concerns for appropriate resource utilization contributed to their conviction that long-term ventilation is in general not recommended for patients in this child's condition, the mother wished all possible support for the child to be continued. The particulars of the case led them to a decision at odds with their reasoned presuppositions about what should be done. Considering several general considerations against long-term ventilation in such cases, the physicians concluded that none of them was sufficient to override the parent's wishes in this case. The absence of consensus and the impossibility of finding criteria which can be consistently applied across cases left them dissatisfied with the decision they had reached in this troubling case.

In her response, philosopher Anita Silvers tacitly praises their resolution while faulting their method of reaching it. Arguing for the desirability of case-sensitive ethical decision making and the moral importance of relationships, Silvers suggests that they might have been less conflicted about the resolution they reached had they not been distracted by their belief that they needed justification in terms of general principles. Silvers' expansive discussion of morally relevant considerations in medical decision making reiterates the important role of families and others with emotional ties to patients. It is a contribution as well to the theoretical debate in philosophical bioethics about appropriate methods of ethical reasoning in clinical ethics.

If there is a single diagnosis which should strongly support withholding or withdrawing life-sustaining treatments, brain death is that diagnosis. In Chapter 6 Lorry Frankel and Chester Randle introduce an unfortunate child who sustained a cardiac arrest and was brain dead. Complicated family considerations led to a situation where parents' wishes to continue ventilating the child were accommodated, despite the physicians' strong feeling that it was inappropriate to do so. The case presents an extraordinary concatenation of considerations, ranging from the parents' unwillingness to see a brain-dead child as "dead," overseas relatives traveling to support the grieving family, transfer of care, invocation of legal advice from the hospital attorney, and complications surrounding organ donation.

In his commentary Amnon Goldworth takes the occasion to meditate upon the considerations which have led to the development of the medical and legal category of brain death, and the conceptual and practical difficulties of applying it in contested situations. In cases like the case of "brain death," where terms of art with specific and clearly defined parameters are superimposed upon ordinary-language (and richly symbolic) terms like "death," the meanings and expectations of one group, the physicians, can diverge widely from the expectations and understandings of the non-professional family members trying to meet their own needs of grieving.

4.1 Letting go: a study in pediatric life-and-death decision making

Lawrence H. Mathers

Introduction

No prospect is more terrifying for parents than being asked to consider the possibility of withdrawing aspects of medical care being provided for their child. Their decision may result in the child's death (Farrell and Levin 1993). Family beliefs, religion, medical science, social values, and the ongoing debate over the importance of individual human life will interact, and sometimes clash, during the process which will culminate in a decision (Luce 1997a, 1997b). The following case illustrates many of the questions which arise, and the difficulty of choosing a clear course of action.

The case of JM

A three-year-old male, JM, wandered into the back yard while his mother was answering the doorbell and fell into the family swimming pool. It took the mother about five minutes to conclude her business with the visitor at the door. When she returned to the back yard, it took her another two to three minutes to notice that JM was missing. She searched the house rapidly, and eventually made the tragic discovery that her son was lying motionless at the bottom of the pool. Initially she panicked, then retrieved him from the water, laid him on the side of the pool, initiated mouth-to-mouth breathing, and then dialed 911 in order to summon help. When the EMS personnel arrived, the child was pulseless and cyanotic. It was believed that he had spent somewhere between 10 and 15 minutes in the water. They performed CPR with a bag-valve-mask device with 100% oxygen. The emergency medical technician intubated the trachea and satisfactory breath sounds were auscultated bilaterally. The child continued to need chest compressions

Ethical Dilemmas in Pediatrics: Cases and Commentaries, ed. Lorry R. Frankel, Amnon Goldworth, Mary V. Rorty, and William A. Silverman. Published by Cambridge University Press. © Cambridge University Press 2005.

despite positive pressure ventilation with 100% oxygen. Epinephrine and atropine were administered through the endotracheal tube, and an intraosseous needle was placed in the left tibia. Additional doses of epinephrine were administered through the intraosseous needle. Resuscitation continued en route to the hospital. The patient recovered a spontaneous pulse, at a rate of 30–40 beats per minute.

Upon arrival at the emergency room, JM exhibited irregular spontaneous gasping movements. His core body temperature was recorded at 34 °C, his spontaneous heart rate was now 55–60 beats per minute, and he appeared to be minimally responsive to painful stimuli. As further resuscitation continued, his spontaneous heart rate rose to ∼140 beats per minute. His blood pressure was 82/44, but his spontaneous respirations were irregular and ineffective.

He was further stabilized and then transported from the emergency room to the pediatric intensive care unit where he was placed on mechanical ventilation, with 100% O_2, and pressures sufficient to produce good movement of his chest. A chest X-ray showed diffuse bilateral patchy infiltrates. Femoral venous and arterial catheters were placed. His initial arterial blood gas indicated significant metabolic acidosis. His pupils were fixed and dilated; he was areflexic, and unresponsive to all stimuli. He was apneic without the ventilator. He required high-dose dopamine and epinephrine to maintain adequate blood pressure. Calcium, bicarbonate, and antibiotics were administered as well.

He remained in the pediatric intensive care unit for the next 24 hours, during which time his blood gases improved; however, his pupils remained fixed and dilated and his peripheral muscle tone flaccid. He began to exhibit repetitive twitching movements of his upper limbs, which progressed to a generalized tonic–clonic seizure. Phenobarbital was administered until a therapeutic level was reached and the seizures stopped.

A neurology consultation was obtained, and an EEG performed. The neurologist interpreted the physical exam to be compatible with brain death. An EEG showed very-low-voltage neural activity throughout the brain, with occasional spike-and-wave activity consistent with suppressed seizure activity. A CT scan of the head showed severe edema of the brain, with elimination of sulci and gyri on the surface of the brain as well as occlusion of the ventricles and cisterns surrounding the brain.

As a result of these findings, a conference was scheduled on the afternoon of the second day (∼30 hours post-immersion), involving the parents, physicians, and representatives from nursing and social services. The parents were accompanied by the maternal grandmother, two aunts, and the family's clergyman. Information was presented to the family that there had been severe anoxic brain injury, with subsequent swelling of brain tissue, resulting in severe and permanent injury. The physicians stated that the child's prognosis was extremely poor, that the brain had been profoundly and globally damaged, and that survival was unlikely, even with intensive medical support. The physicians recommended that support be withdrawn, with the near-certain prospect that the child would die within minutes. The family was offered reassurance that the child was feeling no pain and would not suffer. It was emphasized that the minuscule chance of prolonged survival would only lead to permanent disability, permanent coma, and dependence on medical care for all aspects of life.

Discussion

Frequently, a severely injured patient survives only with the provision of vigorous medical support. In adult medicine, advance directives can express patient wishes about end-of-life issues. Unfortunately, in pediatrics, advance directives are rare. In the case of a child with a chronic illness who has had the opportunity to contemplate death, the child may have expressed his or her wish, but such a wish may conflict with the wishes of a family member or be considered inappropriate by a caregiver.

Debate about continuation of medical care occurs when a patient is biologically alive but with a profoundly limited life. Our legal traditions are quite clear that the taking of another's life, even when the process is accidental, as in a motor vehicle accident, requires legal scrutiny and often leads to the assignment of responsibility and punishment. A person whose action or inaction causes or contributes to the death of another person may be judged to have committed a criminal act.

Why, then, are medical personnel treated differently when, for example, they discontinue mechanical ventilation in a terminally ill patient, resulting in his or her death? This patient is dependent upon the ventilator for continued life, and the physician who discontinues such support does so with certain knowledge that the patient's life will end in a matter of minutes. This is a well-thought-out process in which the consequences are foreseen. However, physicians are not held responsible because of social conventions.

In the medical context, when the matter of quality of life and/or futility are weighed alongside the basic issues of life and death, the physician has historically defined life with reference to objective and measurable parameters (such as heart rate, spontaneous respirations, maintenance of body temperature, consciousness, purposeful movement, and interaction with the surrounding environment, etc.). While there might be little disagreement with employing these parameters to define life, there is profound disagreement about the threshold of life. In patients who are profoundly damaged, our current standards tell us that consideration of the quality of life should be accorded importance equal to life itself.

Conclusion

The debate centering on quality of life/futility has created a problem about when medical care and support can legitimately be terminated. Many states now recognize two criteria to determine death: cardiopulmonary and brain death. Despite the objective definitions of brain death enumerated in various states' statutes, the vast majority of cases of severe brain injury fall short of meeting legal brain-death criteria. This forces physicians to consider the issues of life and futility of care.

Those who are willing to approve of the withdrawal of support for the severely brain-injured may be troubled by the possibility that their actions may be premature, or mistaken. Application of criteria for withdrawing support from those still "alive" (but not enjoying a quality of life which would justify continued treatment) arouses fear that today's narrow criteria for withdrawal of support may one day expand to include patients less severely damaged. Therefore, since broadly applicable criteria for withdrawing support are difficult to define, each case becomes a self-contained problem, and abuses of the option of withdrawing support inevitably occur.

The difficulty of dealing with these problems has given rise to the following options to provide support in a profoundly damaged patient:

(1) No support whatever: withhold hydration and nutrition, as well as treatment for infections, fever, etc. – provide warmth, hospital bed, comfort measures.

(2) Provision of most basic support only: warmth, hydration, nutrition, antibiotics, and comfort measures.

(3) Provision of all but intensive care: "do not resuscitate" status, and provide warmth, nutrition, and treatment of infections, fevers, and serious complications – tracheal intubation, cardiac stimulants or vasopressors, hemodynamic support, chest tubes, or other invasive procedures are not offered.

(4) Full medical support including resuscitation: patients are to receive the full range of medical treatment, with no consideration given to opinions about their long-range quality of life, although certain forms of treatment (e.g., surgery) may be deferred due to the patient's fragility.

In our experience, difficulties such as described in our case are dealt with through meetings with the family. This includes the communication of medical facts and prognoses, and reassurance that decisions about the future medical treatment of their child are and will remain a matter of dialogue and consensus amongst the treating medical professionals and family. Should the medical team perceive intransigence on the part of the family, or perhaps one member of the family who seems to have strong influence over positions that the family ultimately takes, it is wise to avoid any impression of impatience or intolerance of such views, and never to approach deliberations in a threatening or confrontational manner.

Medical professionals often become frustrated with families who do not agree with them. The nursing staff, who work long hours at the bedside with such seriously ill patients, often feel the frustration of the seeming pointlessness of continued support. Medical professionals must act with great circumspection when the family is faced with the possibility of the withdrawal of treatment. They will generally not appreciate or accept the imposition of a decision based on the supposed superior knowledge and understanding on the part of the medical professionals. Reaching consensus with a family in this circumstance is not easy.

When it first becomes clear that the family is going to take a position counter to what medical professionals recommend, it is essential that respect for the family's views and their right to assert them be made clear. Information should continue to flow, with daily updates on their child's condition. Even if the medical professionals feel that the patient's situation is irretrievable, they should not be perceived as browbeating. It is exceedingly rare that a family will continue to be unreasonably optimistic for an extended period. It may take several days or even weeks for a family to fully appreciate the information presented by the medical professionals. We should not expect families to see the permanent damage resulting from a patient's tragic illness as quickly as our experience enables us to do. It is important that the medical professionals should not display any disagreements amongst themselves when they present such information to a family.

We must give the family members all the time they need to process and examine the information put before them. Even when a cogent argument is made that continued support for a patient demonstrably beyond all hope of survival is indefensible, continued care for even a few days may be indicated. Especially when dealing with the impending death of a child, our role must be to provide the best in medical care to our patient and simultaneously to recognize and honor the individual predilections of each family's way of dealing with such circumstances. Modern pediatric intensive care medicine rests on carefully developed scientific treatment protocols, and consistent application of such treatments. In the area of life-and-death decisions involving children, however, such protocol-driven approaches are often not effective, and risk the destruction of the trust between the family and physicians.

FURTHER READING

Avery, G. B. Futility considerations in the neonatal intensive care unit. *Seminars in Perinatology* **22** (1998), 216–222.

Bock, K. R., Teres, D., and Rapoport, J. Economic implications of the timing of do-not-resuscitate orders for ICU patients. *New Horizons* 5 (1997), 51–55.

Rhodes, R. Futility and the goals of medicine. *Journal of Clinical Ethics* 9 (1998), 194–205.

Scribano, P. V., Baker, M. D., and Ludwig, S. Factors influencing termination of resuscitative efforts in children: a comparison of pediatric emergency medicine and adult emergency medicine physicians. *Pediatric Emergency Care* 13 (1997), 320–324.

4.2 Near-drowning, futility, and the limits of shared decision making

Simon N. Whitney

Introduction

Suspended between life and death, this child is caught between his parents' hope and his physicians' growing despair. We know the facts of how he came to this point, but next to nothing about how his parents are coping with this sudden turmoil or to what dreams they still cling, nor are we shown how this particular drama ends. We do not know if this initial disagreement is resolved through further negotiations, as is almost always the case, or if it evolves into a stalemate, with family and physicians holding firm to conflicting positions.

Dr. Mathers gives a clear description of the process through which he helps families agree to withdraw life support for irreparably injured children. He clearly believes that responsibility for these important decisions should be shared between clinicians and the family. His concern for the well-being of the family is evident, and many clinicians could profit from his description of the importance of patience in negotiating with families. Nonetheless, the case history shows confusion about the roles of family and physicians. A careful look at the ethical and legal circumstances of the case suggests a better approach.

In this essay, I discuss the various forms of clinical decision making and conclude that the decision about discontinuing life support for JM must rest solely with the family, and in that sense is not shared at all. Nonetheless, the medical staff has an important role to play in ongoing discussion with the family, a discussion that may yet unite family and staff. Let me make it clear at the outset that I understand the difficulties the physicians face, respect their commitment to this patient and his family, and would never want to keep my own child alive in this condition. In fact, that is part of the problem: our experiences as physicians, as parents, and as members of the community provide us with only a vague sense of the legal framework that

Ethical Dilemmas in Pediatrics: Cases and Commentaries, ed. Lorry R. Frankel, Amnon Goldworth, Mary V. Rorty, and William A. Silverman. Published by Cambridge University Press. © Cambridge University Press 2005.

binds our lives. Our legal nearsightedness is ordinarily of no moment, but when the parents reject JM's physicians' advice, legal unclarity leads to confusion about where decisional authority resides. Untutored experience and unexamined intuition serve us poorly in atypical and extreme circumstances.

Most physicians in the United States agree that patients with severe brain damage and no realistic hope of recovery should be allowed to die quietly, although the degree of clinical certainty and expected disability required to trigger a recommendation that life support be withdrawn varies between and within institutions. When it is clear that an unconscious patient will not recover, physicians raise with the family the question of withdrawing life support. Although families sometimes draw back from this suggestion, the medical staff assumes that time and continued explanation will reveal the good sense of this path and its advantages over continuing care that the professionals consider futile. This consensus view is the unwritten subtext of the case history, one that I would phrase thus: "The struggle ahead is long and, we know from experience, hopeless; the best we could hope for is survival with overwhelming disabilities. Therefore, it is best, although painful, to withdraw life support and permit death. Reasonable families will agree, given clear explanations and time to adjust."

This analysis is understandable but things are not so simple. In a context of concern over healthcare expenditures, there are powerful economic arguments for terminating life support with patients like JM. But although economically it is sound, ethically it is debatable, and legally it is wrong. A family that refuses permission to turn off the ventilator in these circumstances should be met with more than mere patience. To understand why this is so, it will be helpful to review the theoretical models of how authority is divided in clinical decision making before we see how they pertain to specific situations.

Three models of clinical decision making

Clinical decision making may be divided into three general models, based on the allocation of authority between patient (or surrogate) and physician. The first model is *paternalism*, with the physician assuming full responsibility for decisions without authorization from the patient. This historically common mode is now in bad odor, although there is reason to believe that both patients and physicians sometimes find an element of paternalism to be not only acceptable but desirable (Schneider 1998).

The second model is one of *patient autonomy*, in which the physician's only role is to provide information and carry out the patient's decision; this has been called the "patient sovereignty" model (President's Commission 1982: 38). As Brock describes it,

The physician's role is to use his or her training, knowledge, and experience to provide the patient with facts about the diagnosis and about the prognoses without treatment and with alternative treatments. The patient's role in this division of labor is to provide the values – his or her own conception of the good – with which to evaluate these alternatives, and to select the one that is best for himself or herself. (Brock 1991)

This model, emphasizing the autonomous choice of the patient or his or her surrogate, finds its strongest support in the law of informed consent. However, it is not always clear how to implement this approach, since many observers feel that it is not possible for the physician to provide information that is free of his or her own values. This model has been criticized as not only idealized and unrealistic, but also undesirable (President's Commission 1982, Brock 1991, Emanuel *et al.* 1992, Engelhardt 1996) since most families need and want the active involvement of their physicians in these choices.

In the third model, both patient and physician participate in making decisions. This model has been given a variety of names but it is most commonly referred to as *shared decision making* (President's Commission 1982, Emanuel and Emanuel 1992) (although that name has also been applied to the second model, in which all authority is vested in the patient [Brock 1991]). When Dr. Mathers says the family should be reassured that "decisions about the future medical treatment of their child are and will remain a matter of dialogue and consensus amongst the treating medical professionals and family," he is almost certainly invoking this model.

The general concept of shared decision making has great appeal. It recognizes our conviction that patient and physician are making common cause against illness and suffering and does not relegate the physician to the role of technician. It conforms to the reality of how difficult decisions are usually made in practice, and the phrase "shared decision making" certainly has a satisfying feel. This approach, with various refinements, is widely acknowledged as a reasonable middle ground (President's Commission 1982, Katz 1984, Brock 1991, Emanuel and Emanuel 1992).

Ethical and legal considerations in shared decision making

Just what *is* shared decision making? Do patient and physician share equally in the actual decision itself, or do they share in the process that leads to the decision, each playing his or her own role (the physician primarily providing information and the patient making the decision, with guidance from the physician)? Imprecise use turns the phrase "shared decision making" into a slogan.

The Committee on Bioethics of the American Academy of Pediatrics (AAP), in a statement on decision making in pediatrics, has commented, "Decision-making power or authority is increasingly seen as something to be shared by equal partners in the physician–patient or physician–surrogate relationship" (American Academy of Pediatrics Committee on Bioethics 1995). The Committee also says, "For many patients and family members, personal values affect health care decisions, and physicians have a duty to respect the autonomy, rights, and preferences of their patients and their surrogates" (American Academy of Pediatrics Committee on Bioethics 1995). The Committee does not say that respecting the preferences of parents necessarily requires deferring to them in the decision-making process. Taken in the context of the report as a whole, I believe the Committee is urging physicians to be respectful of the values of parents while physicians and parents try to reach decisions that are acceptable to all concerned. This is only a statement of their desire, one that describes the world the Committee wishes to create, not the one we now inhabit. Shared decision making is not now and likely will never be obligatory.

Two questions are critical in understanding the meaning of shared decision making in any given case. First, which interventions may legitimately be contemplated? The Committee's statement clearly implies that an intervention that the treating physicians do not propose or no longer recommend (such as continuing life support for a patient who is not expected to recover) falls outside the scope of appropriate choices: "Society recognizes that patients or their surrogates have a right to decide, in consultation with their physicians, which *proposed* medical interventions they will or will not accept" (American Academy of Pediatrics Committee on Bioethics 1995, emphasis added). The AAP, then, supports the decisional authority of parents so long as the parents choose from the options that the physicians consider appropriate. This is precisely concordant with the views of JM's physicians.

The second question is just how the actual decision is to be reached. It is easy to permit the family an active role in the final choice if the family may select only from a menu of choices offered by the physicians, all of which the physicians consider acceptable. But what happens when the family wants an intervention that the physicians feel is inappropriate?

Decision making in context

When patient and physician disagree – as is the case when JM's physicians recommend withdrawing life support and his parents resist – many physicians think that their response should be further negotiation and provision of information rather than simply accepting the family's preference. As noted earlier, Dr. Mathers reassures families like this that "decisions about the future medical treatment of their child are and will remain a matter of dialogue and consensus amongst the treating medical professionals and the family."

This approach is widely supported in the literature of medical ethics, but I believe that there are cases where it is inappropriate and that this is such a case. As some commentators have pointed out, medical decisions need not be made by consensus: "Although the patient and physician *may* reach a decision together, they need not" (Faden *et al.* 1986: 279, emphasis in the original). Legally, the choice is the family's alone, and their choice will have the strong support of the legal system. As seen in the patient-sovereignty model, sole authority here rests with the family. Professional organizations have every right to expound their views of optimal decision-making processes, but they have no right to expect their opinion to eclipse the long-standing legal rights of patients and families. This is the legal situation.

Ethically, this case is more complex. In the most straightforward view of the situation, the family is vested with making the decision unless it is clearly acting contrary to the best interests of the child or contrary to some distinct and identifiable other interest, one weighty enough to outweigh the parents' wishes. Some might argue, for instance, that the physicians' own moral values, including a repugnance toward providing care they perceive to be valueless, are infringed in this kind of situation. Whether or not one finds this argument persuasive in cases like this, the key point is not ethical dissensus but legal consensus.

The scope of family decisional authority

Families have many different reasons for wishing to continue life support, some of which seem more reasonable than others. They may have been told by a physician friend of the family that it is too early to be sure; they may sense that the staff doesn't like them; they may be concerned that the physicians are giving up too soon. They may have had a prior experience in which a physician foretold the inevitable death of a family member who later recovered fully. They may not trust these physicians, or this hospital, or the medical system as a whole, and they may be right.

A family's religion may require continued life support. Secular physicians sometimes forget the role of religion in the lives of patients. Even in the case of brain death, life support is discontinued only on secular grounds that need not persuade parents who believe that one respects the sanctity of life by continuing life support for a child whose heart beats and whose skin is pink and warm to the touch. There are religious traditions, such as Orthodox Judaism and some Japanese and Native American branches, within which the concept of brain death is alien (Gervais 1995: 548). Physicians have a duty of respect to these important value systems, although they may also point out that some of these traditions do permit withdrawal of treatment once the patient is actually dying (see the concept of *goses* in Orthodox Judaism) (Vanderpool 1995: 555).

But family authority goes beyond this, for families are entitled to ask that treatment be continued for unreasonable or irrational reasons. Perhaps they are not ready to say goodbye. Perhaps they have seen a movie or television program in which a similar situation ended in miraculous recovery (Diem *et al.* 1996). Perhaps they can provide no justification for their position. That is all right, for no justification is required of them. The whole point of decisional authority is not that the surrogate has the authority to make "good" decisions, but that he or she can make decisions with which the physician sharply disagrees. Of those reasons that the treating physicians deem inappropriate, some will be altered by gentle persuasion and time, others will not.

Family authority is not utterly without bounds. For example, when a surrogate's decision appears driven by psychiatric illness, or when the decision cannot be considered as in the patient's best interests no matter how charitably viewed, outside help or intervention (by a consultant or the ethics committee, for instance) should be sought. These cases are uncommon.

Decisions for this child

With this background, we can look more carefully at JM's situation. There is not a single decision to be made, but a series of decisions, decisions to continue life support for another hour, another day. For the purposes of discussion these can be condensed into two decisions, immediate and delayed.

The immediate decision concerns turning off life support in advance of more definite knowledge of JM's eventual outcome. The delayed decision will be reached if this child survives long enough to stabilize. The case history explains that survival is possible, although unlikely. The range of possible outcomes includes traditional (cardiorespiratory) death, brain death, permanent coma, persistent vegetative state (PVS), and, perhaps, survival with some regained consciousness although with severe impairment. In PVS, a portion of the lower brain has survived enough to produce wake–sleep cycles, but because of devastating injury to the centers of consciousness the patient is not aware even when awake. This was the condition of Karen Ann Quinlan and Nancy Cruzan, and patients may live in PVS for decades. It is not clear if the clinicians hold forth hope for any restoration of consciousness in JM, so I will assume that PVS is the least impaired outcome for which we can hope.

The delayed decision, then, turns on whether or not this family has the authority to request continued life support if JM enters a vegetative state and becomes stable in that condition. If the family may decide that they wish JM to be kept alive even in PVS, a fortiori it is permissible for them to insist that aggressive care be continued so that their child can attain that condition. So, does the family have the right to decide that they would wish JM to be kept alive in a vegetative state that may become permanent?

When the question is asked in this way, the answer is obvious. This family is at liberty to see PVS as an acceptable outcome for JM. The Consensus Panel of the American College of Chest Physicians and the Society of Critical Care Medicine explicitly noted that "the existence of a persistent vegetative state alone . . . should not dictate the withdrawal of life support" (American College of Chest Physicians/Society of Critical Care Medicine Consensus Panel 1990). Although most people would not want to be kept alive in the PVS (Emanuel *et al.* 1991, Malloy *et al.* 1992, Gillick *et al.* 1993, Reilly *et al.* 1994), no one else can dictate how JM's family should value this condition for their child (Engelhardt 1996). Tresch and co-workers looked at the families of patients in PVS, and found that most who had decided to maintain their relatives on life support felt that this decision was right for them (Tresch *et al.* 1991).

This decision may be right for the family, but clearly it is not welcome to the clinicians. The case history suggests that these clinicians feel firmly that the continuation of life support serves no medical purpose, and if the family continues to insist on its continuation, we enter the unsettled territory of futility. I am sympathetic to the frustration of physicians and nurses who are forced to provide care that they consider pointless, particularly when the patient is suffering, but the process of developing generally applicable approaches to these issues will be long, the path difficult, and the outcome unpredictable. This is not the place for a comprehensive discussion of futility, and the debate over futility has little relevance to JM, either now or in the foreseeable future. Ethicists themselves have varying views of the suitability of withdrawing life support in cases that are generally considered medically hopeless (Fox and Stocking 1993).

What if the physicians cannot persuade the parents to withdraw life support, and if outside assistance (such as members of the clergy or of the ethics committee) fails to break the deadlock? The physicians and hospital have the option of turning to the courts. However, the view of the law with regard to this case is clear. A judge would see the role of the physicians in clinical decision making as providing information, not coercion, to the parents. In the case of JM, the absence of brain death would provide strong support for the family's view. If the hospital were to bring JM's case to court, asking that a surrogate guardian be appointed who would approve the discontinuation of life support, the judge would almost certainly reject this request and support the parents' desire to continue aggressive care.

A recommended approach

The physicians' approach in situations like this must be appropriate for families of all kinds, including families who believe it is obligatory to continue life support at all costs, and who are deaf to the mainstream values reflected in the staff's recommendations. In this circumstance, the decision making follows the patient-sovereignty model. This model brings the power of the law squarely into the parents' corner. However, if taken by itself, it also reflects an impoverished view of what physicians can and should do, and in most cases is not what parents want. Once the family's decisional authority is recognized and incorporated into the staff's thinking and communication, the physicians' obligations can be seen more clearly. They have these duties:

Support the family

For every family that is sure from the beginning what they want in a case like this (a certainty that will usually stem from deep religious conviction about the meaning of life), there will be many that struggle with warring emotions and values. These families will welcome more involvement by the medical staff. For families that do not have firm views, the accumulated wisdom of the intensive care unit has tremendous power to guide them to a decision that will be right, not in any absolute sense, but in terms of how most ordinary people come to feel about children like JM. As Schneider (1998) has shown in his review of the empirical research on decision making, most people look to their physicians for help in making choices, and that assistance can improve the decisions that are made.

The family thus holds sole decisional authority, but most families will want active, ongoing assistance as they bear this responsibility. The law shelters families from those who would share in their decisions unbidden, but leaves them entirely free to accept advice and persuasion from those they trust. This help must be given with the clear understanding that the decision truly is the family's. The staff provides the family with information, analysis, and their own predictions of what the future will hold. The family assimilates all of this as it reassesses its own values and its beliefs as to what the child's situation is and may be. Over time, we expect to see most families persuaded by the staff's conviction that continuing life support serves no useful purpose. In all of this the distinction between persuasion and coercion must be preserved (Faden et al. 1986), a distinction that is here grounded in the staff's willingness to share the burden of the decision while recognizing that the family may not consent to this sharing. The staff may stumble at times as they counsel the family – this is a human undertaking and will be imperfectly implemented – but it is something that the staffs of intensive care units generally do well.

None of this talk about legal rights and ethical theories is meant to fault the good intentions and reasonable judgment of JM's physicians. Their approach works well in the vast majority of cases, and in fact this collaborative approach to decision making is usually appropriate, as most families want help in making difficult choices. Prendergast and Luce (1997) observed the termination of life support in a large series of patients in an intensive care unit, and found that the family or surrogate first raised the question of its withdrawal only 12 percent of the time. The responsible physician should not wait for the family to raise the topic or make the suggestion; families usually don't know when it is appropriate to turn off the respirator. In so doing, the physician is not asserting decisional authority, but rather exercising what might be called decisional *priority* (Whitney *et al.* 2004), accepting responsibility for making the suggestion that life support be terminated and offering to share the burden of deciding to allow life to end.

Maintain clear communication

What else can be done to help this family reach an appropriate decision? Clear communication is critical in avoiding conflicts with families in the intensive care unit (Dunn and Levinson 1996). Misunderstandings can arise from a variety of sources. The family may not understand the basic facts of the case. Commonly physicians believe they have provided a clear explanation but it is so loaded with jargon and statistics that it is impenetrable. Other physicians avoid technical terms but their vocabulary may be difficult and their sentences complex. We do not know the actual words used by the physicians in this case, but not every family understands the words "minuscule" and "coma" or the implications of the phrase "dependence on medical care for all aspects of life." Sometimes descriptions are not enough, and it can be helpful to arrange for the family to visit a long-term care facility so that they can see the likely reality of their child's future if they do not withdraw life support.

Even when the physician's language is clear, the family may have difficulty absorbing the information it hears. On the day of his admission, JM's family began the day in their normal routine; it ended in the intensive care unit with JM's life hanging by a thread. It would be an unusual family that could hear, understand, and process what the physicians are saying at that point. Before the family will be able to make reasoned decisions, it must get over the initial shock. This is one of the reasons it is helpful to have less-intensely involved relatives and friends participate in discussions with the clinicians, if possible; they may be able to hear and remember more of what the professional staff are saying.

For patients like JM, the treating team should inform the parents from the beginning of the clinical facts, of the team's reasoning, and of the range of outcomes and the most likely result. Brody (1989) has pointed to the importance of explaining the reasoning behind physicians' decisions in primary care, and it is equally applicable here.

Early prognostic information is helpful in preventing the family's appreciation of the situation from lagging behind the staff's (King 1992). Communication should not be restricted to the clinical facts and a comment that the prognosis is "uncertain." King has pointed out, in the analogous setting of the neonatal intensive care unit, that physicians early on sometimes provide parents with many data but no predictions. When the physicians in her study later suggested withdrawal of life support, they were surprised when parents were not yet prepared to accept this recommendation (King 1992). At the time JM was admitted to the intensive care unit, the physicians took every possible measure to increase the likelihood of his intact survival. This is of course right, and what parents expect; but if we had the opportunity to talk with the physicians in private, we would find they had a plan that included reassessment the following day. More likely than not, based on his obvious severe neurologic injury, they anticipated approaching the parents at that point with a suggestion that life support be discontinued. It is always helpful to sketch out for families both what is happening now and what they must be prepared for when tomorrow comes; this is part of preventive ethics (McCullough and Chervenak 1994). Ongoing communication, avoiding surprises, involving all members of the staff, all these will reduce the chance of future disagreement. The physicians should be certain to listen to the family so that they know how the family perceives the situation.

The parents need help, help that can best be provided in the context of respect for the fact that they are the ones who have known and cared for this child and who continue to be responsible for him. The ICU staff must recognize not only the reality, but the *validity*, of the family's near-absolute decisional authority and the fact that the staff advises but need not share in the decision, unless invited. This slight adjustment in attitude, conveyed through the staff's intonation and choice of words, can make a significant difference in the family–staff relationship. Families respond better to encouragement than pressure. I believe an approach that recognizes the responsibility of the family to make these decisions will result in less prolonged negotiations. Further, it will eventuate in better relations between family and staff in those uncommon situations in which the family resolutely insists on continuing life support. An analogous situation occurs in the context of prenatal diagnosis. The professional who does not assume that every fetus with Down syndrome will be aborted should maintain better rapport with deeply religious parents.

Beyond this there should be no change in the normal interactions between professionals and family. Frequent communication, honest answers, and an opportunity for the family to express grief and ventilate feelings of rage and betrayal will ease the family's progress through this difficult period.

Recommend psychological help

One more aspect of this family must be mentioned: they live in hell. The mother is experiencing guilt of an intensity that few people must endure. Over and over she replays what happened; where was her intuition, she may wonder, is there something wrong with her as a mother that she did not sense danger sooner? She panicked initially – what harm did that delay cause? And why did she not look in the swimming pool the moment she realized she did not know where her son was? And the father – how can he not blame his wife when she blames herself?

Any marriage can be strained by a child's serious illness or injury. Nixon and Pearn (1977) interviewed the families of children who suffered immersion injuries in the past. Among families in which the child survived, none of the parents were separated; among families in which the child died, 24 percent (eight of 29) separated or divorced. Nixon and Pearn found that stress within the families often persisted for years after the accident. Among siblings of drowning victims, they found guilt and sleep disorders; among parents, anxiety, sleep disorders, nightmares, and increased use of alcohol. Parental suicide has occurred (Zamula 1987).

This family needs help. It is good to read of the grandmother, aunts, and clergyman who attended the family conference, but even if these participants are all supportive, I would recommend family counseling. Many PICUs have social workers, who can play an important role, but they do not usually provide ongoing care. Some clergy are quite capable of providing this counseling themselves; when they are not, referral to another professional is appropriate. Another invaluable resource is the bereavement support group. There are a variety of support groups available; some hold meetings, some have internet discussion groups, and some do both. One group of this type is the Compassionate Friends (http://www.compassionatefriends.org), which hosts email discussion groups and has chapters worldwide.

Pediatricians always have a responsibility to promote family well-being, and that responsibility is particularly apparent when the child is beyond saving.

When family and physician disagree

How should physicians respond to a family that refuses to withdraw life support? First, of course, by reconsidering the facts of the case and the range of medical opinion. If the facts are clear and there is consensus of professional practice in similar situations, then the reasons for the family's objection should be gently explored.

The case history does not tell us why the family initially insists that life support be continued. This critical datum will help identify the optimal approach to the family. Perhaps they are acting on the belief that their religion requires continuing life support; if so, they may be correct, as would be the case for some conservative Christian denominations in this situation, or it may be incorrect. Catholics, for instance, are permitted to forgo therapy that is judged to be burdensome in relation to the expected benefit (Kelly 1951), but not all Catholics are aware of this important point. Perhaps this family has not come to terms with the fact that this child's life is essentially over; grief moves at its own pace. It is my belief that allowing them more time (as Dr. Mathers is clearly willing to do) is not only humane but may improve their long-term adjustment to this loss.

Although patience is desirable, delay can also cause problems. If some brain-stem function returns, this child may survive and enter a permanent vegetative state. If this happens he will no longer be ventilator-dependent. That will be good news if the parents wish their child to live, no matter how severely disabled. It will be bad news if the parents feel they cannot withhold or withdraw other life-sustaining support (such as a feeding tube); this can happen when families believe, or are advised, that it is morally appropriate to withhold or withdraw extraordinary therapy, such as a ventilator, but not ordinary therapy, such as a feeding tube. The distinctions between withholding and withdrawing treatment modalities, and between ordinary and extraordinary treatments, are out of favor in contemporary ethical thought, but they persist in some physicians, family, and clergy.

When the family and the professionals cannot reach agreement, it is sometimes helpful to bring in outside assistance. This could be, for instance, a member of the clergy or a member of the hospital ethics committee. As Dr. Mathers points out, it is rarely necessary or appropriate to turn to the courts to resolve these disputes. His description of patient, respectful dialogue with the family is marvelous and echoes published suggestions for negotiation with the family (Dunn and Levinson 1996).

In the end, most families consent to the withdrawal of life support (Prendergast and Luce 1997). If they have come to see this as the right course, this is a satisfactory outcome. If they simply yield to pressure, I worry that they will always regret not standing firm (this might also lead to exacerbated intrafamily tensions). However inwardly impatient the physicians may be, the family needs enough time.

The case history does not mention money. A family may wonder if the physicians are trying to save money for the institution or the insurance company, or to acquire organs for transplantation. Money is certainly germane to these decisions. ICU care costs thousands of dollars a day; if life support is continued, there is a decent chance that the patient will be alive, but still unconscious, 40 years on. The costs for institutional care for a severely injured child were estimated in 1988 to be $90 000 to $100 000 per year (Wintemute 1990). A 1987 Consumer Product Safety Commission report estimated the cost of home care supplies at $30 000 per year, and the cost of adequate babysitting and nursing at an additional $60 000 per year (Present 1987). These figures would be higher today.

The responsibility for using our resources prudently begins with society as a whole. Oregon made a valiant but failed effort to rationalize its system. Isolated federal initiatives, such as the move to diagnosis-related groups (DRGs) and the crackdown on Medicare fraud, have been predictably unequal to the task of slowing healthcare spending. The role of the individual physician in saving money is debatable, and it would be counterproductive to raise the topic with JM's family or in making decisions about him at this point. Fried (1975) has made a strong case that the individual physician's obligation is to his or her own patient, not to society's need to conserve resources. If society as a whole chooses to limit its spending for patients with particular medical conditions, it is free to do so through the usual legislative processes. JM's parents should be assured that the recommendation to withdraw life support is not being made to save money.

There is one case in which resource allocation decisions must be made at the local level. If a bed in an ICU (or a hospital) is needed by more than one patient, then a decision specific to that situation is unavoidable. In that case, the choice should be made, if possible, by a physician who is not involved in the care of any of the patients who are candidates for the bed.

On doing everything

Even when the situation is hopeless, the family will sometimes ask the physicians to "do everything." Adapting comments by David Pisetsky (1998), the physicians cannot do everything; they can only adjust the medications and the respirator settings. I tell parents in this situation that only they can do everything, for only they can hold this child, and tell him how much they will miss him. Only they can promise him that they will honor his memory by continuing to love each other. These words can be whispered to him only by this man and woman who will never forget him and will always love him.

ACKNOWLEDGMENTS

I am grateful for the editorial assistance of Anna Kieken, Ph.D., and the helpful comments of Dan W. Brock, Ph.D., Mary M. P. King, J.D., and Laurence B. McCullough, Ph.D.

4.3 Topical discussion

Futility

Despite wide recognition that it cannot be meaningfully and univocally defined, the term "futility" is sometimes invoked in medical cases where there is reason to doubt (1) the medical efficacy of the treatment ("it won't work"), or (2) whether it will improve quality of life ("it's not worth it"). Its ordinary-language connotations make it very difficult to convert the term into a technical term with a specific and limited meaning, but since its first introduction in 1987 in connection with CPR it has been used with increasing frequency as a shorthand for a variety of scientific and subjective reasons for not offering, or for suggesting withdrawal of, medical therapies.

The court cases related to futility are of two kinds. In the first kind, if the family or surrogates wish to withhold or withdraw life-sustaining treatments, they may do so (with evidence of patient preferences, as in the Quinlan case of 1976), including withdrawal of medical nutrition and hydration (if the state allows it, as in the Cruzan case of 1990). In the other kind of case, surrogates wish to institute or continue care that the team or facility considers ineffective or inadvisable. If the team are unable to reconcile themselves to offering life-sustaining treatment, they must transfer the patient to an alternative physician or facility which will provide the care (as happened with Baby Ryan Nguyen in 1994) or, if that facility is not equipped for emergency care, must continue to provide the care themselves (as occurred in the Baby K case).

On its objective pole it may be correlated with predictions of efficacy for various patient groups, via such scales as the APACHE, or statistics about outcomes in previous similar cases. Schneiderman *et al.* have suggested that "when physicians conclude . . . that in the last 100 cases a medical treatment has been useless,

Ethical Dilemmas in Pediatrics: Cases and Commentaries, ed. Lorry R. Frankel, Amnon Goldworth, Mary V. Rorty, and William A. Silverman. Published by Cambridge University Press. © Cambridge University Press 2005.

they should regard that treatment as futile." "Potentially ineffective care" has been recommended by the AMA as substitute language in this context. The AMA assures physicians that "they are not ethically obligated to deliver care that in their best judgment will not have a reasonable chance of benefiting their patients," and that denial of treatment can be justified by reliance on "acceptable standards of care." This recommendation may offer solace to perplexed physicians, but it is difficult to apply, for it presumes consensus on what are "acceptable standards of care," and occludes difficulties with medical uncertainty and the unpredictability of individual variation.

The term is also invoked as a value judgment, that a patient is suffering or has a quality of life such that their continued life is of negative value, or that continued treatment is just prolonging the inevitable. There are categories of patients to whom the term in this sense is most frequently applied – patients in PVS, anencephalics, or terminally ill patients – but according to whose values is that judgment made, and who is to decide? As Whitney makes clear in his response to this troubling case, the law is very clear about who has the ultimate authority to decide in the case of infants: the parents as surrogate decision makers.

Although there is uncertainty in predicting outcomes of medical interventions, parents are not likely to challenge the probability assessments of their child's physician. But the assessment of the value of outcomes is a different matter. Where the physician may see only a child of extremely limited capacity and therefore place a very low value on further treatment, the parents may judge the treatment, if successful in saving their child's life, of such enormous value that the small possibility of success is ignored or dismissed. Uncertainty of scientific predictability, conjoined with acknowledged differences in values, makes determination of futility a Gordian knot with implications for both cost and resource utilization. Outcome studies, procedural guidelines, and consensus building and measuring offer the only hope of progress in resolving some cases, but the ethical challenge presented by this concept is not going away.

Quality of life

While quantity of life is its length, quality of life is a multifactorial and contextual evaluation by an onlooker about a patient's experience, and is generally agreed to be difficult to objectively measure. Because of its complexity, quality of life has been described as one of the most morally controversial issues in modern medicine (Hastings Center 1987). It is widely agreed that scientific medical assessments require added consideration of their effects on the patient's subjective condition, experience and value system, but that is inaccessible to third parties. The more capable a patient is of making his own evaluations, the more likely they are to express that patient's experience. In pediatrics, where such judgments are being made for a young incapable patient, the judgments are also subject to a second level of subjectivity by the extent to which they are influenced by the values and capacity for imaginative projection of the evaluator. For infants such as the child in this case, there is little opportunity for first-person evaluation of quality of life.

Most attempts to evaluate quality of life take into consideration a range of factors from the physiological to the social. Dimensions typically included in quality-of-life evaluations for infants and children are the absence of pain and capacity to feel pleasure, the level of physical functioning and associated appropriate behaviors, capacity for social relationships, and degree of consciousness and self-awareness. The positive or negative evaluation of quality of life is relational, in that it takes as its baseline what a given patient (or surrogate) might expect at best, and measures positive or negative quality of life in terms of the gap between those expectations and the actual present experience, capacities, or functions.

There is considerable concern in the larger society that quality-of-life considerations not be used as a justification for discriminating against people with disabilities, as is seen in the history of the Baby Doe laws of the mid-1980s, and more recently in the Americans With Disabilities Act passed in 1990. While Baby Doe laws initially excluded all quality-of-life judgments in treatment decisions, it was quickly realized that such a rigid exclusion was unfair to the experience of patients, the expertise of physicians, and the decisional rights of families, and that the proper place for treatment decisions was at the bedside, not in the courts. In clinical practice concern about biases may be controlled for by asking whether a given intervention would be considered in a patient with the same presenting problem without similar background disabilities.

While decision makers sometimes invoke quality-of-life judgments in deciding whether a proposed treatment is in the patient's best interest, there is currently no ethical support for using quality-of-life judgments in rationing decisions, despite considerable pressure on physicians to take a more active role in bedside rationing.

Family authority

The legal recognition of the ultimate authority of parents as surrogate decision makers seems to beg the question of whether parents are always ideal decision makers – informed, unbiased, and aware of the consequences of their decisions. Caregivers are responsible for providing the information about condition, care options, probable prognosis, and future course to the parents, who bear the financial, emotional, and rehabilitative burden of the child's care. Although there has been some discussion in recent ethics literature about whether the best interests of the entire family, rather than just the best interests of the patient, should figure in "family-centered" decision making, conceptual difficulties in such an approach make it an unlikely candidate to replace the current patient-centered ethic, especially in pediatrics, where surrogate decision making is the norm.

Pediatrician philosopher Lainie Friedman Ross argues that the "best interest" standard does not adequately consider the right of families to perform "intrafamilial trade-offs," maximizing in care decisions values which may vary across different families, providing that the basic needs of child family members are secured. She describes her alternative as a model of "constrained parental autonomy."

Shared decision making

Decision making in pediatrics involves physician experience and expertise, and parental preferences and responsibilities. Whitney's discussion of three models of clinical decision making delineates a continuum between medical paternalism, where the decisions are made virtually unilaterally by the physician, and patient sovereignty, what another physician has called being "a technician to our patients' desires." Both extremes seem undesirable; but finding the proper point on the continuum in a given case is a challenging exercise in ethical judgment. The call for shared decision making acknowledges the importance of as comprehensive an exchange of information as possible – the physicians contributing their medical knowledge, the parents their situation and values. The idea of shared decision making is as much an ideal as a description, as Whitney notes, with the desired goal a consensus among those with a stake in the case about how to proceed in situations of uncertainty.

FURTHER READING

Bradlyn, A. S., Varni, J. W., and Hinds, P. S. Assessing health-related quality of life in end-of-life care for children and adolescents. In *When Children Die*, ed. M. J. Field and R. E. Behrman (Washington, DC: National Academies Press, 2003), pp. 476–508.

Buchanan, A. E. and Brock, D. *Deciding for Others: the Ethics of Surrogate Decision Making* (Cambridge: Cambridge University Press, 1989).

Cantor, N. L. Twenty-five years after *Quinlan*: a review of the jurisprudence of death and dying. *Journal of Law, Medicine and Ethics* **29** (2001), 182–196.

Caplan, A. Odds and ends: trust and the debate over medical futility. *Annals of Internal Medicine* **125** (1996), 688–689.

Drane, J. F. The quality of life concept and the best interest standard. In *Clinical Bioethics: Theory and Practice in Medical Ethical Decision-Making* (Kansas City, MO: Sheed and Ward, 1994).

Lantos, J. D., Singer, P. A., Walker, R. M., *et al.* The illusion of futility in clinical practice. *American Journal of Medicine* **87** (1989), 81–84.

Ross, L. F. *Children, Families and Health Care Decision Making* (New York, NY: Oxford University Press, 1998).

Schneiderman, L. J., Jecker, N. S., and Jonsen, A. R. Medical futility: response to critiques. *Annals of Internal Medicine* **125** (1996), 669–674.

Youngner, S. J. Who defines futility? *JAMA* **260** (1988), 2094–2095.

5.1 Long-term ventilation in a child with severe central nervous system impairment

Ronald M. Perkin, Robert Orr, and Stephen Ashwal

The case

The following question was brought for ethics consultation. Is it appropriate to initiate long-term ventilation for a child with severe neurologic compromise in order to avoid repeated respiratory exacerbations which necessitate transfer from his long-term care facility to a tertiary intensive care unit?

This case involved a 26-month-old male who was healthy at birth but developed a severe case of bronchiolitis caused by respiratory syncytial virus at two months of age. This illness resulted in apnea which was followed by cardiac arrest. Although he was successfully resuscitated, he did not recover neurologically and at the time of writing, approximately three years after his cardiac arrest, he was in a persistent vegetative state that was judged to be permanent.

The child was transferred to a chronic care facility at five months of age (three months after his cardiorespiratory arrest). He had a tracheostomy as well as a fundoplication and gastrostomy tube performed prior to his long-term placement. Once established in the long-term care facility the child required 23 transfers and admissions to a tertiary care facility over a 20-month period for episodes of hypercapnic respiratory failure. The child's respiratory drive was not consistently maintained and each time his respiratory drive failed he required admission to the pediatric intensive care unit (PICU) and mechanical ventilation for 7–10 days. Consideration of long-term ventilation at the chronic care facility was suggested to avoid these repeated transfers and to decrease his overall costs of care. His mother requested that all therapies be provided, including long-term ventilatory support.

Ethical Dilemmas in Pediatrics: Cases and Commentaries, ed. Lorry R. Frankel, Amnon Goldworth, Mary V. Rorty, and William A. Silverman. Published by Cambridge University Press. © Cambridge University Press 2005.

Discussion

Long-term or chronic ventilation evolved from experience with the poliomyelitis epidemics of the 1940s and 1950s, from increasing experience with long-term tracheotomies, and from advances in the care of critically ill children and newborns. Respiratory failure that could be managed by long-term ventilation in childhood arises from diverse causes including spinal-cord trauma, neuromuscular disease, central ventilatory control failure, bronchopulmonary dysplasia, and various congenital abnormalities. Although chronic mechanical ventilation is technically feasible in all these conditions, it has generated debate because of ethical, medical, economic, and psychological concerns.

Absent from the list of indications for long-term ventilation is the child with severe central nervous system impairment, including those with severe mental retardation or in a permanent vegetative state. Chronic ventilation has generally not been offered to such patients not because of futility but because of value decisions made at a policy level by the providers of this service.

The benefits of mechanical ventilation have been one of the outstanding successes of modern medicine. It is commonly and most appropriately used as a temporary bridge until patients can maintain adequate and independent respiratory function. However, many patients receiving ventilatory support are never successfully weaned, either dying while receiving ventilatory assistance or dying when it is withdrawn. The use of mechanical ventilation raises important ethical issues when it supports the patient with irreversible disease and when there is no hope of gaining awareness (Todres 1992). Recent surveys have found that more healthcare professionals are concerned about the inappropriate use of ventilators than any other life-sustaining treatment, including cardiopulmonary resuscitation and artificial nutrition and hydration (Solomon *et al.* 1993, Faber-Langedoen 1994).

One of the difficulties in making management decisions on behalf of profoundly brain-damaged patients relates to the incomplete understanding or misunderstanding of the term vegetative state and a general lack of experience in working with profoundly brain-damaged patients over the long term (International Working Party 1996). Concern has also been expressed about the use of the terms persistent and permanent in the terminology of the vegetative state (International Working Party 1996).

The vegetative state is characterized by unawareness of the self and the environment, with preservation of brain-stem autonomic and hypothalamic function. According to the Multi-Society Task Force on the Persistent Vegetative State, both children and adults are considered to be in a permanent vegetative state three months after non-traumatic and twelve months after traumatic brain injury. Recovery to consciousness is extremely unlikely in correctly diagnosed patients in the permanent vegetative state and the life span of such patients is markedly reduced (Multi-Society Task Force on PVS 1994, Ashwal *et al.* 1994).

Many individuals and groups have expressed opinions about the use of invasive and expensive technology to prevent death in patients who are in the vegetative state. The Society of Critical Care Medicine Consensus Task Force considered intensive care for vegetative patients futile and recommended that vegetative patients should not be maintained in the intensive care unit to the exclusion of other patients who could derive more benefit (Society of Critical Care Medicine Task Force on Ethics 1990). A similar position was taken by the Bioethics Task Force of the American Thoracic Society which considered care futile if it would not restore sentient function (American Thoracic Society Bioethics Task Force 1991). The Hastings Center (1987) concluded that providing intensive care to patients in a persistent vegetative state is generally a misuse of resources, and the President's Commission (1983) stated that such patients should be removed from life support if such action is necessary to benefit another patient who is not in a persistent vegetative state.

Life-sustaining therapy for patients in the vegetative state is not futile in the physiologic sense because it may stabilize a patient's vital signs. Nevertheless, such therapy cannot benefit the patient as a whole because sentient function cannot be restored.

In spite of the growing consensus not to provide life-saving therapy to patients in a persistent vegetative state, demand for such therapy continues to occur, as in our case. Although it has been stated that "patients or surrogates may not compel a physician to provide any treatment that, in the professional judgment of the physician, is unlikely to benefit" (Luce 1995), little information exists to guide the physicians when families demand therapy for patients whose vegetative state is judged to be permanent (American Medical Association Council on Ethical and Judicial Affairs 1991). The medical community and numerous courts have recognized that permanent unconsciousness – devoid of self-awareness or human interaction – is a dismal status that most people would prefer to avoid; it is hopeless, undignified, and entails a burden upon family and care providers (Cantor 1996). However, the surrogate does not have to reach that conclusion (in the absence of advance instructions from a competent patient).

The central issue in this dilemma is the scope of a surrogate's authority to act on behalf of an incompetent patient. In such situations, the surrogate (usually the child's parents) is empowered to act consistently with the child's "best interests." Preservation of life is normally deemed consistent with best interests – a fitting presumption in a society that has traditionally revered human life (Cantor 1996, Sprung and Eidelman 1996). Some see biological existence – even without the possibility of human interaction – as good, or at least they do not see permanent unconsciousness as intolerably demeaning.

For this reason, when a child is chronically ill with minimal or no cognitive ability, healthcare professionals almost always follow parents' wishes for or against life-sustaining treatments. Parental decisions are challenged only when it appears that they are not acting in the child's best interests.

However, assessing the "best interest" of a child in the vegetative state is problematic in that they do not have personal interests. Family requests for aggressive therapy in patients in a permanent vegetative state reflect their interests and their values; it does not reflect patient autonomy but rather it reflects family autonomy. Conflict, if it develops, concerns physician or caregiver integrity and family autonomy (Halevy and Brody 1996). Physician or caregiver integrity may lead to a judgment that the request for long-term ventilation in patients in a permanent vegetative state is unseemly, represents an inappropriate stewardship of resources, or both (Halevy and Brody 1996).

The physician has the right to discuss, explain, even attempt to persuade; however, in the last analysis, the goals and beliefs of the patient or surrogate are most often respected (Jonsen 1986, Sprung *et al.* 1995). Sprung believes that a patient or surrogate request need not be honored and physician autonomy should prevail *only* when there are well-established and accepted medical criteria and standards for not providing interventions. These criteria are few and include brain death and cardiopulmonary resuscitation in certain circumstances (Sprung *et al.* 1995).

In this case, the patient's mother chose as a primary goal the survival of her son regardless of the treatment required. This goal of survival was technically feasible but required either frequent ICU admissions or long-term mechanical ventilation at the chronic care facility.

It may rarely be justifiable to withhold or refuse therapy which is requested by parents for their children and which is technically feasible. Refusals are typically based on physician's opinion that the treatment is futile, non-beneficial, unreasonable, cruel, wasteful, or not in the best interests of the patient (Morreim 1994). The use of these subjective labels as objective medical facts may not convince a family to change their minds (Sprung *et al.* 1995). However, the wise physician recognizes that these value-laden terms often stem from an underlying conviction that the patient has minimal personal status. At worst, these subjective labels may be used as medical facts to manipulate the decision maker; at best, they may be used as a way to discuss conflicting values attached to unconscious life that are present.

The following specific arguments for not providing long-term ventilation were considered in this case:

(1) *The therapy causes the child great suffering with little observable benefit.* Long-term ventilation of this patient at a chronic care facility would not cause disproportionate suffering; in fact it might decrease his burden of frequent transfers.

However, discussion of benefits versus burdens of therapy for patients in a persistent vegetative state is not logical or appropriate. Patients in a vegetative state are by definition unaware of self and the environment and therefore have no personal interests and cannot recognize pain or suffering. Such patients cannot recognize benefit or burden.

(2) *The proposed therapy is outside the standard of medical practice.* Even though there may be an emerging theoretical view that doctors do not have to provide "useless" therapies requested by patients or their families, there is presently no professional or societal consensus on the issue (Morreim 1994). The question is whether physicians may simply refuse requests they deem medically inappropriate or whether, in an era of enhanced patient and family autonomy, they are required to provide more specific and detailed justifications of their decisions (Prendergast 1995). If they must provide specific justifications, what sort of reasoning justifies physician discretion when the alternative to treatment is death?

A strong societal consensus should be developed that maintenance of non-interactive biologic life with mechanical ventilation, cardiotonic drugs, or dialysis is inappropriate (Truog *et al.* 1992, Frader and Thompson 1994). A societal consensus, however, may not be reached quickly. The lack of consensus may, in part, be an expression of societal bewilderment and confusion as technological developments overtake our capacity to control or understand them (Marshall 1992). In addition, there is a wide gap between ethical thought and technological possibility. Healthcare professionals have been expected to continue or provide life support demanded by surrogates, despite the objection that the care is "inappropriate." Efforts to resolve the conflict between surrogate and healthcare professional must continue.

(3) *The therapy is precluded by institutional, regional, or payer policy.* Specific institutions may make policy decisions rationing expensive or scarce resources. No such policy existed which precluded long-term ventilation of this patient.

A way to confront aggressive treatment of patients in a permanent vegetative state is by development of "futility" policies. Healthcare professionals and the public can work together within communities to forge consensus regarding futile or inappropriate treatment (Murphy and Barbour 1994, Prendergast 1995, Tomlinson and Czlonka 1995). What appears to be critical is that communities must work together to implement policies regarding treatment limitations. One or two hospitals acting alone cannot be expected to make appropriate changes. The risk of bad public relations and litigation is probably too great for any institution acting alone. However, if the majority of institutions in a community adopt similar policies, the risk of bad public relations and litigation is reduced (Murphy and Barbour 1994). Recent approaches utilize an open and fair process of determining futility which balances patient autonomy with professional and institutional integrity (Prendergast 1995).

. (4) *The therapy is not financially feasible.* The allocation of considerable sums to permanently unconscious patients or to severely debilitated, end-stage patients is a serious concern. The cost issue has not been faced in cases litigated to date (e.g. *Wanglie, Baby K*) (Cantor 1996). Cost is frequently mentioned as a reason for not providing long-term life support; however, in this particular patient, long-term ventilation would most likely decrease the overall cost of his care by decreasing transport costs, emergency department evaluation costs, and tertiary ICU costs.

As a group of authors we believe that patients in a permanent vegetative state should not be chronically ventilated; it is treatment which provides no benefit for the patient even though it may comfort the family and it represents inappropriate stewardship of resources. A similar opinion was expressed by Mallory and Stillwell (1991).

Even though we had these beliefs, for the reasons outlined above, no compelling reason to not provide long-term ventilation could be formulated to combat the mother's firm stance.

Long-term ventilation was initiated at the chronic care facility. Since that time the child required only one readmission to the tertiary ICU in two and a half years, and it was decided to transfer to home mechanical ventilation.

5.2 Autonomy, community, and futility: moral paradigms for the long-term ventilation of a severely impaired child

Anita Silvers

Introduction

Principles and practice

Casuistry, or case-based reasoning, is the preferred methodology for clinical ethics. Broadly speaking, this practice of thinking through the ethical aspects of medical decisions gives the particularities of each case primacy over appeals to principle. Emphasizing the details of and differences between cases in this way has proved to be a welcome heuristic against excessively abstract principles and impersonal institutional policies. Furthermore, case-based disquisition not only respects, but emerges out of, the experience-enriched perspectives good clinicians bring to their practice.

In the execution of moral deliberation, however, it can be difficult to discern whether principle-directed, or instead case-based, moral reasoning is being attempted. That is because both methodologies incorporate reference to model cases, albeit in very different ways. But arduous as it may be to disentangle these approaches, the utility of doing so is evident. For where the methodologies have been scrambled, cases will prove themselves resistant to our expectations about how they should be resolved, and will leave a residual puzzlement and dissatisfaction about their outcome. Furthermore, this lack of closure may precipitate premature calls for policy making.

Prior to yielding to pressures to promulgate policies, however, it is prudent to gain a better understanding of what values difficult cases bring into play. Doing so helps to predict when a prospective policy is liable to clash with the values of the broader community. To illustrate, let us explore why, after having successfully executed "long-term ventilation in a child with severe central nervous system impairment," Drs. Perkin, Orr, and Ashwal continue to find the case an irritant. There is an ethical

Ethical Dilemmas in Pediatrics: Cases and Commentaries, ed. Lorry R. Frankel, Amnon Goldworth, Mary V. Rorty, and William A. Silverman. Published by Cambridge University Press. © Cambridge University Press 2005.

principle that the authors are convinced should have governed their actions in this case. They articulate their principle categorically: "As a group of authors, we believe that patients in a permanent vegetative state should not be chronically ventilated." Nevertheless, in practice their principle failed to apply, or at least they failed to apply it.

Acting on principle

Why did they fail to find sufficient reason to act on their conviction? As they state their conclusion, it was because "no compelling reason to not provide long-term ventilation could be formulated." They suppose that their principle failed them because it could not generate reasons forceful enough "*to combat the mother's firm stance*" (emphasis added).

What in their view could furnish their position with sufficient strength to prevail against a mother's objections, and, consequently, to secure their self-determination of their own actions? Note that they frame their discussion in the language of power, as if moral deliberation is an occasion for struggle between physicians and the representatives of their patients. They describe cases like the one they discuss as "conflicts" between physician integrity and family comfort. If such cases are interpreted as threatening professional standards, physicians may seek to establish institutional policies that will shield them. Furthermore, the power accruing to consensus can fortify them in adhering to their principles. In this spirit, the authors invite the establishment of coalitions of providers sufficiently numerous to lessen the risk of "bad public relations and litigation." They seek to forge a consensus of professional judgment that "patients in a permanent vegetative state should not be chronically ventilated."

In my view, however, the solution to their problem does not require the politics of forging a coalition forcible enough to overcome the obstacle they identify, namely "a mother's firm stance." Their casting the mother in a role oppositional to their own may be neither perspicacious nor helpful. For it is improbable that a mother's preference alone would have prevailed over three physicians' principles, as they report its having done, if the sole decisive factor were the exercise of power. Accordingly, it is unlikely that the addition of further professionals, in the form of a coalition of providers, will resolve the issue simply by the weight of numbers. For this reason, identifying the additional factors that forestalled the physicians from acting on their principle is important.

Classical ethical theory typically traces failure to act on one's principles despite having the power to do so to one of two causes: weakness of will, or the formulation of the principle itself, that is, its imprecise articulation and the consequent uncertainty about where it applies. I propose that it is neither the authors' will nor their principles, but instead confusions traceable to their method, that occasion their remaining disquiet about this case. Their plan to restore power to their principle disregards important characteristics of the case by attempting to assimilate it to a dissimilar paradigm. So I will consider whether, from a moral point of view, their proposal is advisable, and will argue for the prudence of proceeding with great caution. Imposing a political process where case-insensitive "quality of life" principles prevail over case-attentive sensibilities calls for thoughtful focus and discriminating adjustment if we are not to further erode public confidence in the decency of professional health care.

Principle-directed and case-based moral reasoning

Like case-based moral reasoning, principle-directed moral decision making assigns exemplary cases an important role. Because principles are barren, in the absence of illustrations of how they are applied, well-chosen cases show us what it means to live by each principle.

Typically, our confidence in any principle's strength and intelligibility is influenced by our having found the doctrine enlightening and effective in its applications to cases we consider paradigmatic. These exemplary and illustrative paradigm cases have a variety of sources. They may be drawn from personal experience, or they may be commonplace in the professional climate in which an individual practices, or they may have stimulated sufficient conversation to have gained prominence in the broader political, social, and cultural environment.

In contemporary medical practice, the litigation of cases such as *Conroy* (Supreme Court of New Jersey, 98 NJ 321, 486 A. 2d 1209, Jan 17, 1985) and *Cruzan* (US Supreme Court, 58 LW 4916, June 26, 1990), and the publication of others such as Dax (Liever 1989, Cowart and Burt 1998) and Diane (Quill 1991) are presumed to exemplify powerful principles both by those who introduce them into the literature and by those who subsequently cite them as precedents. These are paradigms that invite extrapolation beyond themselves. In other words, they invigorate principle-directed moral reasoning by authorizing categorical action of the kind they illustrate.

What then distinguishes principle-directed ethics, where paradigmatic cases merely illustrate exemplary judgment, from case-based ethics, where paradigmatic cases create exemplary judgment? In deliberations about medical ethics, principle-directed extrapolation and case-based intuition often rely on the same cases. But the two methodologies disagree about the force of these paradigms. While the paradigms appealed to in principle-directed reasoning are generalized to the extent of their being idealized, those central to case-based moral consideration tend to be idiosyncratic. One way of characterizing the contrast between principle-directed and case-based moral methodology thus is in terms of their dissimilar tolerance for divergence between paradigm cases and the ordinary cases to which they are compared. Principle-directed ethics creates very broad categories of application and treats the relevant principle as categorical albeit defeasible – that is, as holding in all cases but the few that manifest certain specified conditions which defeat or curb it. Consequently, within its proper scope, each established principle is presumed to be compelling, if not exactly dispositive or necessarily decisive, in respect to newly encountered cases.

Case-based ethics, on the other hand, is much more conflicted about extrapolation. Case-based ethics relies on our being able to derive guidance from the resemblance our immediate case bears to its exemplary predecessors. Central to this practice is the systematic examination of the differences between each new case and its purported paradigms. Our intuitions about whatever new case is before us thereby assume a much greater weight in case-based practice than they bear in principle-directed decisions. Our intuitions constitute a sort of a-posteriori standard in that, on this approach, we expect either that the conclusion of our reasoning in a case will accord with how we intuitively respond to it, or else that our intuitions will have been transformed in the course of our deliberations.

It is not per se the reference to paradigms which confuses the physician authors in the case described, since both case- and principle-based moral reasoning rely on paradigm cases; but instead, the role paradigms play in their reasoning. So it will be illuminating to follow the play between established paradigms and immediate intuitions in considering how Perkin, Orr, and Ashwal decided whether to initiate long-term ventilation in a two-year-old patient. Doing so will disclose why this case confounded their acting on their own principle against ventilating patients in a permanent vegetative state. In this instance, the compelling particularities central to case-based ethics deflected the categorical application favored by principle-directed ethics.

Values relevant to ventilating

Three values are central to most discussions about imposing, withdrawing, and refusing treatment. Those values are (1) respecting autonomy, (2) furthering community, and (3) avoiding futility. Each has its familiar paradigms which may or may not be apposite to the particulars of a case. Perkin, Orr, and Ashwal explicitly refer to some of these values. Others are evoked by examples whose influence is felt because they have become prominent signposts in the evolving conversation about physicians' obligations to treat or to refrain from treating. What will become evident is that its similarities to, and differences from, these paradigms actually were more important to the disposition of the authors' case than was their principle.

Paradigms of autonomy

The differences between adults and children contraindicate the application of certain moral paradigms in pediatric cases. For example, it is questionable that children, especially very young ones, fully possess some of the central morally relevant properties of persons, such as the capacity for rational self-determination that we call "competence" and take to be a necessary condition for a patient's being within the scope of the principle of respect for autonomy. As a result, principles for which autonomy figures as decisive, or at least as weighty, may not be applicable to pediatric cases like this one. A collection of well-known legal cases, followed closely in the popular press and analyzed fully in the biomedical ethics literature, offer the initial paradigm for the role of autonomy in cases of discontinuing life-sustaining treatment. The cluster of cases, of which the stories of Karen Quinlan and Nancy Cruzan are probably the best known, are part of the background of any discussion about assisting the physical functioning of an individual in a persistent vegetative state (Arras 1991). The legal cases that shape this paradigm focus on the contrast between the vital way the patients formerly lived and their currently inert and unresponsive existence. Arguably these patients were not the same people they once had been because their cerebral cortical functioning, the brain activity correlated with reflective experiencing, had ceased. Such a way of speaking about them is figurative, but nonetheless forceful.

Should they continue to be treated with interventions that stand between their bodies' life and death? In acknowledgment of their autonomy, competent citizens have a right to self-determination that includes the control of their own bodies. As the Supreme Court reaffirmed in *Cruzan*, in light of this principle a competent person has the right to refuse medical treatment when she construes that doing so is in her interest, and surrogates can act on her behalf to do so as well. A competent individual's decision equating her own interest with the withdrawal or refusal of treatment is usually to be given precedence over the collective interest in privileging practices that preserve life. But to establish that an incompetent patient's enduring her present state is an individual harm great enough to outweigh the collective interest in preserving life, there must be evidence of the patient's conviction, when she was competent, that a state like her present one is intolerable.[1] Indeed, the court in the Cruzan case made clear that it takes decisive evidence of the patient's rejection of her current way of life, evidence that refers to the views she articulated when she was competent, to override the state's interest in preserving life. Notice that this paradigm establishes how references to the best

---

[1] But see Dresser and Robertson (1989) for an argument that third-party assessments of the demented patient's present interest sometimes prevail over the patient's earlier predictions about what she would want if she became demented.

interests of individuals who are in persistent vegetative states are to be made meaningful.

Drs. Perkin, Orr, and Ashwal think it is problematic to cite the interests of children in vegetative states because "they do not have personal interests." This is the case, but it is so because they are children and thus cannot be reconstituted as competent persons, not because their being in a vegetative state negates their having interests. That is, we have developed a paradigm which permits us to act to comply with the personal interests of people in vegetative states. The paradigm takes the historical person who has become the individual now in a vegetative state as the person whose judgment must be respected. It is a virtual person – the person who was – who decides. Ideally, we have the historical person's very words, written or uttered in advance of her incompetence, to direct us. However, in the absence of such a specific document, other evidence of an incompetent patient's past convictions and contentions often will do. (In some states, for instance, testimony or other documentation of the individual's orally expressed wishes is sufficient.) Similar processes of historical reconstruction are deployed by the courts in areas from estate law to Congressional intent in order to establish purposes that have been formed in the past.

It is important to understand how case-based reasoning operates here. The case-based method compares the relevant paradigms with the instance at hand and searches for differences that detract from or dispute its relevance. The model for establishing whether a currently incompetent individual previously believed he or she should not be made to endure a state like the current one interprets the absence of clear evidence as being evidence to the contrary. That is, if neither written declarations nor credible reports of clearly confirming behavior sustain the decision to refuse treatment, the model presses us to assume that the competent person identifies his or her interest with continued life.

But the patient in this case lost cerebral cortical function after only 60 days of life. He never was capable of considering, let alone articulating, whether he believed being in a condition like his present one was a harmful state. Consequently, he has no history that can be used to anchor an account of his personal interest. The paradigm of the formerly self-determining individual who was persuaded of the personal harm attendant upon being in a vegetative state, as well as the formerly self-determining individual who was not so convinced, simply can not be a paradigm for children.

Because the model is not appropriately applied to children, autonomy cannot be at issue in the case considered here. The authors understand that there is no question of the child's being autonomous, but nevertheless they claim that "family autonomy" conflicts with "physician integrity." But from the model we see that families cannot impersonate the patient in exercising his or her autonomy. The duty of someone who is a surrogate for an autonomous patient is to gather evidence of how the patient would speak, if he or she could, not to speak in lieu of the patient. If the patient has never been autonomous, as in the case under discussion, no one who speaks for the patient should be thought of as speaking in terms set by the paradigm of patient autonomy.

Community

However, families, friends, and caretakers who have emotional attachments with the patient appropriately do speak to another value, namely the connectedness the individual continues to have with other people. For even an individual who cannot interact may be considered part of a community. Unlike autonomy, which issues from the patient's claim to self-determination, community is a value that is projected onto the patient by others. Why does the value of furthering community play so small a role in Perkin, Orr, and Ashwal's satisfaction with their resolution of this case? The answer may lie in the nature of the paradigm for community.

What is the paradigm for a patient's connection to community? In answering this question we need to keep in mind that the medical view may not match the conception that prevails in the wider society. In particular, medical professionals place a premium on mental function. Commenting that medical professionals place a premium on functioning minds, Mary Mahowald, a clinical ethicist at the University of Chicago's Pritzker School of Medicine, offers the following illustration:

A little boy named Chris suffered a prolonged umbilical cord prolapse at birth. The event left him completely immobilized from the head down. He was also blind, and possibly deaf. At 3 months of age Chris remained prone in a hospital crib, depending on medical technology for all vital functions, including respiration and nutrition. There was no realistic expectation that he would ever be weanable from his dependence for survival on extensive medical technology. In the past, his caregivers, in accordance with parental wishes, had removed life support from infants whose basic bodily systems were functional but had suffered severe brain hemorrhages predictive of massive and irreparable cognitive damage. With Chris, the situation was the reverse, leaving his caregivers much more ambivalent than they were in the other cases about whether to continue his treatment. "He has a good brain," one said. "How can we let him go?" (Silvers *et al.* 1998)

Mahowald's story shows us how, on the medical model, the body has come to be thought of as a service system for the brain. Figures like Stephen Hawking and Christopher Reeve have accustomed the public to ventilator-dependent individuals who go about their business in the community. As the case authors point out, our familiarity with ventilator-dependent individuals has been developing for nearly 50 years. They note that "long-term or chronic ventilation evolved from experience with the poliomyelitis epidemics of the 1940s and 1950s." A child's head emerging from an iron lung was the initial image of ventilator dependence. A very few post-polio patients have been continuously dependent on mechanical breathing assistance for as much as five decades, and there are spinal-cord-injury patients who have lived this way for almost as long. Other post-polio individuals began to use mechanical breathing assistance decades after the onset of the disease. Many in this last group use breathing assistance only for part of the day. Like the authors' young patient, mechanical assistance in breathing is not a mortal need for many of the post-polio patients. But whether mechanical assistance with breathing is medically necessary in these latter cases is of less interest for our purposes than the fact that it is quite readily prescribed.

The authors do not see how the paradigm centered on post-polio patients resembles their case. Granted, their patient is like some of these paradigmatic ventilator users in that, although he was maintaining without long-term mechanical ventilation, long-term ventilation alleviated the incidents of respiratory distress that necessitated emergency treatment. Nevertheless, the authors deny that long-term ventilation can benefit their patient as it does the paradigmatic ones. Their thought is that he cannot experience (and so cannot appreciate) heightened well-being from this intervention, nor likewise experience harm from its absence. He is indifferent; therefore, there is indifferent value in their intervening.

However, this decision on their part retains the individualistic focus on reflective self-determination, a paradigm emphasizing patient autonomy that we have already seen to be inapposite in pediatric cases. We need to look for an alternative paradigm of community involvement with patients, one that construes patients in terms other than as speaking participants in dialogical interactions. There is another, very powerful paradigm that focuses on caring for, rather than communicating with, patients. It is the influence of this paradigm that commits the community to caring for incompetents.

This model for community concern about the medical care of severely impaired individuals, especially children, has been authoritative since the early twentieth century (Trent 1994). Concern for such individuals is not exclusively a role for healthcare professionals. Everyone in a community that emphasizes connectedness between people is concerned about the most vulnerable members. Because citizens generally feel such concerns, journalistic exposés of the physical ill-treatment of intellectually impaired individuals become the stuff with which Pulitzer Prizes and other accolades are won.[2] On this communitarian paradigm, the collective well-being has more importance than personal well-being. The collective interest is enhanced by practices which protect the least competent among us, and is

---

[2] See Lempinen (1997) for an example. This series, which continued to run through most of 1998 in the *San Francisco Chronicle*, was nominated for a Pulitzer Prize.

threatened by practices that do not. The paradigm provides that treatment of individuals who may not themselves appreciate elevations and degradations of their well-being nevertheless contributes to the well-being of the community members who interact with them.[3]

What we should notice about the community model is that a patient's intellectual impairment is not accepted as defeating that individual's claim to the care needed to maintain corporeal health. A public outcry would ensue if it became known that a provider refused to set a fracture, or prescribe an antibiotic, simply because the bodies to be treated served persons with a very limited capacity for interpersonal interaction. Should such a person suffer a fracture or an infection, there would be no hesitation on the part of physicians in treating it. Similarly for the ventilator-dependent incompetent individual. There is no community agreement that patients with impaired or absent cerebral cortical function should have their fractures or simple infections go untreated. This is because personhood on the community model is not like personhood on the autonomy model, for the community acknowledges those who depend on it as well as those who contribute to it.

It is useful to notice that the community paradigm we have been invoking conforms to the understanding of disability that informs the 1990 Americans With Disabilities Act (ADA). This legislation prohibits providers from discriminating against people with disabilities by offering them inferior services. The ADA does not privilege people with disabilities by requiring that they have access to experimental or unusual treatment. Nor does the ADA run counter to the practice of refraining from futile interventions, that is, to interventions that will be ineffective because of an individual's disability. (To protect people with disabilities from false theories about the limitations their impairments impose, the ADA shifts the burden of proof to the provider, who must demonstrate, rather than merely suppose, that the procedure or medication will be ineffective in the individual in question.) But it does prohibit denying them the usual medical services if the reason is an unsubstantiated supposition that their impairments inhibit their being benefited.[4]

Avoiding futility

The medical conceptualization which characterizes humans as entities whose physical functioning is in the service of their intellect also places the value of self-determination, or autonomy, at the center of deliberations about the responsibilities and responsiveness of physicians to their patients. So it is understandable that the

---

[3] See MacIntyre (1998) for an argument to this effect.
[4] See Brock (1995, 2000) and Orentlicher (1996a, 2000) for discussions about how the ADA affects the rationing of health care.

authors are inclined to approximate their case to the autonomy paradigm rather than to the community paradigm. The inappropriateness (not the failure) of the former to guide them in this case partly explains why the authors remain disquieted about its outcome.

In addition to the authors' worries about the unseemliness of prolonging life without mind, a second consideration – the (mis)use of resources – prompts their position. And there can be no doubt that the non-wasteful allocation of healthcare resources is a significant collective concern. The authors worry that it is futile to provide long-term ventilation to a child for whom no improvement is foreseen. In support of this worry, they cite documents such as the Hastings Center's *Guidelines on the Termination of Life-Sustaining Treatment and the Care of the Dying* (Hastings Center 1987) and the report of the President's Commission for the Study of Ethical Problems in Medicine and Biomedical and Behavioral Research, titled *Deciding to Forego Life-Sustaining Treatment* (President's Commission 1983). These introduce rationing proposals directed at a variety of situations which, for the most part, are assimilated to a triage paradigm.

The triage model requires medical personnel to determine who will receive the greatest benefit from a scarce resource. So, for instance, the President's Commission recommends that patients in a persistent vegetative state should be removed from life support if such action is required so as to free resources to produce similar benefits in a competent patient. However, it should be noted that most cases of rationing, including the case under consideration, differ importantly from this paradigm in that there is no direct transfer of a scarce resource from one to another patient. Moreover, in non-emergency situations, where full deliberation is not merely permitted but is required, we cannot escape some notorious moral and political difficulties. For instance, grave problems occur in attempting to determine whether a successful outcome in one person would be of greater or lesser benefit to that individual than an equally successful outcome would be to some other person who is competing for access to the procedure. Perkin, Orr, and Ashwal attempt to avoid these problems by declaring individuals in permanent vegetative states to be non-persons, and therefore non-competitors. But their reasoning is faulty because they inappropriately assume that autonomy is the pre-eminent value in their care, when in fact it is not relevant to their care.

There is need to explore what articulations of principled rationing will be helpful when cases are evaluated on the community rather than on the autonomy paradigm. It is unlikely that a satisfactory formulation can be predicated simply on the denial of services to certain sorts of individuals, or even on the denial of certain services if such a practice has a disparately negative impact on any group protected by the community. For instance, the theory that life as a person with a disability is of lesser value than life as a non-disabled person influenced the ranking of services in the

Oregon Health Plan. In this form, the Plan was ruled in violation of the ADA (Brock 1995, 2000). Futility is a characteristic of pointless unsuccessful interventions, not of interventions that succeed in respect to their usual end but secure that result for the wrong kind of individual, one whose life is imagined to be of lesser value. So treating a patient who is intellectually disabled is not per se medically futile.

Currently, the quite different question of which sort(s) of individuals should be privileged over others to receive treatments often is decided with respect to who has access to generous, and who to restricted, healthcare plans. The randomness introduced into physicians' practice by this kind of determinant clearly disturbs the authors, who make a point of commenting that their patient's insurer did not prohibit long-term ventilation (which, after all, reduced medical costs to the insurer). Rather than calling for a political consensus among professionals to stand against those who value protecting the most vulnerable patients, a course which undoubtedly will clash with adherents of the community paradigm, it is more useful to seek forms of rationing which enjoy widespread community acceptance and conform to the community paradigm that emphasizes connectedness among individuals.

Conclusion

In instances in which the nature of the illness, the patient's status, and the patient's connectedness to other people all interact so as to heighten moral complexity to a troubling degree, appeal to moral paradigms should be case-sensitive rather than principle-driven. Perkin, Orr, and Ashwal propose to assign categorical principles primacy over the details of their patient's situation. They invoke the value of autonomy. But paradigmatic instances of respecting autonomy differ significantly from their present case.

Subsequently, they misconstrue the import of this difference, imagining that the absence of a fit between the paradigm and their immediate case means they are dealing with the absence of a person. They mistakenly believe that their patient thereby fails to qualify for treatment. When their view does not prevail in practice, they call for increasing the number of professional caregivers who, through their institutions, are committed to promoting this view.

I analyze their encounter and its outcome as being the product of an inapposite model of ethical reasoning that cannot be made more compelling by politicizing adherence to principles. Their focus on principle persuades them to disregard important characteristics of a case in which moral value is collective rather than atomistic. Even if there is no autonomous individual patient, there is in this case a locus of benefit, namely the interpersonal connectedness served by improving how the patient is maintained.

Facilitating the collective value of interpersonal connectedness by facilitating the mother's connectedness with the child is the point of providing long-term ventilation in this case. Patients need not be competent or capable of self-determination to be connected to those who care for them. However, case-based reasoning also warns against simple extrapolation from this to other cases, that is, against imagining that, on principle, family desires to maintain connectedness should categorically prevail. Case-insensitive judgment on principle obscures this important value for Perkin, Orr, and Ashwal. Further, it disposes them to appeal to triage criteria, although there is no other individual who is competing with their patient for the contested treatment. Analysis suggests that confidence in the responsiveness of healthcare practice is incompatible with imposing a political process whereby case-insensitive "quality of life" principles prevail over case-attentive sensibilities.

5.3 Topical discussion

PVS

Intense debate persists about the terminology, clinical diagnosis, and criteria for decision making for patients in vegetative states. The acronym PVS technically refers to persistent vegetative state, but as noted by our authors "persistent" vegetative state typically becomes "permanent" vegetative state after a period of time, and diagnosis of the state cannot be absolutely certain. Various court cases in the USA have established parameters for bases on which to consider forgoing life-sustaining treatment and who has the moral (or legal) standing to make such decisions, but it is not the case in the USA, as it is in some other countries, that all such decisions must undergo judicial review. Support for patients in PVS involves patients, their families and friends, the organizations providing the care, the organizations funding the care, and the individual care providers, and while some cases proceed with little disagreement, as in this case, there is considerable opportunity for disagreement and ethical quandary.

There has been a spate of literature discussing the "minimally conscious" state, a description of patients for whom the criteria of PVS are not met. The medical discussion is bedeviled by the difficulty of drawing a bright line in a continuum of conscious states, and the ethical discussion by the inevitable fact that an argument for treating (or withdrawing) at any point on that continuum can equally well justify the same course of action for the case next to it on that continuum – a conundrum sometimes called the "slippery slope."

Standards for decision making

There are several standards for medical decision making that have evolved legally and ethically. If the patient has previously expressed wishes (verbally, or in writing,

Ethical Dilemmas in Pediatrics: Cases and Commentaries, ed. Lorry R. Frankel, Amnon Goldworth, Mary V. Rorty, and William A. Silverman. Published by Cambridge University Press. © Cambridge University Press 2005.

via an advance directive), the *substituted-judgment* standard applies, where the proxy strives to approximate the decision the patient would make if competent. Evidence of the patient's own wishes is the substance of this standard, and it derives its legitimacy from its connection with self-determination.

In cases where the patient has never been competent, as in this case, or when the patient has never expressed an opinion or the opinion is not known, the standard that applies in many cases is the *best-interest* standard, which involves weighing the benefits and burdens to the patient of a possible course of action, considering such factors as relief of suffering, preservation or restoration of function, and quality and extent of the life sustained. The best-interest standard is problematic in its application to the early infant because in practice it is being applied to the family, not the child.

In pediatric cases the proxy decision maker is typically the parent, although in cases where the clinician has reason to believe that the surrogate is not deciding in the best interests of the child, by reason of conflicts of interest, conflicting interests, or incapacity, the matter may be pursued through further discussion, ethics consultation, or, as a last resort, through the courts.

Cost as a factor in ethical decision making

Individual and organizational care providers have always had to consider costs and balance their responsibility for providing care with their need for economic sustainability, but until recently such decisions were "internal" matters within the healthcare system. With recent changes in the patterns of reimbursement for healthcare delivery in the USA, many of which are explicitly directed toward cost constraint, it is not possible to ignore the question of who pays for desired care, often raising difficult and unresolved questions of distributive justice on the individual, institutional, and broader social level. Cost may require that some needed care is unable to be delivered; but social justice requires that so far as possible cost restraint should not contribute to discrimination on vulnerable or disadvantaged groups. The role of recent anti-discrimination legislation in maintaining fairness in access to care is introduced by Silvers in her commentary on this case. The United States is virtually unique among western democracies in not having any provision for a universal healthcare system, a fact that must be kept in mind in any deliberations about what would constitute "fair" distribution of social resources.

Cost is not the only form of limitation on resources. In this case it was not necessary to consider how to choose between two possible candidates when only one ICU bed (or ventilator, or organ for transplantation) was available, but such "rationing" decisions that require choosing between persons competing for healthcare services are virtually an everyday occurrence in healthcare institutions.

Most healthcare organizations have developed prospective patient selection policies for ICUs and emergency-room triage, and such policies need to be regularly reviewed and scrutinized for potential conflicts of interest and for fiscal accountability.

Methodology and cases

In the literature surrounding ethics consultation there is extensive discussion of what factors are to be taken into consideration when determining the ethical issues at stake in a given case. In her commentary on this troubling case Silvers warns against top-down applications of principles to cases, or even the use of principles as ordering categories for grouping issues to be considered, unless familial and in some cases broader community values are given standing among those principles. Principles tend toward universalization and universalizability, while relationships, in their brute particularity, may have an ethical weight that defies universalization.

In the bioethics "methods" debate increasing attention is being paid to "care," suggested as a balancing principle to (potentially universalizing) justice. It is invoked in the name of partiality and relationships, suggesting that there may be good reasons for distributing goods in ways that do not, for instance, maximize the greatest good for the greatest number, or represent the best possible use of resources. Intimate relations and special obligations are morally relevant considerations as well. As one commentator noted, "Family members", for instance, "are not replaceable by similarly (or better) qualified people" (Nelson and Nelson 1995: 74). Considering the family, consulting their preferences, and taking into account the well-being of all family members, is standard practice in pediatric medicine.

FURTHER READING

Ashwal, S. and Cranford, R. The minimally conscious state in children. *Seminars in Pediatric Neurology* 9 (2002), 19–34.

Giacino, J. T., Ashwal, S., Childs, N., *et al.* The minimally conscious state: definition and diagnostic criteria. *Neurology* 58 (2002), 349–353.

Lantos J. D., Singer, P. A., Walker, R. M., *et al.* The illusion of futility in clinical practice. *American Journal of Medicine* 87 (1989), 81–84.

Marshall, M. F. Patient selection: tragic choices. In *Introduction to Clinical Ethics*, ed. J. C. Fletcher, P. A. Lombardo, M. F. Marshall, and F. G. Miller, 2nd edn (Frederick, MD: University Publishing Group, 1997), pp. 227–238.

Marshall, M. F., Schwenzer, K. J., Orsina, M., Fletcher, J. C., and Durbin, C. G. Jr. Influence of political power, medical provincialism, and economic incentives on the rationing of surgical intensive care unit beds. *Critical Care Medicine* 20 (1992), 387–394.

McLean, S. Legal and ethical aspects of the vegetative state. *Journal of Clinical Pathology* 52 (1999), 490–493.

Wade, D. T. Ethical issues in diagnosis and management of patients in the permanent vegetative state. *BMJ* **322** (2001), 352–354.

Weijer, C., Singer, P. A., Dickens, B., and Workman, S. Bioethics 16: Dealing with demands for inappropriate treatment. *Canadian Medical Association Journal* **159** (1998), 817–821.

Youngner, S. J. Who defines futility? *JAMA* **260** (1988), 2094–2095.

6.1 Complexities in the management of a brain-dead child

Lorry R. Frankel and Chester J. Randle Jr.

First of all I would define medicine as the complete removal of the distress of the sick, the alleviation of the more violent diseases and the refusal to undertake to cure cases in which the disease has already won the mastery, knowing that everything is not possible to medicine.

Hippocratic corpus (Lloyd 1978: 140)

Introduction

The management of the brain-dead individual moves physicians beyond the traditional boundaries of medicine. The physicians are confronted with an assortment of moral, professional, and psychological problems whose effects are deeply felt by both family members and healthcare providers. To vividly illustrate how such cases can play out in practice, despite all preparations of protocols and policies, we present a case which focuses upon the problems encountered once a four-year-old child is diagnosed as fulfilling brain-death criteria. We focus upon the medical interventions and the psychosocial support that were required in the care of this patient, and in addition we address the ethical dilemma caregivers faced while caring for this patient in a critical care unit.

The case

The patient was a four-year-old female who was transferred to a tertiary pediatric intensive care unit following a cardiorespiratory arrest. Prior to this event she was bed-ridden with Pierre-Robin syndrome (an autosomal recessive disorder characterized by a small jaw [micrognathia], retracted tongue [glossoptosis], and upper airway obstruction) and severe developmental delay. Because of poor airway control

Ethical Dilemmas in Pediatrics: Cases and Commentaries, ed. Lorry R. Frankel, Amnon Goldworth, Mary V. Rorty, and William A. Silverman. Published by Cambridge University Press. © Cambridge University Press 2005.

and gastroesophageal reflux, she was fed via a surgically placed gastric tube. She had frequent episodes of aspiration pneumonia which were likely the result of her inability to control her oral secretions.

During a home visit, the home health nurse found the child cyanotic, with no spontaneous respirations. The paramedics were called and provided CPR. Multiple attempts to intubate her in the field were unsuccessful, and she was ventilated by bag and mask and taken to the emergency department of her local hospital.

Upon arrival to the community hospital she required multiple doses of epinephrine, atropine, and bicarbonate. Her initial arterial blood gas on 100% oxygen showed a severe acidosis. Her pupils were dilated to 5–6 mm and fixed, but she had spontaneous respirations. Her trachea was finally intubated in the emergency department of the referring hospital. During her 30- or 40-minute period in this department, a part of a rubber nipple was found in her posterior pharynx. She was then transported to our regional pediatric intensive care unit.

While in our PICU, she initially had only occasional spontaneous respirations and minimal response to deep painful stimuli. She had no pupillary response to light and no gag reflex. Because of the prolonged period of hypoxia, the difficulty of the resuscitation efforts, and the results of her initial neurological exam, the family was informed that her prognosis for any meaningful recovery was extremely poor. In the ensuing days her neurological status continued to deteriorate. By the third hospital day her electroencephalogram was isoelectric, supporting evidence of brain death. On the fourth hospital day spontaneous respirations ceased and she developed diabetes insipidus. Clinical examination, performed by both the attending neurologist and pediatric intensivist, determined that she was brain dead. The intensivist repeated the exam in 12 hours and confirmed the diagnosis of brain death.

The presence of brain death was determined according to current criteria by both the child's attending intensivist and the neurologist on duty, based upon physical examination. They used multiple physical examinations and one EEG. This included detailed physical examinations which included neurologic assessments and the apnea test. An observation period occurred which did not reveal any changes in physical examination. As per our institutional policy and the guidelines for the determination of brain death in children as set forth by the American Academy of Pediatrics (1987), brain death was declared. This included the coexistence of coma and apnea, absence of brain-stem function (no pupillary reflexes, absence of eye movement to oculocephalic and oculovestibular testing, absence of gag, cough, sucking, or rooting as well as absence of spontaneous respiratory efforts despite an elevated carbon dioxide level [$PaCO_2 > 60$ mm Hg] and flaccid muscle tone). In addition the patient maintained normal blood pressure and temperature throughout her hospital stay.

Several hours before she was declared brain dead the pediatric intensivist had extensive discussions with the family about the meaning of brain death and about plans for termination of cardiac and ventilatory support. In this hospital, the usual practice is to repeat the exam within a 12- to 24-hour period, and then discontinue support. On rare occasions, life support will be continued for a few more hours, pending arrival of other family members. As an alternative, patients whose families request organ donation continue to receive ventilation and pharmacological support to perfuse vital organs while awaiting organ retrieval. However, they are pronounced dead at this time, and are only sustained in order to harvest the vital organs.

Although these parents had no questions about the diagnosis of brain death, they were not convinced of the irreversibility of their daughter's condition and they wanted her to remain on life support for a much longer period than the 24 hours protocol suggested. An additional reason for the parents' desire to have prolonged support was their wish to have the maternal grandmother and aunt come (from the Philippines and Hong Kong respectively) to see the child before such support was withdrawn. This was particularly important because these relatives had never seen the child. They could also provide emotional support to the parents, who were quite distraught at the thought of losing their child. The parents at this time expressed no intention to make their daughter an organ donor.

Unfortunately, neither of the relatives had visas to travel to this country, so it would take three days for them to get to the hospital. Although the pediatric intensivist understood the parents' requests and sympathized with their predicament, he felt that prolonged medical support of their child was unjustified. But the parents continued to insist that support continue far beyond the 24-hour period, until their relatives arrived. They went so far as to obtain legal counsel, who was prepared to obtain a court order to prevent the withdrawal of medical support.

The hospital administrator on call was notified of these developments. In addition to contacting a hospital attorney, the administrator notified the hospital vice-president for medical and legal affairs. The latter suggested that some way be found to address the needs of the family, and asked that an ethics consult be obtained. The pediatric intensivist felt that to continue medical interventions for an extended period of time was difficult both for him and for the ICU staff, and that he would do so only under duress.

The following day, which was 36 hours after the child was first declared brain dead, another intensivist in the medical group volunteered to take the first intensivist's place. However, unsure of the legal issues, the second intensivist sought legal advice from the hospital attorney about the legality of withdrawing cardiovascular support. The attorney informed him that although brain death was legally recognized in the state, the physician's responsibility for the brain-dead child was unclear and it was advisable that he and the family should reach a mutual agreement about terminating care. The attorney believed that because withdrawal of life support was an irreversible decision, a judge would likely not allow it unless a negotiated agreement with the family to that effect were reached. In addition, the attorney believed that the family would succeed in obtaining a court order that would compel continuing support. She advised the intensivist to make all efforts to avoid a court action.

The brain-dead child was continued on mechanical ventilation and received a low-dose dopamine infusion and vasopressin to control urine output. The second attending intensivist and the vice-president for medical and legal affairs met with the parents on a daily basis in order to encourage them to agree to discontinue support. Contrary to the parents' wishes, the arterial line was removed on day 6 and the child was transferred to a less acute area within the pediatric intensive care unit.

Although the hospital was able to accept referrals of all critically ill children at this time, there was a list of 11 children waiting for elective admission to the hospital. The possibility existed that critically ill infants and children in need of critical care services would need to be transferred to another facility because of high census and acuity.

On day 9, after the child's aunt had arrived, the parents altered their position and decided to donate their child's organs. The child was taken to the operating room where the organs were harvested and mechanical ventilator support was withdrawn.

Ethical issues

How is brain death determined? The determination of brain death is a matter that requires a great deal of care. The invocation of an institutional policy in addition to the American Academy of Pediatrics guideline was in response to the variability found among clinicians in the determination of brain death. Mejia and Pollack (1995) reviewed a prospective cohort study from 16 PICUs which included 248 deaths of which 93 (37%) were secondary to brain death. However, not all of the patients' brain-death examinations conformed to the guidelines established by the American Academy of Pediatrics. For example only 75% underwent an apnea test (less than one per patient), and the mean $PaCO_2$ was 63 ± 17 mm Hg. Also, there appeared to be inadequate documentation by both the nurses and physicians. This variability among physicians in the determination of brain death and the need for organ procurement may result in rather hasty decisions made regarding the pronouncement of brain death.

Although the parents were informed from the beginning as to the dismal prognosis and the potential diagnosis of brain death for their daughter, they maintained an optimistic attitude. Once the diagnosis of brain death was made, the treating physicians encountered significant reluctance on the part of the family to accept this diagnosis. Even after the second brain-death exam, which was repeated in the presence of the parents, their denial and refusal to accept the fact that their daughter met brain-death criteria created further barriers in the ongoing management of their daughter. The intensivist on clinical service attempted many times to work with the family through the social workers, to no avail. The case was then referred to a second intensivist, who was brought into the situation only to deal with this complex matter. This enabled the initial attending to care for the other critically ill patients within the PICU. The new attending spent many hours and days working with both the family and the hospital administration to facilitate the child's removal from life support. Eventually, the family consented, not only for the removal from life support, but, surprisingly, they opted for organ donation. This was a significant turnaround which required many hours and days of negotiation.

Should the attending physicians have pursued another strategy in the care of this child? They felt that they had limited options. If they had further challenged the family with a court order, it was unlikely that a reasonable compromise would have been achieved. On the other hand, had the physicians withdrawn life support immediately following the second brain-death exam, they would have been confronted by the family and their legal counsel. This clinical situation, although rare indeed, speaks to the question of physician autonomy and what is perceived to be the best medical practice, versus the rights of the parents to dictate medical care.

6.2 The moral arena in the management of a brain-dead child

Amnon Goldworth

Introduction

In the management of the brain-dead child discussed by Drs. Frankel and Randle we encounter descriptive anomalies and problems that are intimately connected with our moral posture toward brain death. I will discuss these anomalies and problems, and then consider whether brain death should continue to serve as the criterion of death, and whether the brain-dead individual should simply be called dead.

Descriptive problems

Let us consider some descriptive problems connected with this case. Notice that in describing this situation, the phrases, "prolonged medical support," "medical interventions," "attending physician," and "life support" were employed. Indeed, it was difficult to do without them, since they are part of the conventional terminology.

Is the brain-dead child dead? Most physicians would say yes. (It is less clear whether an ordinary person would agree.) A human being, particularly in the early period of death, is also called a corpse (Pallis 1982, Annas 1996). If so, do we then believe that it is sensible to speak of ventilatory support of the brain-dead child as ventilating a corpse? If not, can we consider such support a form of treatment?

One response might be to point out that physicians treat organs, as well as people. But it is normally the treatment of the organs of the living, rather than those of the dead, patient. If we extend the use of the term "treatment" to the organs of the brain-dead, we may be giving credence to the view that the brain-dead individual is, in some sense, alive.

Ethical Dilemmas in Pediatrics: Cases and Commentaries, ed. Lorry R. Frankel, Amnon Goldworth, Mary V. Rorty, and William A. Silverman. Published by Cambridge University Press. © Cambridge University Press 2005.

An alternative approach is to maintain that, so long as the heart continues to beat, the brain-dead child is not dead. This view permits us to be intelligible in speaking about the physician "treating" the brain-dead child, or about the parents insisting on continuing support. All of the conventional adjectives employed in medical descriptions are then applicable. But then heart transplantation would, as a result, be murder.

The moral obligation of the physician

The medical profession has moral obligations to treat the sick: to cure or to offer palliation. Over the course of time, medicine has offered succor to the living. It has established and proclaimed the roles of curer and caregiver through codes of ethics and oaths of initiation. But what moral obligation does the physician have toward those who are dead? It is a commonplace to speak of the need to respect the dead. However, there is nothing in this general injunction, other than a prohibition against desecration, which identifies a particular obligation on the part of the physician toward the dead.

But suppose that an individual who is dead is on cardiopulmonary support. Does a physician have a moral obligation to continue such support so long as the organs continue to function? This cannot be justified by merely pointing to the fact that support is already being provided. Although there may be a psychological difference between withholding and withdrawing, it has been persuasively argued that there is no morally significant difference between the two. The same sort of reasons that justify the former apply to the latter (Brock 1989).

Suppose we create a new category of patient whom, to use Willard Gaylin's term, we will call neomorts (Gaylin 1974). Neomorts will be managed by physicians called thanatologists. Since the sole function of the thanatologists is to maintain the cardiopulmonary function of the dead, there will be no conceptual confusion concerning the nature of this role. Furthermore, all of the moral obligations associated with medical support will now be applicable. But for parents to accept the fact that their child is a neomorph is to acknowledge, as the parents in our case refused to do, that their child is really dead. Thus, descriptive difficulties can be resolved completely only when all concerned parties accept brain death as death, and when the medical management of the dead is institutionalized.

But, to return to the present-day setting, it is not the dead child, but rather the parents who need care, given their need to come to terms with the death of a loved one. Is such care a moral requirement for the physician? To answer this question, we need to distinguish between being obliged and being morally obligated. We may feel obliged to provide a clean sheet of paper from our writing pad to someone who asks for it because it is a considerate action. But, we are not morally obligated to do so. A physician may feel obliged to take care of the needs of the parents because it is a considerate action. But he is not morally obligated to do so, since the parents are not his patients.

Distributive justice

The presence of the brain-dead child in the pediatric intensive care unit may have precluded the care of another child in her place. Although we are told that no severely ill child was deprived admission, any one of 11 children who could have profited from being immediately admitted were excluded. This raises the moral question concerning the priority between ventilating the dead child and treating a living one. This question can be approached from two moral perspectives:
(1) Deontological. Does the dead child have any moral rights?
(2) Teleological. What consequences follow from choosing each of the options?

From a deontological perspective, the dead child has the right to be treated with the dignity and respect that befits her link to her past existence as a living human being. From the teleological perspective, we need to consider what good or bad consequences would follow from providing cardiopulmonary support for the dead child. Serving the best interests of a living child would be teleologically justified. But this might not apply to the dead child, since she has no interests. In addition, there are bad consequences that follow from extended artificial support for the dead child if such support prevents treatment for another living patient. Thus caring for the brain-dead child, which entails the use of expensive medical resources, can not be justified under either of those approaches.

Professional problems

In our case, one of the problems for the attending physicians was the requirement that they continue to act as if they were physicians treating a patient when they believed that the brain-dead child was dead. They judged this to be a threat to their professional integrity and an expenditure of a scarce resource in the form of time which might have been better spent on the care of other critically ill children. It was also psychologically disturbing, since it required the physicians to apply their professional expertise to a situation for which it was not intended (Luce 1995).

At a grand-rounds discussion of this case it was suggested that in order to avoid threats to professional integrity or the psychological stress generated in managing the brain-dead child, physicians should continue to use the conventional terminology that would be appropriate for a living child. Metaphors such as "patient," "medical treatment," and "life support" can serve as a kind of security blanket. Unfortunately, such metaphors, extensions of our usual usage, may result in misleading forms of communication.

Another predicament for the physicians stems from legal ambiguity. If it is unclear what the legal responsibility of the physician is toward the brain-dead child, then it is unclear whether or not the physician can be successfully sued for malpractice in managing such a child. Thus, along with burdens to integrity and psychological well-being, the physician is now faced with prudential considerations that may very well conflict with them.

Appearances and medical judgment

A dead child who requires cardiopulmonary support will show outward signs of life: a heaving chest, color in the cheeks and bodily warmth. The child has the appearance of being asleep. Appearance belies the medical determination of death. Under normal circumstance, outward signs are good indicators of inner states. But, in this instance, they are not. Thus, parents and others will vacillate between judgments based upon appearance and those relying upon medical judgment. The psychological confusion generated by this bifurcation needs to be addressed with sensitivity. Providing cardiac and ventilatory support for a short period of time can legitimately be described as an act of compassion toward family members. However, it is not compassion, but a violation of human dignity, when, as has occurred in some cases, such support extends for months (Annas 1996).

Brain death as a social construct

For centuries, death was determined by certain cardiopulmonary signs, and the description of the condition of the individual as dead was accepted by both the physician and the public. Modern medical technology has given us the ability to provide nutrition and hydration, maintenance of ventilation, circulation, and the elimination of waste matter in an organism whose entire brain has ceased to function. It has also provided the means by which organs from the brain-dead can successfully be transplanted. It was the latter development that contributed to the emergence of the brain-death criterion of death. This criterion has been widely accepted by western physicians, but apparently less so by the public. One of the reasons for this, as suggested by James Bernat *et al.* (1982), is "the practical difficulty of reconciling this [brain dead] standard, which includes a new understanding of death, with the more popular [cardiopulmonary] conception of death." Another reason is offered by Raymond Devettere (1990): "Decades after whole-brain death has been publicly accepted as medical and legal policy, much confusion still continues. People, including some health care providers, may know on one level that a totally brain dead person on life support is actually dead, but insist on thinking at another level, unless reminded of the facts, that death occurs when life support is removed." Thus brain death is not as well established a social construct as the earlier cardiopulmonary criterion of death. One result has been a willingness to accommodate (in the states of New York and New Jersey) those who, for religious reasons, do not accept brain death as death.

Should brain death continue to serve as the criterion for death?

Given the continuing debate about brain death and the difficulties that attach to its use as the criterion of death, why not dispense with it and return to the traditional cardiopulmonary criterion? There are those who deny that death occurs when the organism as a whole ceases to function. For these individuals, the continued functioning of the heart and lungs, as produced by the use of mechanical ventilation, is evidence that the individual is alive and must be respected and protected as other living human beings are (Bleich 1989). The traditional criterion is indeed satisfactory in the absence of artificial support, since brain death soon follows interruption of cardiac and pulmonary function. But when artificial support is present, heart and lungs continue to function in the absence of any brain activity. Perhaps we should judge an individual to be dead if removal of support would result in cardiopulmonary arrest. But this is unsatisfactory, since those on such mechanical support as cardiac pacemakers would then have to be considered dead (Truog and Fletcher 1990).

Since being machine-dependent does not rule out cases where it is desirable to continue considering the person to be alive, we need to examine the issue of life and death when the patient is brain dead and is being given cardiopulmonary support. We also need to recognize that although the irreversible loss of awareness and cognition are the loss of what is essentially significant to the nature of the human being (Veatch 1986), an individual may be unable to think and yet still be alive. The loss of cerebral activity alone cannot be the criterion of death, otherwise individuals who are in a persistent vegetative state would have to be considered dead.

What is needed is a definition of the biological death of an organism that incorporates these concerns and an associated criterion of death. This has been provided by James Bernat and his colleagues:

We define death as the permanent cessation of functioning of the organism as a whole. We do not mean the whole organism, for example, the sum of its tissue and organ parts, but rather the highly complex interaction of its organic subsystems. Also, the organism need not be whole or complete, it may have lost a limb or an organ (such as the spleen), but still remain an organism. The spontaneous and innate interrelationship of all or most of the remaining subsystems and the interaction of the perhaps impaired organism with its environment is to be regarded as the functioning of the organism as a whole. (Bernat et al. 1981)

This is followed by the criterion of death:

The criterion for cessation of functioning of the organism as a whole is permanent loss of functioning of the entire brain. This criterion is perfectly correlated with the permanent cessation of functioning of the organism as a whole. It integrates, generates, interrelates, and controls complex bodily activities. A patient on a ventilator with a totally destroyed brain is merely a group of artificially maintained subsystems, since the organism as a whole has ceased to function. (Bernat *et al.* 1981)

Cardiopulmonary indications of life when artificial ventilation is being supplied, such as color in the cheeks or heaving chest, or tests for respiration and circulation, are misleading, not because of the use of mechanical support, but because what was at one time an integrated organic system is one no longer.

It is clear that the whole-brain death concept and the use of mechanical ventilation has facilitated organ transplantation (Ad Hoc Committee 1968). But the use of mechanical ventilation has also been defended by some because any human life is perceived by them to be of intrinsic value. As long as the heart and lungs are functioning, this position holds, the individual is alive and must be respected and protected as other human beings are (Bleich 1989). Any effort to accommodate to the diversity of beliefs that are held in our heterogeneous society is in keeping with our democratic standards. But such accommodation is unwarranted when a belief is instrumental in harming others. As noted by Alexander Capron,

society has a basic interest in defining for all people a uniform basis on which to decide who is alive – and consequently subject to all the protections and benefits of the law – and who is dead. The public's interest is great enough to override individual scruples even when based in religious beliefs, just as statutes authorize autopsies without familial consent in cases of concern to the public. (Capron 1978)

The extent to which the public interest is served by a uniform definition of death can be gauged by the following list of legal issues:

All wrongful death actions, whether or not they involve special situations such as transplantation or cessation of extraordinary care, can be brought only after death. Similarly, death is a prerequisite to a successful prosecution for homicide . . . Numerous property and wealth transmission issues raise death questions. When may an estate be probated? When may property of a testate or intestate decedent be distributed? When does a life state end? When does property pass to a surviving joint tenant? When do life insurance benefits become payable and health insurance benefits cease to accrue? When may property escheat? And when do banks become liable for admitting persons to safe deposit boxes and paying money out of accounts? When is an estate tax due? And perhaps most importantly, who dies first in the event that persons with interests in one another's estates perished in a common disaster? Status relationships often turn on whether someone is dead. For example, whether a person who remarries is a bigamist . . . Coroner's obligations and the mandatory contents of death certificates require determinations of the time of death. (Dworkin 1973)

The above list should dissuade anyone from believing that having more than one definition of death or permitting exceptions to a single definition of death is in the public interest. But why not adhere to the traditional conception of death that is based on cardiopulmonary signs? Why not forgo brain death?

This has been recently recommended by Robert Truog (1997). He believes that the concept of brain death is incoherent and confused in practice and that we should therefore separate the definition of death from the issue of organ procurement. The latter should be based not on the issue of death, but on whether organ donation which has been consented to would harm the potential donor. However, he does acknowledge that

the most difficult challenge for this proposal would be to gain acceptance of the view that killing may sometimes be a justifiable necessity for procuring transplantable organs. (Truog 1997)

Truog believes that a return to the traditional cardiopulmonary approach is something which all cultures and religions would find agreeable. Perhaps so. But it is surely not the case that there would be widespread acceptance of the proposition that killing was a justifiable necessity for procuring organs even if donor consent was given. Even if all were finally convinced that such killing was morally justified, what should be done in the meantime? Since organ transplantation and the diagnosis of death are presently linked, and since the traditional view maintains that a brain-dead individual on artificial support is alive, we must either declare a moratorium on present transplant practices or continue these practices on the basis of brain death.

After the Harvard Ad Hoc Committee justified the brain-death concept by saying that "obsolete criteria for the definition of death can lead to controversy in obtaining organs for transplantation" (Ad Hoc Committee 1968), Paul Ramsey counseled that

if no person's death for this purpose be hastened, then the definition of death should not for this purpose be updated, or the procedure for stating that a man has died be revised as a means of affording easier access to organs. (Ramsey 1970)

To abandon the traditional concept of death so as to facilitate organ transplantation appeared to Ramsey to violate Immanuel Kant's dictum: never treat a human being solely as a means by which to achieve the ends of others. But Kant had the living human being in mind, and this depends on an acknowledged view of when a human being is alive or dead. That is clearly what is at issue here. Death is a subjective concept that is shaped by the needs and values of the times. Let us see how this applies in two time periods: one in the past and one in the future.

According to the cardiopulmonary criterion, in which the heart and lungs make possible the flow of "vital" fluids, if someone who is neurologically dead is considered alive because his heart and lungs are active, then heart transplantation as supported by the brain-death criterion violates Kant's dictum. But if we turn to the period of the Enlightenment, in which the distinction between life and death was blurred, so that until a body suffered rigor mortis or putrefaction, someone who was neurologically dead and whose heart and lungs were no longer active was considered alive, then our current practice of transplanting kidneys or a cornea, as supported by the cardiopulmonary definition of death, would also violate Kant's dictum (Farrell and Levin 1993).

Now consider recent events in Japan concerning transplantation. Japanese law, supported by religion and culture, defines death as the moment at which the heart ceases to beat. Because of this view, heart, lung, and liver transplants are not possible. As a consequence, many Japanese die who are unable to afford a transplant operation elsewhere. Notwithstanding these legal and cultural barriers, in June 1997, the Japanese parliament approved a bill that would permit heart and lung transplants. Although this bill does not set aside the standing legal definition of death, an individual with a non-functioning brain can be defined as dead if prior consent for donation has been given. In addition, polls indicate that approximately 50% of the Japanese population approves of classifying an individual as dead who is brain dead (Anon. 1997).

We see then that a definition of death is not "writ in stone." Nor is it susceptible to proof in any strict sense. It is a method of classification that is affected by values and pragmatic considerations. And these, at present, favor the neurological definition of death. Once this is recognized, it becomes sensible to put aside the expression "brain death" in favor of the term "death."

By referring to the absence of brain activity as death, rather than brain death, the following desirable effects are likely to occur. It will eliminate the suggestion engendered by the qualifying word "brain," that there is another kind of (non-brain) death. It will likely have the salutary effect of making healthcare providers and those who talk and write about healthcare matters more cautious in their use of descriptive terms and phrases that are appropriate for the living but not for the dead. Concomitantly, it will result in the use of less misleading terms and phrases such as "management" (as in our title) rather than "treatment" of a dead child. It will discourage physicians from using psychologically comforting but misleading terms such as "life support," when referring to the management of a dead child. And finally it may facilitate the transition from false hope to acceptance, from illusion to reality, by persuading parents that their child is dead.

6.3 Topical discussion

Brain death

Clinical criteria have been established for determining brain death, which differs from PVS in that brain-stem function is absent. The Uniform Determination of Death Act (1981) incorporates the Harvard criteria: (1) coma, demonstrated by total unreceptivity and unresponsivity to stimuli; (2) absence of spontaneous breathing; (3) absence of reflexes; and (4) a flat or isoelectric electroencephalogram. It states, "An individual who has sustained either (1) irreversible cessation of circulatory and respiratory functions, or (2) irreversible cessation of all functions of the entire brain, including the brain stem, is dead." The American Academy of Pediatrics in 1987 established guidelines for the determination of brain death in children, but they are thought to be determinative only where the child is above the age of six, because of the unpredictable effects of the recuperative capacities of young children.

Because of the continuing disparity between the number of donated organs available for transplantation and the number of potential recipients of donated organs, there has been continued discussion of refining the criteria for brain death, including some suggestions that "higher brain death," the absence of cognitive functions, should count as the death of the person. The extensive and continuing discussion about what constitutes permanent vegetative states, and minimally conscious states, as well as the infrequent but widely publicized cases of "locked in" syndrome, reflect the difficulties associated with third-party determination of subjective states.

Despite the relatively clear criteria and the clinicians' agreement that this case met those criteria, the distraught parents rejected the diagnosis and threatened legal action, perhaps for reasons having to do with varying degrees of acceptance of brain death in other cultures, perhaps with the incongruity of a declaration of

Ethical Dilemmas in Pediatrics: Cases and Commentaries, ed. Lorry R. Frankel, Amnon Goldworth, Mary V. Rorty, and William A. Silverman. Published by Cambridge University Press. © Cambridge University Press 2005.

death despite the appearance of life discussed by Goldworth. No communication issues comparable to those encountered in the case in Chapter 2 bedevilled this case, but the difficulty in reaching an agreement about how to proceed was similar. The desirability of avoiding a legal case was perceived by the hospital's legal staff. Had the case progressed to a legal one, the institution would have had a strong case, but the decision to continue to accommodate the parents' wishes while working for resolution had as much an ethical as a legal rationale. The response by Simon Whitney to the earlier case, where brain death was not clearly a factor, suggests that even in cases of brain death, the family is typically perceived by the courts as having the final say in the care of a child, and the problematic case of Baby K in Virginia in 1993, where courts mandated continued treatment of an anencephalic child, confirms his view.

An alternative to brain death

Defining death as brain death has generated a number of debates. One of them, noted by Goldworth, concerns the relationship between brain death and the more conventional cardiopulmonary definition. Another challenges the adequacy of the brain-death definition, which depends on the loss of all functions of the brain. Claims that an individual has suffered brain death may be undermined by evidence that isolated collections of brain cells continue to survive. Rather than attempting to qualify the whole-brain criterion of death, it has been suggested that a better alternative is to define death as the irreversible loss of higher-brain functions. Robert Veatch is an important advocate of this approach. Opponents invoke versions of the "slippery slope" argument, arguing that if irreversible loss of cognitive function were sufficient to qualify as "dead" the category might be gradually extended to include the profoundly retarded or senile, as well as people in PVS, and point to the danger of widening the gap between clinical death and death as ordinarily understood.

Cultural difference

The time required to locate far-flung family members in this case suggests that the parents may have been recent immigrants or foreign nationals. The issue of possible cultural difference was not emphasized in this case or in its commentary, but differences in ethno-cultural background between caregivers and recipients of medical care can affect a variety of issues, including the meaning ascribed to illness, the language used to discuss sickness and death, the symbolic value of life and death, the care of the body after death, appropriate expressions of grief, the role expected of the healer, and background models of how families ought to make decisions.

To presuppose the values and attitudes of others on the basis of their membership in a given culture is a form of cultural reductionism that can easily lead to stereotyping. On the other hand, culture, language, or national origin can alert caretakers to explore further possible individual differences in values, expectations, and presuppositions that might affect clinical decision making. Goldworth's discussion of the difficulties surrounding the language of brain death suggests that even within relatively homogeneous communities the attitudes and understanding of medical personnel and medically unsophisticated community members can differ.

Organ donation

Ever since its inception, transplantation has been a subject of intense ethical scrutiny, with controversies surrounding all aspects, from the source of organs to their allocation. Even if procurement of organs from deceased individuals, with their prior permission, has been institutionalized, the question of when they are deceased raises questions, as discussed in Goldworth's commentary. Organs for transplantation are a scarce resource – but a resource for whom?

Organ donation in the USA is conceptualized as an altruistic voluntary act, a "gift of life" to another. In the USA, and indeed world-wide, there are fewer organs available for therapeutic transplantation than there are possible recipients. As Siminoff notes, the number of patients waiting for solid organs has increased 70% during the last decade, and children from birth to 17 years of age constituted approximately 3% of those on the waiting lists. While all parties are concerned to minimize the suffering of those left behind when a person dies, there is also a great deal of pressure on the medical community to increase the number of organs available for transplantation. There have been various proposals for increasing the donor pool, including "opt out" (rather than the current "opt in") legislation for donors, and financial incentives for organs, but so far all proposals for change have met with social and ethical resistance.

The Omnibus Reconciliation Act of 1986 requires that all hospitals participating in Medicaid programs refer all potential organ donors to their local organ procurement organization (OPO) when identified. Since 1998 a US government regulation requires that a request for donation to the family if the organs are deemed suitable by the OPO is no longer optional, but obligatory. Still, of 12 000 to 15 000 patients per year declared dead using neurological criteria, only about 6000 become organ donors, and the number of children whose organs are donated by their families remains lower than the number of potential recipients. If families are not donating, it is evidently not because they have not been asked.

Some anomalies in the donation program continue to provide ethical conundrums. Patients without access to reimbursement for the expensive transplantation procedures can be donors, but would not be eligible as recipients for donated organs, raising questions of fairness. Due to a lack of regulatory oversight of tissue banks, there is a competitive, for-profit tissue industry that some potential donors find problematic. And the complexity of policies and procedures surrounding financing, allocation, and distribution of organs calls into question in some cases the extent to which families are operating with information adequate for valid consent. With the growing number of uninsured and underinsured, there is widespread concern that fear of undertreatment or coercive financial considerations negatively influence both donations and public perceptions of organ donation.

The decision of the parents to donate the organs of their brain-dead child in this case seems to have been unexpected, representing one stage in an extended and changing legal terrain associated with transplantation in the USA.

FURTHER READING

AAP Policy Statement. Pediatric organ donation and transplantation. *Pediatrics* **109** (2002), 982–984.

Capron, A. M. Brain death: well settled yet still unresolved. *New England Journal of Medicine* **344** (2001), 1244–1246.

Cook, A. F., Hoas, H., and Grayson, C. Asking for organs: different needs and different values. *Journal of Clinical Ethics* **14** (2003) 37–48.

Koenig, B. A. and Davies, E. Cultural dimensions of care at life's end for children and their families. In *When Children Die*, ed. M. J. Field and R. E. Behrman (Washington, DC: National Academies Press, 2003), pp. 509–552.

Lock, M. *Deadly Disputes: the Body in Death in Japan, North America and Europe.* Doreen B. Townsend Center for the Humanities Occasional Paper 4 (Berkeley, CA: University of California Press, 1995).

Cultural aspects of organ donation and transplantation. *Transplantation Proceedings* **31** (1999), 1345–1346.

Ott, B. B. Defining and redefining death. *American Journal of Critical Care* **4**(1995), 476–480.

Siminoff, L. A., Gordon, N., Hewlett, J., and Arnold, R. M. Factors influencing families' consent for donation of solid organs for transplantation. *JAMA* **286** (2001) 71–77.

Veatch, R. M. The impending collapse of the whole-brain definition of death. *Hastings Center Report* **23** (4) (1993), 18–24.

Wijdicks, E. F. M. The diagnosis of brain death. *New England Journal of Medicine* **344** (2001), 1215–1221.

Part III

Life by any means

Treatment decisions in complex cases depend on a variety of factors: parental (or patient) wishes, informed medical judgment, and the predictions of the physicians about the results of any given treatment. But contextual factors, such as what treatments are available or feasible, are crucial as well. In the three cases in this part, only very complex, invasive, and high-risk interventions can postpone the death of a pediatric patient. The availability of such treatments influences the goals of medical treatment of this patient in this situation. In different ways, each of the authors meditates on the impact that the very availability of such options has on treatment decisions. Two of the three cases in this section involve transplantation, and provide useful insights into the current success rates of various organ transplantations, as well as sensitive discussions of the various factors taken into consideration in the allocation of organs.

The stage is set in Chapter 7 by an English physician, Robert Burne, who introduces William, the sixth of eight children. After what appeared to be a normal birth, William was discovered to have a complicated form of congenital heart disease. His hypoplastic heart was surgically treated, and his parents were informed of his poor prognosis and the likelihood of his developing problems leading to heart failure in his early adulthood. His condition worsened at the age of two following a major stroke, and when he was five his shunt was modified to halt progressive cyanosis. Four years later his condition had worsened to the point that another surgical intervention was becoming necessary. The ensuing discussion between family and physicians concerned the risks and benefits of surgery versus non-invasive procedures. The family chose the latter, concentrating on the quality of William's life. He remained at home with only periodic stays at the hospital until his death at the age of 13.

In his commentary, American physician William Silverman contrasts English practices, where the major decisions made by William's family took place in their home, and where arrangements were made for the boy to die at home, with the comparable practices in the United States, where deliberations most often occur in a hospital setting. Silverman recalls that refusals of life-prolonging interventions for seriously ill children were respected in the USA as in the UK until the 1980s. He then plots the history that reshaped American practice so that home care of the dying patient is difficult to obtain.

Chapter 8 presents a patient with a similar problem – hypoplastic left heart syndrome, or HLHS – but with a very different course of diagnosis and intervention, revealing in a graphic way exactly the differences Silverman noted. Similar contemporary diagnoses in different social and medical contexts are treated very differently. Clifford Chin presents the case of an infant in a high-tech, well-subsidized medical environment, whose heart condition was diagnosed prenatally. Before birth he was already listed as a transplant candidate. Chin wrestles with the dilemmas faced when possibility confronts probability. The parents were asked to decide about the interests of a child yet unborn, and were encouraged, or at least allowed, to opt for a treatment which, in light of the scarcity of donor hearts for infant transplants, was uncertain of success. Because of the course of the disease, the child in fact was treated with the conventional surgical approach.

Chin discusses ethical issues connected with the listing of a fetus for transplantation, UNOS (United Network for Organ Sharing) policy on organ allocation, and counseling for parents who confront surgical or transplantation options for their children. His concern for the scarcity of donor hearts leads him to speculate about the policy against anencephalic donations, and whether chromosomal abnormalities should play a role in eligibility for donated hearts. The theoretical, if not actual, availability of a variety of high-tech interventions, and the speed with which the diagnosis and surgeries progressed, represent end-of-the-century medicine at its best and worst, and one can only wonder what the author of the case in Chapter 7, Burne, would have advised in the situation described.

Commentator Joel Frader responds in detail to the various arguments introduced by Chin, separating those that deal with appropriate treatment from those that concern the appropriate allocation of available hearts. He suggests that functionality, not merely survival, is relevant in choosing between treatment options, and knowledgeably discusses UNOS policy. He acknowledges the volatility of the issue of anencephalic donation, and draws a distinction between various chromosomal abnormalities. As the publicity surrounding a recent case in California showed, denying treatment to trisomy-21 (Down syndrome) children, like the question of anencephalic organ donation, is a matter of wide public concern. Frader believes that the major ethical problem, which Chin fails to address, is the absence of reliable empirical studies which would resolve some of the issues confronting Chin.

The three authors of the case in Chapter 9 describe a radical intervention in a precipitously deteriorating adolescent. As Garcia-Careaga, Castillo, and Kerner note, "intestinal transplantation has not yet attained the success of heart, kidney, and liver transplantation, but offers the only chance for . . . people who would otherwise die." The child described, a 15-year-old with only 12 inches (30 cm) of small bowel, was born with multiple intestinal atresias which had led to removal of most of her small intestine. She was totally dependent upon medically provided nutrition and hydration but was rapidly losing venous access. The initial recommendation of bowel transplant was changed to liver and bowel transplant as her condition continued to deteriorate, and the transplant was performed in her 16th year. The initial euphoria of an apparently successful intervention was followed within five months by sepsis, system failure, and death.

The poignant account of her hospital course conveys the picture of a valiantly supportive family, determined but conflicted physicians, and an adolescent patient who preferred ignorance and optimism to a full and frank exchange of information about her situation and prognosis. Cognizant of the low probability of success of the operation, the authors, in their ethical commentary, wrestle with the question of what justifies such interventions. The answer usually given, "informed consent," clearly fails to satisfy the authors as they recall the attitude and reactions of the adolescent patient, recognize the difficulties of conveying (to patient or parents) the experiential reality of the proposed operation, and speculate on its wider social utility in the face of limited financial resources for medical treatment.

The commentator, philosopher Rosamond Rhodes, concentrates on three of the complex issues raised in the ethical commentary on this case: just allocation of scarce transplant organs, justified paternalism, and appropriate surrogate decision making. Unlike commentator Linda Granowetter in Chapter 10, Rhodes focuses first on the general considerations before turning to the specifics of this case of adolescent decision making, and explores distributive justice in organ allocation; capacity and consent in relation to risk, urgency, and uncertainty; and the conditions which can justify paternalistic action. Her careful consideration of possibly relevant factors, survey of current and traditional literature on autonomy, beneficence, respect for persons, justice and fairness in allocation of scarce resources, and attention to psychological factors make this commentary a useful resource for any person trying to think through the moral implications of decisions in high-stake situations. While supportive of the decisions reached by authors Garcia-Careaga, Castillo, and Kerner, she concludes "transplantation in the pediatric setting is challenging, not only for the many technical problems it presents, but also because of the difficult moral terrain that has to be negotiated."

7.1 Where should a child die?

Roger Burne

Introduction

The case to be discussed concerns the course of illness of William, which began at birth and continued until his death at 13 years of age. What is significant are the values of the caregivers and the family that led them to acknowledge the need for restraint in the care of this child. These attitudes are specifically discussed in answering the following three questions: Who decides? What are the aims of treatment? Where to die?

The case

William was born on August 17, 1984. He was his mother's sixth child. The following year his mother had twin girls. Apart from William all the children were, and are, healthy. A few hours after a normal birth William was noticed to be cyanosed and unwell. He was admitted to the neonatal intensive care unit where he was found to have a complex form of congenital heart disease with hypoplastic ventricles and pulmonary hypertension. A Blalock shunt, which is a palliative procedure, was performed successfully, though he subsequently required a balloon atreal septoplasty.

From the start it was recognized that he had a rather poor prognosis. At the earliest stage this was discussed with the parents by the cardiologist, who offered an opinion that

William's short-term outlook is relatively good. His long-term outlook depends on whether his relatively underdeveloped left ventricle will grow. If not, then he becomes effectively a univentricular heart of the right ventricular type. They tend, unfortunately, to develop significant problems with heart failure in their teens or early twenties. I think we must give the parents a very guarded long-term prognosis. On the other hand, the treatment of congenital heart disease is developing

Ethical Dilemmas in Pediatrics: Cases and Commentaries, ed. Lorry R. Frankel, Amnon Goldworth, Mary V. Rorty, and William A. Silverman. Published by Cambridge University Press. © Cambridge University Press 2005.

so rapidly that by the time he develops a problem we may well have newer methods of dealing with these complex congenital heart lesions. If nothing else, a heart transplant might be a much more acceptable option when he becomes older.

Given within a few months of his birth, this prognosis proved to be a useful guide over subsequent years.

After a somewhat stormy period, things seemed to go reasonably well. William grew and developed satisfactorily. He was prone to become more cyanosed and short of breath during minor illnesses and needed hospital admission on a number of occasions for this reason. Gradually his cyanosis and shortness of breath became more severe. By the time he was approaching his second birthday, it was clear that he would require some further intervention. He was admitted to a major cardiothoracic unit for cardiac catheterization. Following this procedure he collapsed and was found to be profoundly hypoglycemic. He suffered a major stroke. He then required mechanical ventilation for a week. He was eventually discharged to home with a right-sided hemiplegia, cortical blindness and the inability to talk. A head CT scan subsequently showed extensive ischemic damage affecting the territories of both posterior cerebral arteries and the left middle cerebral artery. On the basis of this study it was thought that the primary episode might have been due to embolization or thrombosis rather than hypoglycemia.

Within a few months he had started babbling to himself and was able to answer "yes" and "no" to questions. His vision was slowly recovering, at least for perception of shapes. By his third birthday, he had made considerable progress. His vision had recovered, though he had a very limited field of vision. His general development was thought to be appropriate for about half his chronological age. He could walk and climb stairs. He had learned to use his left hand quite well in preference to his dominant right hand. He had a very short attention span, with a tendency to wander and explore aimlessly with a degree of hyperactivity. He had epilepsy, with predominantly myoclonic seizures that were difficult to control. His speech was restricted to single words, though he understood everyday requests and instructions. This degree of neurological impairment remained with William for the rest of his life. In particular his hyperactivity, his seizures, and his visual impairment needed constant attention. He remained moderately developmentally retarded.

Over the next year he became increasingly cyanotic though his general health seemed to be better. The number of admissions to the hospital was greatly reduced, as well as the outpatient visits. William's mother now preferred to have all regular follow-up visits with the family doctor. This was partly to deliver care through a single physician rather than the numerous specialists who had some involvement, and also because both William and his mother had developed a strong dislike for the hospital environment.

By five years of age, it was clear that he needed further intervention for his progressive cyanosis. A cardiac catheterization was performed which revealed limited pulmonary blood flow. It was decided to modify his shunt. This surgery took place four months later. The operation was successful, leading to improvement in his degree of cyanosis and less dyspnea. The next few years were medically uneventful except for his hyperactivity and the need for seizure control. Four years following this surgery he became significantly cyanotic and polycythemic. His cardiologist advised that another surgical intervention might be indicated. Assessment for surgery would have necessitated another cardiac catheterization. William's mother was reluctant to consent to this procedure in view of the previous adverse events.

There followed a series of discussions involving William's mother and family, the family physician, and his cardiologist. These discussions centered on William's prognosis, the likely risks and benefits of further surgery, and the possibility of non-invasive evaluations. The conclusions reached were summarized as follows:

The MRI showed that William has quite reasonable-sized pulmonary vessels. A cardiac catheterization would be needed to check the pressures before surgical intervention could be considered. If William were to have a cardiac catheter and if the pressure were low enough then a Fontan procedure might be a possibility. This has a high early mortality but after the initial period 65% do well for a good many years. William's mother wishes to take this decision with William's father and her older children, and she intends to take a week or two to do this. My understanding is that they are more likely to go down the road of symptomatic care but this will need to be confirmed after the family have discussed matters.

The family chose symptomatic care without invasive procedures. Further management concentrated on quality of life for William. He was referred to a children's hospice, which offered periodic respite care. Extra attention was paid to the control of his seizures, which were becoming more severe and causing problems both for William and for his family. His polycythemia was monitored. He gradually became severely cyanotic but his activity level remained good and therefore no further intervention was necessary.

Approximately one year later he collapsed and was admitted emergently to the hospital. Following this episode, it was thought to be advisable to record the management plan in case he should require urgent care from physicians unfamiliar with the medical history. Accordingly, his mother was given a detailed document describing the medical history and clarifying that further surgery was not to be undertaken and that treatment should be focused on seizure control and comfort care. Copies of this document were placed with his family doctor and the hospital.

He continued to be cared for at home with regular admissions to the children's hospice. Over the next couple of years he gradually became less energetic. He had a number of episodes of syncope and was readmitted to hospital on several occasions. It was uncertain whether these episodes were cardiac or epileptic in nature. Since he recovered from these episodes, no further diagnostic studies were performed.

However, it was apparent that he was deteriorating. At 13 years of age he had another syncope episode while at school and was taken to the hospital. During this admission, he was clearly very ill. The physicians decided that there was nothing further to do for him in the hospital. Remarkably, he sat up and looked better when the possibility of going home was mentioned. At home he was comfortable. However, he quickly developed pneumonia. It was decided to provide comfort care. He was given morphine for his distress. A few hours later, he died in his sister's arms.

Ethical implications of the case

I have written at some length about the medical problems present during William's life and the practical steps that were taken to resolve these problems. So far there has been no explicit mention of ethics. I suppose that we grappled with ethical issues from the moment William was diagnosed. The decision-making process we went through over the years of William's illness and death can perhaps be discussed in the form of answers to three questions.

Who decides?

William's parents clearly had the right to give or refuse consent to treatment. By the age of 13 most children would also be capable of giving their opinions about treatment. For William his neurological damage prevented him having any under-standing or the ability to express his opinion. Even so, his dislike of the hospital environment was a factor which influenced to some degree the decisions which were made.

A lot of time and effort was spent discussing options between William's mother and the relevant doctors. Importantly, this included discussion of possible investigations and the consequences which might flow from them, as well as of the treatments themselves. In the end the family made the major decisions jointly in the privacy of their own home.

What are the aims of treatment?

At the earliest stage, it was recognized that while treatment could be helpful it might not be curative. At this young age death did not figure in our thinking. Rather, the judgment was made that he should have the best and most intensive treatment in the hope that in time he might benefit from a heart transplant. At this point there was not much for anyone to debate. Then tragedy struck. William was still William, much loved and central to the life of his family. He continued to be mobile, active, and happy. Yet, the unwritten contract that modern medicine can cure anything was broken. His cardiac disease was not any different but his neurological status changed everything. It might have been possible to argue that he should still receive the most intensive treatment aimed to cure; however, others might argue that following his stroke he was so neurologically damaged that he should have been allowed to die. Neither extreme view seemed to be correct. In any event, he lived for just over 13 years, having a variety of treatments including two cardiac surgeries. As time went by, the judgment of the family and the doctors was that treatment should be aimed at maintaining William at home with the best quality of life that could be achieved. Length of life became a secondary consideration. The unacceptable alternative was to subject him to additional time in the hospital. William did not like the hospital environment because of the exposures to painful and difficult procedures with little chance of ultimate success.

Where to die?

In some ways my main theme proves to be the easiest question to answer. Once it had been accepted that he would die, William was always going to die at home. This was the family's wish on each occasion it was discussed. This seemed to have dealt with the issue. All that was left was to wait for events to take their course. But real life is more difficult than that. For William to die at home, his entire management had to be organized. Everyone involved needed to understand and accept that cure was no longer an option, and that the aim of all treatment was to ensure his comfort. William did die at home, as had been planned, with his family providing the necessary comfort and support during this process. Perhaps he made his own choice in his own very special way.

FURTHER READING

Black, D. Coping with loss: the dying child. *BMJ* **316** (1998), 1376–1378.

Gillis, I. When lifesaving treatment is not the answer. *BMJ* **315** (1997), 1246–1247.

Goldman, A. *Care of the Dying Child* (Oxford: Oxford University Press, 1994).

   ABC of palliative care: special problems of children. *BMJ* **316** (1998), 49–52.

Royal College of Paediatrics and Child Health. *Withholding or Withdrawing Life Saving Treatment in Children: a Framework for Practice* (London: Royal College of Paediatrics and Child Health, 1997). This report defines five situations where the withholding or withdrawing of curative medical treatment for children might be considered:

   (1) The brain-dead child

   (2) The permanent vegetative state

   (3) The "no chance" situation

   (4) The "no purpose" situation

   (5) The "unbearable" situation

7.2 Where should a child (in the USA) die?

William A. Silverman

> The most important feature of [western political] culture is a belief in individual human dignity; that people have the moral right – and the moral responsibility – to confront the most fundamental questions about the meaning and value of their own lives for themselves, answering to their own consciousness and convictions . . . Making a person die in a way that others approve, but that affronts his own dignity, is a serious, unjustified, unnecessary form of tyranny.
>
> Ronald Dworkin (1993)

American physicians and parents reading Roger Burne's moving account of the life and death of young William in Britain will be startled, I suspect, by the striking difference expected had a real-life drama of similar circumstances been enacted in the USA. When the parents and William said, in essence, "Enough!," the unwritten moral code of professional behavior in Britain sanctioned their doctors' humane self-restraint, as well as the positive action taken by the doctors to make the necessary arrangements for the child to die at home. Moreover, the importance of family's private domain stands out prominently in the story from Burne's side of the Atlantic. The most crucial decisions taken by William's family took place on their own "turf." Unlike too many situations in the USA, the family's deliberations in Britain did not take place in a court of law; and not in a hospital surrounded by well-meaning experts, who are, nonetheless, strangers.

Dr. Burne tells us that when William was nine years old, after years of complex treatment and iatrogenic complications, the risks and benefits of further cardiac surgery were explained to his mother. At this time, he reports, "[she] wishes to take this decision with William's father and her older children, and she intends to take a week or two to do this." In the end, the family did indeed choose "symptomatic care without invasive procedures." It is interesting to see this evidence of respect for parents' refusal of life-prolonging treatments for their seriously disabled offspring

Ethical Dilemmas in Pediatrics: Cases and Commentaries, ed. Lorry R. Frankel, Amnon Goldworth, Mary V. Rorty, and William A. Silverman. Published by Cambridge University Press. © Cambridge University Press 2005.

in the UK; the situation was very much the same in the USA until the actions taken by a determined and highly vocal minority after a series of widely publicized events in the 1980s.

As I have noted elsewhere (Silverman 1998), the remarkable change in the USA was set in motion in 1981 with the broadcast of the decision of parents to decline surgical treatment for their infant born with major neural-tube defects (spina bifida, hydrocephalus, and microcephaly). Right-to-life zealots sought to overturn the parents' decision in a court of law, but this was thwarted by a judge who affirmed that "a most private and most precious responsibility is vested in the parents for the care of their child." The ruling accepted the premise that the choice to forgo surgery. (after consultation with neurosurgeons, social worker, and clergy) was made with love and thoughtfulness. A lawsuit to dismiss the primary responsibility of these parents was dismissed as an "offensive action."

This incident was followed by another highly publicized controversy in 1982 involving a newborn infant with Down syndrome complicated by esophageal atresia and tracheo-esophageal fistula. After hearing the conflicting opinions of consulting doctors, the parents refused to give their permission for corrective surgery. The hospital then sought a court order to compel the operation. The judge ruled in favor of the parents: "Mr. and Mrs. Doe . . . have the right to choose a medically recommended course of [non-surgical] treatment for their child." The wide publicity about this passive treatment of "Baby Doe" (who died at six days of age) soon turned the spotlight on similar unhappy situations; and this was followed by loud demands for governmental action. President Reagan, right-to-life groups, and advocacy organizations for the handicapped saw the Baby Doe incident as an example of unfair discrimination against children with disabling conditions. The clamor led directly to a series of regulations designed to require life-preserving treatment for infants with severe impairments.

The bureaucratic actions ushered in a short-lived but bizarre period in the history of American pediatrics; the era is remembered now as the "time of the Baby Doe witch hunts." The courts ruled against most of these outlandish actions, labeling them as "arbitrary and capricious," but the judicial opinions hinted that "some regulation of the provision of some types of medical care to handicapped newborns" might be needed. As a result of these machinations compromise legislation was finally passed in 1984 as amendments to the existing federal laws against child abuse. These so-called "Baby Doe Regulations II" have been interpreted to mean that treatment (including appropriate nutrition, hydration, and medication needed to ameliorate or correct all life-threatening conditions) is mandatory in these situations. Life-preserving treatment can be withheld only when infants are in an irreversible coma or dying, when such treatment would be "virtually futile" and its provision would be "inhumane." The regulations reject a future-quality-of-life standard as a criterion for providing or withholding life-preserving treatment of a severely impaired infant; thereby ignoring the social, cultural, and spiritual diversity that has guided decision making in the practice of medicine throughout history.

In all the fiery debate about "treat versus comfort care," most American doctors overlooked the fact that the new regulations were, in fact, an empty gesture: the statute merely required that individual states, if they wish to receive federal child-abuse protective service grant funds, must have programs that respond to reports of medical neglect (as defined in the stated guidelines). Unfortunately, doctors concluded that the guidelines themselves defined a new legal standard: that is to say, an enforceable law that required virtually unlimited medical action in all of these complex situations. Thus, American parents experienced an abrupt loss of power over their lives as a direct result of the everyday misinterpretation of the new legislation. The momentous decisions that determine the well-being over the full lifetime of every family member are now made in the hospital – an unreal theater-like setting in which the actors are doctors, ethicists, and, not infrequently, judges.

These dramatic events in the USA have made it increasingly difficult for families who want to bring their fatally ill children home to die. As one medical sociologist has noted (Dicke 1996), "the way people die [in the USA] is shaped by the exigencies of hospital organization. You die the way the hospital is prepared to have you die." A parent wrote movingly about these highly artificial strictures (Alecson 1995): "to die in our culture is to be a failure; and to discuss dying is increasingly taboo. This lack of open dialogue and expressed feelings," she wrote, "makes living in these modern times ever more inauthentic." Similarly, a ten-year-old child with a rare and incurable immune-system disorder, struggling with the terms of his life and acceptance of death, recognized the irrationality of received wisdom when he declared (Shillington 1995), "The doctors try to take care of you. But I was thinking if there's going to be no hope for me, no cure, and I was dying, why should I live [in the hospital] on a respirator and dialysis and stuff?"

Criticism of overall care given at the end of life by physicians in the USA has been severe. For example, an observational study reported in 1995 examined the care received by a large cohort of patients with life-threatening disease admitted to adult ICUs (Moscowitz and Nelson 1995). This was followed by a parallel-treatment trial in which gravely ill patients and their physicians were randomized to receive either a resource-rich intervention or usual medical management. "Bluntly put," the researchers finally concluded, "the intervention failed . . . to achieve any improvement that was at all substantial or unambiguous." Additionally, the Institute of Medicine (1997) issued a scathing report of end-of-life care in the USA. After four years of comprehensive study, a committee of the IOM concluded that "medical culture . . . tolerates and even rewards the misapplication of life-sustaining technologies while slighting the prevention and relief of suffering. Humane care for those approaching death is a social obligation from those directly involved."

Doctor Burne tells us that William's loving family were permitted to make the most important decision about where he should die; and this eminently humane resolution was respected by the British medical system. Compare this with the current situation in the USA. The verdict was proclaimed by George Annas, an American attorney and ethicist. It is plain spoken (and would be understood by William's family). "If dying patients want to retain some control of their dying process," he said, "they must get out of the hospital if they are in and stay out of the hospital if they are out" (Annas, quoted in Miller and Fins 1996).

7.3 Topical discussion

Palliative care

Palliative care has been defined as care that seeks to prevent, relieve, reduce, or soothe the symptoms produced by serious medical conditions or their treatment, and to maintain patients' quality of life. Ideally it is a part of the treatment plan from diagnosis on, but if it is considered an alternative rather than supplement to curative medical interventions and identified only with end-of-life treatment it can pose ethical dilemmas to physicians and families. If it is necessary to accept that death is imminent for a child with a life-threatening or chronic illness, introducing palliative care might be seen as a decision to "abandon hope" and thus may be resisted, both by families and by caregivers who have an emotional stake in the success of their treatment, risking undertreatment of pain and inadequate communication and discharge planning.

In the USA this bifurcation is resisted by considering palliative care to include end-of-life care planning and inpatient or outpatient hospice care, as well as pain management, but there are reimbursement obstacles as well as conceptual ones that make it difficult to more tightly integrate palliative care with mainstream medical therapies. As a result, palliative care is more likely to be a focus in children with terminal illnesses than in children facing chronic or life-threatening illness. It is to be hoped that the growing presence of multidisciplinary palliative care programs in US hospitals, as well as increasing emphasis on pain control and end-of-life care in medical education, will eventually mitigate this compartmentalization and bring the USA more in line with standard practices elsewhere.

Pain management has been seriously studied in the USA since the 1950s, and the founding of an international Association for the Study of Pain in 1973 has improved professional communication on pain relief, including increasing attention to

Ethical Dilemmas in Pediatrics: Cases and Commentaries, ed. Lorry R. Frankel, Amnon Goldworth, Mary V. Rorty, and William A. Silverman. Published by Cambridge University Press. © Cambridge University Press 2005.

non-pharmacological techniques for pain management. While pain control is an important part of the support the ill child and the family may require, emotional comfort, marshaling of community resources, and strengthening communication between the care team and the family are important as well. Palliative care includes ongoing discussion with families of long-term as well as short-term goals, care strategies, and available resources, all of which need to be considered in discharge planning.

Hospice

Hospice is better entrenched in Great Britain than in the United States, and more children there die at home, although statistics reveal that the number of ill children dying at home has risen slightly in the USA in the last decade. Hospice programs typically provide out-of-hospital care for terminally ill patients, either at home or in dedicated institutional settings, and are less common in the United States than in some other countries. Pediatric hospice programs are rare. While there are about 2500 hospice programs for adults, there are only about 250 specifically aimed toward children, according to a 1999 survey.

The original conceptualization of hospice programs intended them for the last few weeks of the patient's life, but the understanding of palliative care has broadened from end of life, to include respite for family caregivers and home care support for children with chronic illnesses.

Regulations governing reimbursement for hospice, and modest support for home care in comparison with intensive care, contribute to the cultural differences noted by Burne and Silverman. The history of Baby Doe regulations, also discussed by Whitney in Chapter 2, has had a strong, if ambiguous, effect upon pediatric medicine in the USA.

Distributive justice

If we were blessed with unlimited medical resources or received all the medical care that we wanted because we were so constituted as to want exactly what we got, then distributive justice would not be an issue. Unfortunately we live in a world in which demand cannot be fully met by existing resources, and we are not happy with these limitations. Distributive justice in the medical setting is concerned with the question of who should receive medical care when not all can? More exactly, what is a fair distribution of limited resources?

The Baby Doe regulations alluded to in Dr. Silverman's essay identified the high-risk infants for whom life-preserving treatment was to be given or withheld. This was an attempt to separate those infants who should receive treatment from those who should not. It did not do so by considering limited resource issues. But any criteria that are used to identify a subset of needy patients to be treated from a larger class could be employed to solve allocation problems. Whether we would want to use such regulations at all is a matter of their adequacy. And here it should be noted that they have been extensively criticized as ambiguous or inconsistent.

A comprehensive analysis of resource allocation should include the issue of equal access or fairness, an examination of cost or efficiency criteria, such as cost-benefit or cost-effectiveness, and the application of ethical criteria, such as the right to health care. A major difficulty with applying the norms generated by these concerns is that they are not compatible with one another. In addition, adopting such norms may also determine who counts as a decision maker and who does not, and this, in turn, may have a bearing on doctor–patient or doctor–family relationships.

Comparative health care

As Silverman's commentary emphasizes, national culture and judicial and legislative requirements make a great difference to what it means to practice medicine in a given country. The balance between cost and quality of care is met by different nations in different ways, as are the competing demands of access and rationing. Countries with national health insurance can provide universal access to a range of treatments but may limit the availability of some high-cost interventions. Although healthcare coverage in many countries is also undergoing change, study of such exemplary systems as Canada, Great Britain, Germany, or Singapore provide many thought-provoking alternatives to the sporadic coverage and market-driven inequalities of the US system.

Different national histories create different cultural expectations. By immigration and short-term stays, by international exchange and multinational projects, US health care becomes less parochial and places higher demands on those involved to be explicit about their expectations and open to learning about those of others. Health-related research is creating some of the most troubling ethical issues in international and multinational medicine, because of the patchwork of regulations (and expectations) about what is due research subjects.

FURTHER READING

American Academy of Pediatrics. Palliative care for children. *Pediatrics* **106** (2000), 351–357.

Childress, J. F. Who shall live when not all can live? *Soundings* **53** (1970), 339–355.

Daniels, N. Health care needs and distributive justice. *Philosophy and Public Affairs* **10** (1981), 146–179.

Field, M. J. and Behrman, R. E. (eds.) *When Children Die: Improving Palliative and End-of-Life Care for Children and their Families* (Washington, DC: National Academies Press, 2003).

Gold, M. R., Siegel, J. E., Russell, L. B., and Weinstein, M. C. (eds.) *Cost-Effectiveness in Health and Medicine* (New York, NY: Oxford University Press, 1996).

McGrath, P. J. and Frager, G. Psychological barriers to optimal pain management in infants and children. *Clinical Journal of Pain* 12 (1996), 135–141.

Rhoden, N. K. Treatment dilemmas for imperiled newborns: why quality of life counts. *Southern California Law Review* 58 (1985), 1283–1347.

Stephenson, J. Palliative and hospice care needed for children with life-threatening conditions. *JAMA* 284 (2000), 2437–2438.

Wolfe, J. Suffering in children at the end of life: recognizing an ethical duty to palliate. *Journal of Clinical Ethics* 11 (2000), 157–162.

8.1 Infant heart transplantation and hypoplastic left heart syndrome: what are the ethical issues?

Clifford Chin

The case

Ms. L was pregnant at 37 years of age. Amniocentesis, performed because of her advanced maternal age, revealed a normal 46 XY chromosome analysis. At 34 weeks estimated gestational age she underwent a routine obstetrical ultrasound which revealed an abnormal four-chamber image of the fetus' heart. A complete fetal echocardiogram revealed a small left atrium and ventricle with mitral atresia, and a hypoplastic aorta without forward flow from the left ventricle to the ascending aorta. The coronary arteries and head and neck vessels were supplied by a widely patent ductus arteriosus. A diagnosis of hypoplastic left heart syndrome (HLHS) was made.

As HLHS carries a grave prognosis if untreated, the parents were given the following options: (1) no treatment, (2) conventional surgical approach (Norwood procedure), or (3) heart transplantation. After much discussion with the pediatric cardiologists at the local children's hospital, the family opted for heart transplantation and the fetus was placed on the heart transplant waiting list at 36 weeks gestation. If an appropriate donor heart became available, Ms. L would undergo a cesarean section, the infant would be immediately resuscitated and started on prostaglandin to maintain ductal patency, and would then undergo the heart transplant operation.

Ms. L gave birth at 38 weeks estimated gestational age. A complete neonatal team was present in the delivery room and observed that the neonate was cyanotic with an oxygen saturation of 80% in room air. The umbilical vein was cannulated and prostaglandin therapy instituted. For three weeks, the infant remained in the neonatal intensive care unit on prostaglandin. Because of the development of hemodynamic instability, dysfunction of the right ventricle and frequent

Ethical Dilemmas in Pediatrics: Cases and Commentaries, ed. Lorry R. Frankel, Amnon Goldworth, Mary V. Rorty, and William A. Silverman. Published by Cambridge University Press. © Cambridge University Press 2005.

episodes of desaturation, as well as the lack of an appropriate heart donor, he underwent the first stage of the Norwood palliation (a series of operations to compensate for the anomaly). In the operating room evidence was found of hypoplastic left heart syndrome with an atretic ascending aorta and left ventricle. The heart itself was dilated and the pulmonary arteries were large. In addition, evidence of pulmonary edema and pulmonary hemorrhage were also noted. The operation was done without complications and the chest wall was closed at the end of the procedure.

The infant's immediate postoperative course was uneventful but he subsequently developed seizures which required treatment with anticonvulsants. A left-side cerebral lesion was found by CT which was felt to be secondary to a middle cerebral artery infarction. The neurologists felt that the child was at low risk for either recurrent seizures or worsening seizures. One month after his operation he was discharged home with his parents. At six months of age, he underwent the second stage of the palliative correction, a bi-directional Glenn shunt. He has done well since and is awaiting the third stage of the surgical procedure.

Analysis

The prognosis for infants born with HLHS is poor without surgical intervention. Over 95% of these patients die within the first month of life (Fyler *et al.* 1981). Since 1987 infant heart transplantation has become an acceptable alternative to other innovative surgeries for infants with intractable heart disease due to certain types of congenital heart lesions and cardiomyopathy. According to a recent registry report (Boucek *et al.* 1997), the one-, five- and ten-year survival for all pediatric heart transplant recipients (<18 years of age) is 80%, 65%, and 50% respectively. However, the results of infant survival after cardiac transplantation is just under 70% at one year. Five-year survival in patients who were transplanted in the infancy period is under 60%. The Pediatric Heart Transplant Study Group (Morrow *et al.* 1997) reported that the outcome for heart transplantation in infants of less than six months of age was poor, with an unacceptably high rate of mortality while waiting for an appropriate donor. The risk of death was highest in the first three months after listing. Infants with HLHS were notably at highest risk.

By contrast, the Norwood surgical procedure for HLHS is possible with good results (Norwood *et al.* 1992, Iannettoni *et al.* 1994). Depending upon the surgical center, the one-year survival after an infant heart transplant is comparable to the first stage of the Norwood procedure. Early survival after the first stage of the Norwood procedure has been reported between 77% (Kern *et al.* 1997) and 85% (Iannettoni *et al.* 1994), with one-year survival of 69% (Iannettoni *et al.* 1994) and four-year survival of 61% (Kern *et al.* 1997). Infant survival reported by the Pediatric

Registry (Boucek *et al.* 1997) for heart transplantation is comparable, with one- and four-year survival approaching 70% and 60% respectively. Surgical palliation, such as the Norwood procedure, potentially requires two additional stages, namely the Glenn and Fontan operations. Both of these operations carry their own risks. Similarly, although additional surgical interventions are very rarely performed after a heart transplant, survival continues to diminish over time secondary to infection, organ rejection, coronary artery disease, and nonspecific graft failure (Baum *et al.* 1991, Pahl *et al.* 1989).

Ethical issues

When should a fetus be listed for heart transplantation? Early listing is not appropriate until the fetus is viable by cesarean section. Although many premature infants under 30 weeks estimated gestational age (EGA) are delivered with excellent outcomes, the United Network for Organ Sharing has adopted a policy of defining "viability" as no less than 32 weeks EGA UNOS (1992). Transplant centers began listing fetuses because of a known donor shortage and high mortality encountered by those infants on the waiting list. UNOS has determined that a gestational age of at least 32 weeks is required in order to list for transplantation, even though a fetus delivered prior to 32 weeks may be viable.

The average waiting time before transplantation for infants under six months of age is approximately one month. Fetuses could theoretically accumulate additional time and thereby improve their likelihood of obtaining an appropriate donor heart. Ethically, could this practice place those individuals listed later as infants at a disadvantage? An understanding of organ allocation policies is necessary to answer this question. Preference is given to those patients based on status, with those at status I given priority over status II patients. Status I patients include infants under six months of age, regardless of the severity of illness. Once these children reach six months of age, they are automatically transferred to status II. Children older than six months can remain or return to status I if they require intravenous inotropic support.

A complicating issue is the consideration of time on the waiting list. Patients accumulate time on the list so that those individuals (in each status stratum) who were listed first have first priority. However, UNOS has established a policy to "restart the clock" at birth if patients were not transplanted *in utero* (UNOS 1992). Although a fetal patient may have accumulated time on the waiting list, at the time of birth that infant would be reclassified as if he or she were listed at birth (that is, there would be no accumulated waiting time on the heart transplant waiting list). These patients, therefore, do not have an unfair advantage over infants listed after birth.

Another ethical issue resolved by UNOS was the allocation policy of organs to fetuses versus infants (UNOS 1992). Clearly, the fetus is at a survival advantage while waiting, as the maternal–placental unit protects the fetus. After birth, the prospective recipient requires warmth, fluids, and nutrition, but must demonstrate spontaneous respirations. Life support may be required and then careful neurologic evaluation is carried out in order to determine the neurologic state of the infant prior to listing as a recipient. Therefore, fetuses are assigned a separate status, whereby organs are allocated to *in utero* recipients only if no appropriate neonatal recipient is identified. What are the implications for the parents who decide to list their unborn child with HLHS for heart transplantation?

In our experience, surgical palliation may be delayed for up to three weeks in some cases because the family chooses transplantation over palliation and hence must wait for an appropriate donor heart to become available. By three weeks of age, the infant may become a poorer candidate for the Norwood procedure secondary to acidosis, failure to thrive, and pulmonary injury related to prolonged intubation, positive pressure mechanical ventilation, and exposure to high levels of supplemental oxygen.

If parents continue to insist upon transplantation, or if the cardiac function is deteriorating beyond the limits of a successful Norwood procedure, a possible option is to place the infant on extracorporeal membrane oxygenation (ECMO) support. ECMO has been used in many medical circumstances, including respiratory distress, sepsis, cardiac dysfunction after surgical repair, and as a bridge to cardiac transplantation. ECMO is often a temporizing measure, used until resolution of organ damage has occurred or as a bridge to transplantation. However, ECMO can be associated with a number of complications, including infection, bleeding, central nervous system injury, and circuit issues, and there is a limited window of approximately 20–30 days while waiting for an appropriate donor to become available. Since the decision to list these patients may have already been made, further cardiac dysfunction, which may require ECMO support (in the absence of other organ damage), should not affect their candidacy.

Thus one is made to delve deeply into the ethical issues of allocating precious organs which are deemed life saving to fetuses and infants. Organ donation is associated with another family's tragedy (the loss of a loved one), as well as uncertain and prolonged waiting periods which may not prove to be beneficial to the recipient or family. The waiting period should be used to assist the family with appropriate counseling, and to provide the infant recipient who is in need of a heart with compassionate and appropriate medical care. The psychological trauma associated with these critical junctures places a great deal of weight on how the medical and nursing teams interact with the family and the patient. In addition, serious discussions need to take place regarding "code status" and other interventions while seriously ill patients are waiting for more definitive therapy.

Should parents of infants with HLHS be counseled toward the Norwood staged surgical approach, and away from heart transplantation? There is a tremendous shortage of appropriate donor organs. Given that patients with HLHS have an alternative form of therapy available to them in the Norwood procedures, and those with end-stage cardiomyopathy do not, one might argue that HLHS patients should be directed toward multi-stage conventional surgical repair. First, results of the stage I Norwood procedure need to be compared with results of infant heart transplantation. As discussed earlier, survival for the two procedures is about the same. Further, Gutgesell and Massaro (1995) utilized the discharge database of the University Hospital Consortium to determine management and early outcome of HLHS in 62 university hospitals. They concluded that patients managed with transplantation had longer hospitalization times and higher costs, primarily due to the lack of donor availability. Since there is an alternative form of therapy with excellent survival, infants with HLHS should be offered the Norwood procedure as the initial treatment option, reserving cardiac donor organs for those with heart disease irreparable by surgery. This conclusion is bolstered by the financial risks associated with heart transplantation compared to traditional surgery. Finally, it does not seem appropriate to delay surgical repair in hopes of transplantation, given the long waiting times on the pretransplant list, the excellent results of Norwood palliation, and the problems that arise in HLHS patients while awaiting an appropriate donor. However, if at any stage anatomical or hemodynamic constraints should be suboptimal for surgical repair, transplantation should be considered as an option for infants with HLHS.

If infant heart transplantation is felt to be an accepted form of medical therapy, and if there is a donor shortage, should the medical, legal, and ethical standards concerning anencephalic infants as organ donors be re-evaluated? The main limitation on infant heart transplantation is due to a limited donor pool. In the late 1980s and early 1990s, UNOS adopted a policy that anencephalic infants could not be considered as organ donors under present standards. Anencephaly occurs in 1–5 per 1000 live births. It is generally accepted that these infants are permanently unconscious but do have some brainstem function. Since brain-death criteria stipulate that brain-stem activity must be entirely absent, anencephalic infants have been excluded from organ donation in the United States.

The vast majority of anencephalic infants die within the first days of life, with only rare cases being reported of patients living beyond one week. In addition, as Walters et al. (1997) observed, brain stems of anencephalic infants are almost completely devoid of any evidence of even primitive functional organization. Since these patients do not have brain function, they do not have thought, emotion, or personality. There is also the further consideration that the parents of an anencephalic neonate often want to donate an organ (Friedman 1990). The act of saving a life can compensate these parents for their tragedy.

One argument against the use of anencephalics for organ donation concerns the difficulty of diagnosing anencephaly accurately. However, the American Medical Association Council on Ethical and Judicial Affairs (1995a) has argued that there are appropriate safeguards to make the diagnosis of anencephaly highly reliable. In their statement, this Council argues that it is ethically permissible to consider the anencephalic neonate as a potential organ donor. It recognizes that these neonates are considered to be alive, but that donation is justified because such infants do not demonstrate any state of consciousness. In light of the above consideration, the medical, legal, and ethical standards should be altered so that anencephalic infants may be made organ donors.

Should infant donor hearts be reserved for those infants suffering from intractable and inoperable heart disease regardless of their chromosomal analysis? Natowicz and colleagues (1988) reported that 12% of cases of HLHS reviewed had an abnormal chromosome analysis. Abnormalities included Turner's syndrome and trisomies 13, 18, and 21. There is a spectrum of cognitive capacity in the population of patients who have trisomy 21, Down syndrome. These individuals range from children who are profoundly retarded to those who may function independently. In the fetal and infancy stages, cognitive capacity may not be able to be adequately assessed. This is of great significance for the transplant community as one criterion used by many centers is whether the Down syndrome patient can care for him- or herself. Although there is no way to predict whether an infant born with congenital heart disease (without a chromosomal abnormality) will be able to care for him- or herself, most with trisomy 21 have cognitive impairment. However, given the unknowns regarding the ultimate functioning of an individual, most centers would still discourage transplantation for such individuals. Further, those with trisomy 21 generally have an increased risk for malignancy. As the general transplant population has at least an 11% risk of developing a malignancy (Baum et al. 1991), those individuals with trisomy 21 may be at much higher risk for the development of tumors. Patients with trisomy 13 or 18 usually do so poorly in the infancy period that transplantation is also not offered as a form of therapy. These decisions may be influenced by the unfavorable recipient-to-donor ratio for heart transplantation.

Conclusion

Considerations of both medical and ethical factors lead us to suggest that individuals with HLHS should be recommended for standard surgical approaches for many reasons. First, survival statistics for the Norwood operation are as good as those for heart transplantation in neonates. Second, the cost of surgery (and follow-up) is lower than that of transplantation. Third, because of a limited donor pool, infant hearts should be reserved for those individuals with intractable heart disease who do not have any surgical alternatives. The scarcity of donor organs also strengthens the argument against heart transplantation in recipients with chromosomal defects. Finally, to somewhat offset the donor-to-recipient disparity, the consideration of anencephalics as donors is justified not only ethically but also morally, medically, and emotionally.

8.2 Infant heart transplantation and hypoplastic left heart syndrome: a response

Joel E. Frader

Introduction

In the case, Ms. L was found to be carrying a fetus with hypoplastic left heart syndrome (HLHS) at 34 weeks of gestation.[1] She and her family, having been informed and having considered the options, elected to pursue neonatal heart transplantation, rather than "palliative" surgery (the Norwood sequence of operations) or a non-surgical approach. (We can only assume Ms. L and her husband had the latter alternative made available to them.)

Unfortunately, the baby did not do as well as do some newborns with HLHS treated with prostaglandin. At three weeks of age, because of a failing cardiovascular system and no available organ for transplantation, Baby L had a first-stage Norwood operation. Seizures some time in the postoperative period led to the diagnosis of cerebral infarction. At six months of age, he had a second-stage procedure and awaited the third stage at the time of the case report. He is said to be "doing very well."

Dr. Chin argues that Baby L should have had palliative surgery in the days immediately following birth, rather than await transplantation. He believes this to be so because (1) survival following the Norwood sequence approximates that following neonatal transplantation; (2) the Norwood approach involves lower (financial) costs; and (3) the inadequate supply of hearts for infant transplantation should be reserved for patients who have no alternative treatments. He also suggests: (4) we should increase the relative supply of hearts for transplantation by denying a transplant to those with chromosomal defects; and (5) we should increase the absolute supply of hearts by using organs from babies with anencephaly. Finally, he

---

[1] A relatively long time has passed since the editors first requested this piece. The clinical care of patients with hypoplastic left hearts has changed somewhat. The addendum at the end of the chapter addresses some aspects of this situation.

Ethical Dilemmas in Pediatrics: Cases and Commentaries, ed. Lorry R. Frankel, Amnon Goldworth, Mary V. Rorty, and William A. Silverman. Published by Cambridge University Press. © Cambridge University Press 2005.

briefly addresses issues regarding fetal diagnosis of HLHS and "listing" fetuses as transplant candidates.

Response

It may help to separate arguments about the appropriate treatment of infants born with HLHS from arguments about more general ethical questions regarding the supply and use of available hearts in infancy.

With respect to the options for those with HLHS, it is true that death while awaiting a donor organ contributes to the overall mortality. Whether this risk is "unacceptably high," as Dr. Chin asserts, depends on several factors. A crucial question, yet unanswered, if not entirely unaddressed, by the community of pediatric cardiologists and cardiothoracic surgeons, involves the long-term *functional* consequences of the surgical alternatives. What is the outlook for the surviving children? Are there differences in neurodevelopment between those who receive a transplant and those who have Norwood operations? For those living beyond, say, ten years, how easily, if at all, can they participate in physically strenuous activities, such as sports? Dr. Chin seems to take the view that survival itself constitutes the only important outcome measure. More likely, patients and families, not to mention healthcare professionals, care a great deal about the quality of life experienced by survivors. Some parents might conclude that current treatments entail so much pain and suffering for children with HLHS, without adequate demonstration of overall benefit, that they prefer to forgo surgery altogether.

We have a small amount of data about the neurodevelopmental outcomes in patients surviving surgery for HLHS. Lynch and colleagues (1994) studied 14 children who received heart transplantation. Eight of the patients had HLHS. One had "slight dysmetria" and normal development at age 20 months. One had hypotonia with "moderate gross motor delay" at 11 months. One had "right hemiparesis, axial hypotonia . . . and moderate global delay" at 16 months. Another child had a normal neurologic examination and a "possible mild expressive language delay" at 23 months. One 16-month-old had a normal neurologic examination "but mild global developmental delays." The others were normal. Rogers *et al.* (1995) studied 11 survivors of staged surgical repair of HLHS. Four of these children had moderate cognitive impairment while three had severe to profound mental retardation. Two more had "suspect cognitive development." Five of the patients had gross motor impairments.

Miller and others (1996) "studied the neurodevelopmental outcomes of 104 consecutive unselected children who underwent open-heart surgery from 1987 through 1989." They found that the median IQ for survivors with HLHS was 66, with only one patient having an IQ above 70. By contrast, the median IQ for those with transposition of the great arteries (TGA) was 109, with only one patient with a score less than 84. That study suggested a relationship between outcome and (1) age (less than one month), (2) prolonged deep hypothermia, as well as a type of congenital heart disease (HLHS versus TGA). It is possible that the HLHS includes a predisposition or vulnerability to neurodevelopmental difficulty. In one report, Bove (1998) noted that 25 out of 49 patients with HLHS were normal after the third stage (Fontan) procedure of the Norwood sequence. On the other hand, Razzouk and colleagues (1996) noted in passing that in HLHS patients surviving transplantation at Loma Linda, "neurologic abnormalities occurred in 10% . . . with dystonia being the most common disability."

Depending upon which study one reads and perhaps depending upon where one's child would receive treatment, a parent could take a pessimistic or hopeful view of proposed surgery. One is certainly hard-pressed to conclude that the Norwood repair produces such compellingly good neurodevelopmental results that it should be preferred over transplantation or even over non-surgical hospice care. Indeed, a report from a German center doing both procedures concludes that "quality of life and physical development are far better in infants after transplantation according to our experience" (Hehrlein *et al.* 1998). One has to take into account other important factors, such as the benefit of having only one major surgical procedure (transplantation) versus two or three (in the Norwood sequence) with the additional physical pain associated with multiple surgeries and the additional risks of brain injury with each period on cardiopulmonary bypass (Rappaport *et al.* 1996). Of course, we have to consider the long-term risks associated with transplantation. These include renal and neuropsychiatric complications of cyclosporin or tacrolimus, infectious risks of immunosuppression, growth failure in patients requiring corticosteroids, and the possibility of developing post-transplantation lymphoproliferative disorder (PTLD), a malignant disease for approximately half of those acquiring it. The good news is that very early transplantation may increase the likelihood of reducing or eliminating the need for immunosuppression (Bailey *et al.* 1989). If that turns out to be important, transplant patients could have the best of both worlds: normal functional anatomy, only one major surgery, and freedom from immunosuppression and its problems.

Would Dr. Chin argue for the Norwood sequence if well-designed comparative clinical trials demonstrated the unequivocal superiority of transplantation? Probably, he would not. Short-term equivalence in survival tells us very little about the wisdom of using one surgical approach to HLHS rather than another. Indeed, at least one large center in the United States continued to do both into the mid-1990s, basing the choice on some anatomical considerations and parental preference

(Bando *et al*. 1996). The current situation does, however, reinforce the need for controlled clinical trials comparing the two treatment regimens on a host of outcome variables beyond survival: quality of life, financial impact, long-term physiologic function, and freedom from complications, such as stroke, cancer, major infections, etc. (Frader and Caniano 1998).

There is not a great deal one can say about the financial costs of transplantation versus staged repair. Unless a heart becomes available immediately, the initial hospital charges associated with transplantation are virtually guaranteed to be higher than for first-stage repair. The need for lifelong treatment with cyclosporin or tacrolimus also suggests greater transplant-related costs. However, the Norwood sequence involves three (or in some cases, only two) bypass procedures. It is by no means clear that the surgery-related costs of transplantation will turn out to be greater. If a substantial portion of infants receive transplanted hearts early and could be weaned from immunosuppression, the continuing financial drain associated with the drugs and their side effects could disappear. Moreover, it is possible that those with normal anatomy (i.e., transplant patients, especially those free of immunosuppression) will have substantially longer lives than those with surgical repair. In that case, the cost per case, amortized over the life of survivors, might be less for transplantation. All of this is merely speculative at this point and it seems unreasonable to make decisions about the favored treatment on the available, quite incomplete, financial information.

Dr. Chin also asserts that the inadequate supply of hearts, given an available alternative to transplantation, itself dictates use of the Norwood approach. The claim seems overreaching. Surely, one must consider the shortage of available organs. However, the discussion cannot stop there. Weighing one path against another must also consider other benefits and burdens associated with each of the options. The kidney transplant community rarely *automatically* rules out end-stage renal disease patients for transplantation simply because they can use dialysis. If the overall morbidity and/or quality of life for HLHS patients were clearly better after transplantation, one would be hard-pressed to steer parents toward reparative surgery just because other patients, who might not have an alternative treatment, could also use the organs. Again, we need much better information, preferably gained in controlled trials, before we make "final" conclusions.

Dr. Chin believes that some HLHS patients with chromosomal disorders should be systematically ruled out for transplantation. Few persons would argue that children with trisomies of chromosomes 13 or 18 should get a heart transplant. Most physicians would support denial of staged repair for HLHS in such patients. While just (fair) use of scarce resources might be an issue in the discussion, the main moral ground for refusing treatment of HLHS under the circumstances would involve the lack of or limitation of benefit for these patients, given their consistently severe to profound cognitive impairment. When it comes to trisomy 21, though Chin may correctly assert "most centers would still discourage transplantation," many find this position morally unsettling. If we acknowledge that patient benefit constitutes the ethical basis for offering treatment (transplantation or staged repair), most pediatricians, policy makers, and ethicists now agree that the majority of persons with trisomy 21 would be better off with successful therapy. It seems unfair to deny treatment to an entire class of patients based on the fact that some (but very few) Down-syndrome patients will not develop sufficient cognitive capacity to appreciate positive operative results. Dr. Chin does not support his suggestion that patients with trisomy 21 would have a "much higher risk" for developing malignancies post-transplantation. Even if we had such evidence, one would still have to weigh the incremental risk and the likely time to development of tumors before finding the information determinative. In addition to doubt about the morality of denying patients with Down syndrome equal access to treatment for HLHS, arguably state laws or regulations enacted after the federal "Baby Doe" law would render such discrimination illegal.

On the matter of anencephaly, Dr. Chin sees potential to increase the supply of hearts. He argues that we may use the organs of patients born with anencephaly because these children are permanently unconscious. (He accepts the fact that such children cannot be declared "brain dead" under current law. The law in each state now requires a donor be dead before removal of the heart, the entire liver, both lungs, both kidneys, all of the pancreas or bowel, etc.) His argument seems to rest on the fact that newborns with anencephaly (1) will die anyway, usually within a few days, and (2) some have parents who favor organ donation. He thus supports a May 1995 opinion of the American Medical Association Council on Ethical and Judicial Affairs (1995a). He neglects to note that the Council withdrew that opinion later in the year of issue, in response to substantial protest.

Discussion of the potential use of organs from babies with anencephaly, similar in many ways to the debate about abortion, stimulates strongly held views. Legal obstacles aside, some feel that the opportunity to save lives using organs from those who cannot themselves benefit from the organs justifies overriding more abstract considerations, such as a prohibition on the merely instrumental use of other human beings. For some, the social and philosophical implications of starting down a "slippery slope" toward discounting the worth of some humans for the sake of others outweighs the possibility of helping a few. A more important point, as with abortion, may well be that the enormous gulf between the two sides makes implementing public policy quite difficult (Walters et al. 1997).

The number of live-born infants with anencephaly in the USA has fallen over the last decades. Some of this may be due to a decrease in the incidence of neural-tube defects (perhaps, in turn, related to better nutrition). Certainly the possibility of detecting anencephaly early in the pregnancy is another factor, since women may choose to abort an affected fetus rather than carry to term. In addition, in 1990, the Medical Task Force on Anencephaly reported that "major defects of the cardio-vascular system" occurred in 4% to 15% of live-born children with anencephaly (Medical Task Force 1990). These preclude use of the hearts for transplantation. Thus, the number of hearts available from this source would be quite small. Given all of this, the position of the American Academy of Pediatrics seems reasonable:

> Even if strong support were to emerge for legislation either defining anencephalic infants as legally dead or allowing retrieval of their organs prior to legal death, serious questions would remain about the wisdom of enacting such legislation . . . sufficient questions exist to counsel extreme caution before adopting a policy permitting organ retrieval from anencephalic infants who retain brain stem function. (American Academy of Pediatrics Committee on Bioethics 1992)

Finally, we should address the question of placing fetuses with HLHS on transplant waiting lists. This issue came to public attention when a mother in Pittsburgh had a cesarean section at 35 weeks gestation in order for her baby to have a transplant when a heart had become available. Transplanters had placed the fetus on a waiting list for a new heart at 30 weeks gestation. It is possible, perhaps even likely, that another baby, already born and waiting for an organ but not listed while a fetus, could have received the heart had it not been for the time the recipient had accrued on the waiting list while *in utero*. The publicity led to reconsideration of the United Network for Organ Sharing (UNOS) policies affecting such matters. A group of us, then at the University of Pittsburgh, attempted to influence the change in UNOS policy; we subsequently published a reflection on the incident and related developments (Michaels *et al.* 1993).

As Dr. Chin states, UNOS policy, in light of the above problem, prohibits placing a fetus on the waiting list until 32 weeks gestation. But the number of weeks has little to do with "viability" (which occurs long before 32 weeks). Moreover, at 32 weeks, the chest of many fetuses would not accommodate many available infant hearts. Thus, allowing listing at 32 weeks seems primarily aimed at allowing the fetus to accumulate time on the waiting list to gain priority when a heart becomes available. Is this morally proper? If accurate cardiac ultrasonographic diagnosis were available to all pregnant women, this practice might not raise questions of fairness. But only about half of pregnant women in the USA get ultrasound examinations and far fewer have "level two" scans, much less examinations by pediatric echocardiographers. As one might imagine, the distribution of testing is not random. Generally speaking, those with better insurance or greater private resources receive the most and the most sophisticated ultrasound examinations. Thus, current UNOS policy continues to perpetuate an injustice.

UNOS policy does appropriately separate listed fetuses from listed babies who have already been born. This practice acknowledges that while *in utero* the fetus with HLHS is relatively well off, compared to the baby on a constant infusion of prostaglandin and other modes of sophisticated medical intervention. The latter patients deserve a "first crack" at available hearts. In addition, the policy helps to minimize placing women at unnecessary additional risk associated with surgical deliveries. The risks involve more than medical implications – they may also entail subtle or overt coercion of women to agree to interventions they would otherwise prefer to avoid. While most pregnant women want to act in ways that clearly benefit their fetuses, one can imagine that some would not see a cesarean section as an unequivocal good, especially if it results in the delivery of a preterm infant.

Conclusion

Dr. Chin argues that doctors should recommend staged repair for infants with HLHS, rather than transplantation. However, he does not demonstrate that the mere fact of an alternative to transplantation alone justifies urging parents to accept the Norwood sequence of operations. The lack of adequate comparative data about the overall benefits and burdens of the two approaches makes it hard to advise parents that they should go along with either choice, assuming they want life-sustaining treatment for their child. The major ethical problem here could be seen as the inappropriate reluctance of the pediatric cardiology/cardiothoracic-surgery community to undertake the needed studies. Certainly we do not now know enough about the financial implications of either pathway to draw conclusions as to the economically preferred approach.

Consideration of organ shortages does not alone suggest answers about whether patients with chromosomal disorders "deserve" transplantation. Rather than using strict (and morally suspect) allocation arguments, the primary concern should be the ability of the patient to benefit from treatment. Patients with trisomy 21 are likely to be able to appreciate the benefits of extended life and systematically excluding them from candidacy for transplantation is wrong. Nor do considerations of shortages once and for all answer reservations about the use of infants born with anencephaly as organ sources. Many have deep philosophical and pragmatic reservations about beginning a policy that permits the use of one class of humans (albeit a severely compromised one) solely to satisfy the needs of others.

Policies for listing fetuses as transplant candidates remain somewhat problematic, though better than before a 1992 UNOS policy revision. The gestational age for listing still fosters injustice and permits situations in which women are vulnerable to coercion regarding otherwise unindicated surgical deliveries. UNOS might be better off working to ensure increases in overall access to transplantation services.

Addendum

The shortage of infant hearts available for transplantation, with the high death rates among those waiting for an organ, has pushed many programs to prefer staged palliation and rarely, if ever, to offer transplantation. As in many areas of medicine, clinicians, and perhaps patients and families, seem to prefer short-term success (survival) over proven long-term benefit. For this reason, the debate represented in this pair of chapters has almost disappeared.

At the same time, another interesting phenomenon has come to light. Kon and colleagues (2003) surveyed US physicians who care for patients with HLHS: neonatologists, pediatric intensivists, pediatric cardiologists, and pediatric cardiac surgeons. They found that while the majority recommended surgery for their patients, the respondents were nearly evenly split among those who would choose comfort care (no surgery), a surgical option, or did not know what choice they would make for their own child diagnosed in the newborn period. (Forty-eight of the sample said they would terminate a pregnancy when prenatal studies diagnosed HLHS.)

Any discrepancy between clinicians' behavior regarding patients and preferences regarding themselves and their families should give us pause. Why should a practice – operations and long-term uncertainty and complications – be "good enough" for patients but not adequately convincing for the physicians personally? Kon's study suggests that perhaps the moral debate about treatment of HLHS has not really ended after all. The lack of commitment among clinicians to examine long-term outcomes through carefully condicted comparative trials among interventions before settling on a "standard of care" constitutes an important ethical problem in its own right.

8.3 Topical discussion

Transplantation

Like the child in Dr. Burne's case (Chapter 7), the infant in Dr. Chin's case suffered from hypoplastic left heart syndrome. The main indication for cardiac transplantation in children under one year of age is congenital heart disease in more than 75% of those infants, and hypoplastic heart is at the top of the list. Overall survival in the pediatric age group after five years is approximately 65%; however, patients receiving transplants at younger than one year of age have a slightly lower survival rate (62%).

Some ethical dilemmas associated with donors and procurement of organs were briefly visited in Chapter 4. Some additional dilemmas associated with recipients and access to organs are raised in this chapter. The scarcity of organs in relation to the number of possible recipients involves considerations of distributive justice. Some of the most complex issues in transplantation ethics surround the distribution and allocation of organs that become available. The competing and sometimes incompatible principles driving allocation are fairness (allowing equal access to transplantation to as many as possible), efficiency (getting the most and best use possible out of the scarce resource), and need (allocating the organs on the basis of medical urgency). From the standpoint of the best utilization of a scarce resource, an available organ might best be transplanted to the candidate who will derive the greatest benefit, in terms such as number of life years extended or extent to which function is improved. A seriously ill person on the point of death arguably has the greatest need for the organ, but may not be the recipient who would get the most and best use of the organ. An additional complication to be factored into this calculus is the established commitment of a given physician to his actual present patient, whose survival may depend upon the receipt of a second organ, or sometimes even

Ethical Dilemmas in Pediatrics: Cases and Commentaries, ed. Lorry R. Frankel, Amnon Goldworth, Mary V. Rorty, and William A. Silverman. Published by Cambridge University Press. © Cambridge University Press 2005.

a third, if the first is rejected, raising questions about fairness. Allocation of organs according to current UNOS guidelines weighs blood group compatibility, medical urgency, and time on the waiting list, in order of weight given to the factor.

In the case recounted by Dr. Chin, the child was listed prenatally – a strategy allowed by UNOS guidelines after 32 weeks gestation, in case an organ becomes available before birth. (The waiting time clock is reset at birth.) For the congenital disease of hypoplastic left heart, transplantation and reconstructive surgical operations have about the same survival rate, about 65%, at one and five years after surgery, including waiting-list mortality. The scarcity of donor hearts and the necessity for lifelong immunosuppressants can weigh in the decision between transplantation and palliative reconstructive surgery.

There is continuing controversy about transplantation as a social practice, some observers suggesting that it is overvalued relative to its personal and economic costs. Cost comparisons of renal transplantation and long-term dialysis favor transplantation, but such calculations cannot be made for situations where there is no life-preserving alternative to transplantation.

Surgical innovation: research or experimentation?

Organ transplantation is now widely accepted as the treatment of choice for a variety of diseases and functional impairments. The early history of organ transplantation represents innovation, risk, and cost to an unusually high degree, and transplantation surgery continues to represent a surgical frontier as a wider range of organs are considered appropriate for transplantation.

Progress in any pediatric surgery involves the diffusion of innovations, often associated with improvements in technology or devices, and typically relies on case series, tracking individual patients and recording their outcomes without comparing the procedure with alternatives. Only a small percentage of surgical investigators use randomized studies of their techniques, and it is only after a new surgical possibility has developed a track record that any comparison between procedures like that represented in this chapter becomes possible. Double-blind or placebo-controlled trials are typically not appropriate (although an unusual placebo-controlled trial of arthroscopic knee surgery, where the knee was cut open without further intervention, revealed results surprisingly similar to actual surgery).

Innovative surgical procedures present different ethical issues than medical or pharmaceutical research. Is innovative surgery clinical practice, or research? If research, what model of research protection is available? Should new surgical procedures be submitted to IRB review, or are institutional committees reviewing individual proposed innovations the best way both to further medical science and to safeguard patients?

Anencephalics as organ donors

The question of whether anencephalic newborns ought to be considered acceptable sources for organs has been intensely discussed but never entirely resolved, and is raised again in the exchange between Drs. Chin and Frader. It is a question driven in part by the disparity between the number of available organs and the number of potential recipients, and in part by a desire expressed by some parents of severely damaged children to turn a personal tragedy into a source of some comfort by aiding other children.

The ambivalence of the medical community on this subject is manifest in the erratic course of the AMA's Council on Ethical and Judicial Affairs, which in 1988 affirmed that anencephalic infants, as both human and alive, were inappropriate sources for organs. In an opinion published in 1995, however, that Council suggested it was "ethically permissible to consider the anencephalic as a potential organ donor, although alive still under present definitions of death . . . because of the fact the infant has never experienced, and will never experience, consciousness." Later the Council reverted to the 1988 position that requires determination of death prior to organ procurement. The larger society seems less willing to consider the question than the professional community, and because of the controversial nature of the question, anencephalics are not considered possible donors in the USA, although there have been recorded cases of transplantation of organs from anencephalics in other countries.

One of the major objections to this proposal is an argument from consistency: any criteria by which the anencephalic might be considered a potential source of organs for transplantation would apply equally well to other classes of unconscious patients, thus equivalent to a move to the controversial "higher-brain" standard of death discussed in Chapter 6. As Frader notes, there are objections as well to any proposal that justifies the "instrumentalization" of one human being in order to advantage another. The difficulty of accurately predicting the life span of anencephalics was vividly illustrated in the case of Baby K, an anencephalic child who lived for over two years and was the subject of a court case in Virginia in 1993.

Disability and transplantation

Candidates for transplantation are evaluated by each center for eligibility to be listed. The evaluation is typically conducted by a multidisciplinary transplant team, including physicians, nurses, and social workers. A candidate must be ill enough to meet medical standards of organ failure, but healthy enough to survive the operation and adapt to a transplant. Further, the candidate must have enough family support, financial resources, competency, and personal stability to manage a complicated post-transplant regimen. According to one source, about 5% of candidates are excluded on psychosocial grounds. The role of mental retardation in such evaluations poses dilemmas for decision makers. The quality of life of an organ recipient, and the extent to which it will be improved by transplantation, is an appropriate consideration. But the laws protecting the disabled are designed to prevent evaluation of the comparative quality of the baseline to which the recipient would be returned in any way that might consistently exclude the disabled from consideration.

Dr. Chin's question about the relevance of chromosomal abnormalities for transplantation might have been answered very differently in the past, and is still an open question, as the disagreement between Chin and Frader on the eligibility of trisomy-21 patients suggests. In a case in California in 1996 publicity concerning the eligibility of a self-sufficient Down-syndrome adult for a heart and lung transplant raised discussion about the impact of the 1993 Americans with Disabilities Act on access to high-risk and high-cost medical procedures. If a candidate is excluded from a medical procedure that would usually be offered, because of a disability unrelated to the source of the medical necessity, or because of membership in a disadvantaged class, the question can be raised whether there is unjust discrimination. In that California case it was successfully argued that it was the candidate's diagnosis of Down syndrome, rather than considerations of her individual ability to carry out a post-transplant regimen, that led to denial of a transplant, and after some publicity the decision was reversed. The national attention that the case drew, however, suggests that such decisions are not yet common. Exclusion of an infant with trisomy 13 or 18 from candidacy would be less controversial.

FURTHER READING

American Academy of Pediatrics. Policy statement: pediatric organ donation and transplantation. *Pediatrics* **109** (2002), 982–984.

Brower, V. The ethics of innovation: should innovative surgery be exempt from clinical trials and regulations? *EMBO Reports* **4** (2003), 338–340.

Caplan, A. L. and Coelho, D. H. *The Ethics of Organ Transplantation: the Current Debate* (Amherst, NY: Prometheus Books, 1988).

Churchill, L. R. and Pinkus, R. L. B. The use of anencephalic organs. *Milbank Quarterly* **68** (1990), 147–169.

Fox, R. and Swazey, J. *The Courage to Fail: a Social View of Transplantation and Dialysis* (Chicago, IL: University of Chicago Press, 1974).

Spare Parts: Organ Replacement in American Society (New York, NY: Oxford University Press, 1992), especially Chapter 8, "Leaving the field," pp. 197–210.

Frader, J. E. and Flanagan-Klygis, E. Innovation and research in pediatric surgery. *Seminars in Pediatric Surgery* **10** (2001), 198–203.

In re Baby K, 16 F. 3rd 590 (4th Cir. 1994).

Kichuk-Chrisant, M. Children are not small adults: some differences between pediatric and adult cardiac transplantation. *Current Opinion in Cardiology* **17** (2002), 152–159.

Moore, F. D. Ethical problems special to surgery: surgical teaching, surgical innovation and the surgeon in managed care. *Archives of Surgery* **135** (2000), 14–16.

Orentlicher, D. Rationing and the Americans with Disabilities Act. *JAMA* **271** (1994), 308–314.

Peabody, J. Organ transplantation. In *Ethics and Perinatology*, ed. A. Goldworth, W. Silverman, D. K. Stevenson, and E. W. D. Young (Oxford: Oxford University Press, 1995), pp. 184–213.

Peters, P. G. When physicians balk at futile care: implications of the disability rights laws. *Northwestern Law Review* **91** (1997), 798–864.

Reitsma, A. M. and Moreno, J. D. Ethical regulations for innovative surgery: the last frontier? *Journal of the American College of Surgeons* **194** (2002), 792–801.

Whitehead, A. Rejecting organs: the organ allocation process and the Americans with Disabilities Act. *American Journal of Law and Medicine* **24** (1998), 481–497.

9.1 Liver and intestinal transplantation

Manuel Garcia-Careaga, Ricardo Orlando Castillo, and
John A. Kerner Jr.

Introduction

In 1959, Richard Lillehei *et al.* were the first to describe the autologous intestinal transplantation of the entire small intestine in dogs (Lillehei *et al.* 1959). The transplanted bowel had an indefinite survival. One year later Starzl and Kaupp successfully transplanted multiple viscera including small bowel in dogs. The surgical techniques originally described by Starzl are employed to this day (Kocoshis 1994).

In the 1960s and 1970s, several reports of human multi-organ transplantation and intestinal transplants were published, but the immunosuppressants used at that time, consisting of prednisone and azathioprine, did not confer sufficient protection against rejection (Grant 1989). The patients did not survive longer than a few weeks. These results were so devastating that intestinal transplantation was discontinued. It was not until the discovery of cyclosporin that attempts at intestinal transplantation were resumed. The introduction of OKT3 and the use of irradiation of the graft yielded encouraging results. In a small series of four intestinal-transplant patients, two of them survived 109 and 165 days. Both of them died as a result of developing lymphoproliferative disorder but not as a result of rejection. With the appearance of newer immunosuppressants like FK506, survival significantly improved, resulting in increased implementation of this potentially life-saving procedure.

From 1990 to 1994, the group at the Children's Hospital at Pittsburgh operated on more than 50 patients of which 32 were children, ranging in age from 6 months to 15 years (Kocoshis 1994). Twenty patients had combined liver and intestinal transplants. Of those patients, 18 were surviving exclusively on oral or enteral feedings 6 to 44 months postoperatively. At the University of Miami, Andreas G. Tzakis *et al.* reported 30 intestinal transplants in 28 patients between August 1994 and May 1997. Overall patient survival was 67% and graft survival was 63%. Actuarial and two-year patient survival was 67% and graft survival 63%. They reported that all mortalities resulted from rejection and its treatment (Tzakis *et al.* 1998). Another drug, mycophenolate mofetil (CellCept), has been added to treat rejection in conjunction with FK506 and steroids. This regimen may lead to improved outcomes. More studies are needed to establish the efficacy of this drug, but at this moment the outcomes are encouraging.

Intestinal transplantation becomes a consideration when there is permanent intestinal failure as a result of disease or loss of a significant portion of the bowel. Patients who suffer from intestinal failure may be permanently dependent upon total parenteral nutrition (TPN). However, TPN may produce chronic liver damage with eventual liver dysfunction and failure. The cost of TPN may run as high as $150 000 per year. Howard and Malone (1996) reported that in 1992 in the United States there were an estimated 40 000 patients on home TPN at a cost of 600 million dollars per year. In addition, the physical constraints of TPN as well as its complexity can affect the quality of life of the entire family of an affected patient.

Intestinal transplantation is indicated in patients in whom TPN has led to severe liver disease with coagulopathy, in patients where venous access is no longer available, and when recurrence of septicemia as a result of central-line infection is a frequent occurrence. Contraindications to intestinal transplant include marked cardiopulmonary insufficiency, aggressive malignancy, advanced autoimmune disease, AIDS, existence of life-threatening intraabdominal or systemic sepsis, severe neurologic impairment, insufficient vascular access, and severe or acquired immunodeficiency (Abu-Elmagd 2003, Beath 2004, Kocoshis 2001).

In the best scenario, surgery for intestinal transplantation may take three to four hours. If the transplant is combined with liver then it may take from eight to twelve hours. During surgery, an ostomy site is created to allow frequent endoscopies with biopsies of the transplanted small bowel to be done to monitor for signs of rejection. As an example, biopsies are taken twice per week for six consecutive weeks and then each month. Enteral feedings are initiated at postoperative days 5 to 7. Patients having isolated small-intestinal transplantation stay in the intensive care unit an average of three to five days. If a combined liver/small bowel transplant is performed, a more prolonged stay may be required. After leaving the intensive care unit, patients go to the post-surgical unit. Once there, the length of the stay depends on the recovery. The major complications include graft rejection, failure of the graft, infection, and respiratory compromise.

The first liver transplant in a child was done by Starzl in 1963. The child succumbed to the attempt. Four more children were transplanted and they met the same fate as the first one. Liver transplantation came to a halt until 1966. Further research led to new attempts that met with better success. As new immunosuppressants emerged, along with better graft preservation and improved surgical techniques, we now expect a survival rate between 85% and 95% five years after transplantation in the major transplant centers in the United States. Intestinal transplantation has not yet attained the rate of success of heart, kidney, and liver transplantation, but offers the only chance for the people who would otherwise die (Vanderhoof 1996).

Case report

The following is a description of the first combined liver and small bowel transplant that was performed at our medical center. The patient was a 16-year-old girl who was born with multiple intestinal atresias requiring resection of most of her small bowel. She was left with 29 cm of small bowel without an ileocecal valve, and was totally dependent on total parenteral nutrition (TPN) for survival. After innumerable complications with parenteral nutrition, small-bowel transplantation was recommended since she no longer had acceptable venous access. Since her liver was functioning well, the recommendation was only for isolated small-bowel transplant.

As is routine in transplant cases, the psychiatry service was consulted. At 15 years of age the patient did not have an understanding of her disease, and she did not want to know about the details of the transplant. She complained of feeling depressed and being anxious. The mother related she had missed all the normal childhood experiences. She had few friends and her peers were cruel to her at school, so she was tutored at home. The mother also felt a lot of guilt and anxiety, especially because she could not stay in the hospital with her daughter because of responsibilities to another young child at home. The mother was a victim of abuse, and she had received body trauma when she was pregnant with the patient. She strongly believed that her frequent physical traumas had caused her daughter to be born with gastrointestinal disease. Several years prior to admission, the family had made the decision to "let her go" when she was very ill. The stepfather felt guilty about this decision because she did recover. The patient's disease was a challenge for the whole family.

According to the mother, during her life the medical staff had consistently treated the patient as a "little girl" and had not shared their thoughts with her. Previously, the patient had complained of doctors not involving her in the medical care. However, when the proposed transplantation was discussed with her, she only wanted to know issues in a very general way and did not want to know all the details of her situation since they "made her nervous." In terms of the transplant, the patient asked very few questions and thought about it in a very concrete way. It was clear that the patient did not understand why she had gastrointestinal problems, but she also showed no interest in knowing why. She fantasized about not having any tubes, but had not thought that she would have to learn how to eat. She also focused on the mention of cancer as one of the possible complications of therapy, but did not ask about other possible complications that were mentioned. She was very defensive and avoided any sensitive issue. She also believed she would be a good and happy patient. She had always taken responsibility for her daily care at home.

During the hospitalization, the patient developed severe hypovolemia due to the extravasation of her central line into the peritoneum. She required volume and vasopressors, and survived another crisis. Given the severity of her illness, the issue of a "do not resuscitate" order was brought up by the parents. It was agreed that if the patient's lungs or heart failed no heroic measures would be instituted. However, she did recover and was discharged 13 days later. She was sent home after direct translumbar placement of a central line into the inferior vena cava. She had a previous placement of a gastrostomy tube but only tolerated minimal infusions of elemental formula. Initially she tolerated the formula well, but soon she developed profuse diarrhea.

For the following eight months she was at her home but her liver function progressively deteriorated. It was then recommended to proceed with a combined liver and small-bowel transplant. Her clinical course turned to a rapid downhill course and she was readmitted to our institution. From this moment on, her only hope was transplantation.

The long-awaited organs arrived and the transplant was performed. It was a major endeavor in a patient with so many previous surgeries. After a series of complications involving necrosis of the bile duct, sepsis, and intra-abdominal abscesses followed by appropriate therapies, she finally stabilized. She was discharged to a transitional area and followed as an outpatient.

Five months after transplant she was transferred to our hospital because of severe anasarca, which her local hospital had no success in treating. Shortly after arriving at our center, she developed hypotension, abdominal tenderness, fever, and myoclonic jerks. She was clinically septic. Her clinical status rapidly deteriorated and the transplant team decided to take her back to the operating room. Very rapidly she became hemodynamically unstable, requiring high doses of inotropics and endotracheal intubation. In spite of these measures, she was not able to maintain adequate blood pressure and oxygen saturation. Her parents decided to discontinue support. She died with her parents and brother by her side.

Ethical issues

(1) Should young adolescent patients be fully informed by their doctors about risks and benefits when the parent refuses to allow them to deliver the grim details? In this case, our patient was fully evaluated by the psychiatry service, which determined that she could accept only general information. They also

found that the patient did not have a full understanding of her disease. We all favor a full informed consent, especially in a patient of an age that might have the capacity to assimilate the information. In this case, the patient's ability and willingness to understand the complexity of her situation was limited, and the parents were very concerned about overwhelming her with too much information. At that point we decided not to deliver more detailed information to the patient.

(2) Was our explanation of the process clear enough for the parents to make an intelligent decision, rather than solely reacting to the real possibility of losing their beloved child, if they did not pursue the last desperate measure – transplantation? Are parents capable of clearly visualizing the possible complications that the patient may incur with high-dose immunosuppresion therapy, and what might happen with graft failure? We presented the parents with a description of the procedure, information about outcomes of intestinal transplant in other centers, our experience in transplantation, the potential complications, and the possibility of death as the result of the latter. They underwent psychiatric evaluation. But perhaps that was not enough, and we needed to make the description more graphic and explicit so that the parents would more clearly understand the commitment they were making for their daughter and themselves.

(3) What is the emotional impact of receiving foreign tissue from a dead person? Other patients express disgust, fear, and curiosity. Our patient did raise this issue, but it was addressed superficially instead of being discussed at length.

(4) Should the desire not to proceed be respected, when the adolescent's refusal is based on the fears that the prospect of transplantation brings? Only after a full psychiatric evaluation of the patient, where we could feel sure that she understood that death was imminent and also understood the process of transplantation, would her refusal to proceed be honored.

(5) Since the possibility of intestinal transplantation leading to death is so high, should we devote large amounts of money to such transplants when those dollars could fund other health services that could reach hundreds of other children with serious health problems? How long will the government be able to pay for the medically indigent population without incurring deficits that result in curtailment of other highly needed services? The impact of this modality of treatment needs to be assessed in terms of how it may affect the resources of primary pediatrics and physical and mental health programs for the pediatric population in the low socioeconomic sectors. There is presently a lack of resources in these centers, with decreased medical personnel, nurses, equipment, and medical facilities. On the other hand, are we going to restrict costly life-saving procedures to those who can afford them? Intestinal-transplant outcomes are not yet as good as other organ transplants, and the cost is exorbitant.

Nonetheless, we have seen enormous progress over the past ten years, especially the last three (Langnas 2004). Better results for patient and graft survival in intestinal transplantation have been demonstrated. The learning process and experience with intestinal transplantation provided by patients such as ours is indispensable to assure the future success of new transplants to come. Steady progress has been the rule with the history of other organ transplants, and we hope that the outcomes of intestinal transplant will continue to improve as experience is gained to reduce its morbidity and mortality. Furthermore, it is expected that the cost involved in intestinal transplantation will fall as outcomes improve.

(6) Finally, should there be medical and ethical guidelines for physicians who inherit the care of short-bowel patients who have little or no chance of long-term survival without TPN?

9.2 Transplantation and adolescents

Rosamond Rhodes

Introduction

Adolescents present pediatrics and transplant surgery with ethically complex cases. The problems relate to the general question of the just allocation of scarce resources and how that issue is affected by two special features of adolescent development: the ambiguity about their decisional capacity and the instability of their commitments to adhere to post-transplant anti-rejection treatment regimens (Slater 1994, DeBolt *et al.* 1995). Combined, these concerns leave pediatricians and transplant surgeons troubled about the allocation of transplant organs to adolescents and troubled about the issue of consent. They are uncertain about when to accept adolescents' agreement to transplantation, uncertain about when to accept their refusal of transplantation, and uncertain about when to accept their decisions to become organ donors. The problems are further complicated when the adolescent is found to lack decisional capacity for making a choice about transplantation. Then the question shifts to determining whether parents should be allowed to decide and determining whether the parents are making an appropriate decision.

Assessment of decisional capacity can be an especially important issue when reasonable people see the proposed transplant as either a good or an evil and, on that basis, choose to go forward with the surgery or to refuse it. Transplantation almost always involves a lifelong commitment to immunosuppressive medications and their side effects, risk of rejection, risk of infection, and immunosuppression-related risk of neoplastic disease. There is also the ordeal of the surgery itself and the postoperative critical care hospitalization. There may also be psychological issues of living with an organ from another person and living with scars. None of these elements is pleasant. Certainly, the likelihood of success and the likelihood and seriousness of complications, as well as the alternatives to transplantation and their

Ethical Dilemmas in Pediatrics: Cases and Commentaries, ed. Lorry R. Frankel, Amnon Goldworth, Mary V. Rorty, and William A. Silverman. Published by Cambridge University Press. © Cambridge University Press 2005.

related risks and likelihoods, must be part of the calculation. Different people could give these factors different weight and reach different decisions about transplantation. In some cases almost everyone would agree that transplantation is the best option. In other cases, where the alternative to transplantation is imminent death but where the chance of success is slim and the likelihood of serious complications is high, the decision seems much more subjective.

The case described by Drs. Garcia-Careaga, Castillo, and Kerner raises the issue of whether to undertake an intestinal transplant for an immature 16-year-old girl. In this case, likelihood of long-term success would be no better than 50%. Her immaturity raises questions about her decisional capacity. On the other hand, her personal history of living with her deteriorating condition and enduring so many hospitalizations and surgical interventions gives her a unique perspective for making an informed decision. The patient's parents are clearly committed to her and concerned about her well-being. But they also feel guilty about their previous decision to allow her to die. In sum, this complicated case of an intestinal transplant for an adolescent brings to the fore the special concerns about transplantation in pediatrics: just allocation of scarce transplant organs, justified paternalism, and appropriate surrogate decision making. In what follows, I will briefly discuss each in turn and then show how our understanding of these several issues can be woven together to provide an ethical framework for thinking about this case.

Just allocation

Given the current rate of cadaveric organ donation and the current state of transplant technology, it is impossible to meet the needs of all patients who could benefit from having an organ transplant because there are not enough organs for everyone who needs one. And whenever someone is chosen to receive an organ those who are passed over and have to wait longer are harmed as they get sicker and in some cases die. Justice and fairness must, therefore, be considered in the distribution of the limited organ supply. Yet the allocation that would be just and fair is not obvious. Complex issues are subtly interrelated so that the theoretical answers are hard to reach and harder still to spell out in the individual cases that must be addressed (American Medical Association Council on Ethical and Judicial Affairs 1993).

Distributive justice

Should everyone who needs a vital organ to live or to live a significantly better life be given the same access to organ transplantation? Or are there some considerations that need to be given special consideration in the distribution? Should social grounds be taken into account or should only medical factors be considered?

Which factors should be counted and how much? Should people be given no more than one organ or should they be allowed multiple organ transplants (e.g., a lung and a heart, a kidney and a pancreas, intestines and a liver)? And if a transplanted organ immediately fails to function or is ultimately rejected after functioning in the recipient for some period of time, should the recipient be given another organ when others on the recipient list have not yet had a chance?

Most countries that perform organ transplantation develop national distribution systems that try to maximize the justice and efficacy of organ allocation for all prospective recipients. By pooling information about donor organs and recipients, a national system can match organs to the special needs of particular recipients and also be more responsive to urgent situations. Because organs must be transplanted within a short period of time after procurement, distance becomes a limiting criterion for organ sharing. In many cases, the advantage of a speedy transplant directs organs to a center that is relatively close to the site of procurement. Urgent need, ideal compatibility, or difficulty in finding an organ that will match a particular donor warrants sharing over greater distance. In the United States, a national organ distribution system, the United Network for Organ Sharing (UNOS), works to provide a just and fair distribution of transplant organs. Its current rules give priority to likelihood of success, to urgency of need, and then to length of time on the list.

If urgency were always the primary consideration, people with the least likelihood of surviving, including some who were in serious danger of losing a transplanted organ or dying regardless of receiving the transplant, would be the most likely to receive a transplant. But because fewer patients would survive transplantation if such a policy were adopted, some alternative scheme would be a better choice for maximizing the effective use of organs.

Triage

Transplant programs typically pay most attention to the medical features of gravity and also likelihood of long-term success. Including the likelihood for benefit among their criteria means that transplantation is denied to patients who have some chance of surviving with a transplant, but are so sick that those chances are not very good. This policy denies treatment to those who need it most but it also improves the overall utility of the distribution system. Such a policy also denies transplantation to those who would be likely to lose an organ because of their post-transplant behavior. Good reasons to expect that a patient would not adhere to necessary post-transplant regimens are good reasons for refusing to allocate a transplant organ.

While it is painful to remove needy patients from the organ recipient list and to triage them out of the possibility of having an organ transplant, the policy is considered to be just. Reasonable people who consider the alternatives would prefer a policy that pays attention to likelihood of benefit over a policy that does not, and therefore would give an organ to someone who dies anyway, while the person next on the list also dies because of the lack of an organ. The triage approach uses the same criteria for patients who need a first transplant, retransplantation, or multiple organ transplants. At each point of assessment the question is not about providing an equal number of chances but about applying the same allocation standards to everyone who needs an organ regardless of their transplant history. In fact, transplant surgeons consider retransplantation an essential component of their treatment. The availability of retransplantation as a therapeutic option makes the overall success rate of transplantation high enough for patients to want the procedure (Rhodes *et al.* 1992).

Social considerations

Critics of the current system complain that it is unjust to provide equal treatment for both those who are ill because of bad luck and those whose previous behavior contributed to their illness. They urge that social criteria should be applied in transplant decisions. Some would like to have taken into account considerations like the patient's previous contribution to society (hence, valuing children less than others), or the patient's future prospects for depleting the stock of social resources (hence, valuing some disabled and some with a poor work history less than others), or the patient's prospects for future contributions to society (hence, valuing children with a good prognosis more than others). And some complain about the unfairness of giving a few recipients more than one organ while others are still waiting for a first chance. Doctors who are committed to equal concern about each of their patients resist social discrimination as an anathema to the profession (Veatch 1989, Cohen and Benjamin 1991, Moss and Siegler 1991, Rhodes *et al.* 1992).

Decisional capacity and paternalism

Adolescents certainly have greater decisional capacity than younger children but they do not yet have the decisional capacity of adults. Uncertainty about the status of adolescent decisions raises questions about whether the decision of any particular adolescent should be accepted, particularly when the implications of the decisions can be dramatically harmful and long-lasting. There are some decisions that, in ordinary circumstances, should be theirs (e.g., choice of recreational activities or attire), other cases where particular options should be paternalistically denied them (e.g., experimentation with cocaine or LSD), and others where the approach will depend upon an assessment of the individual and the particular context. To provide a framework for sorting out when an adolescent's or a younger child's decision should be respected and when paternalistic intervention is well justified, we will need to review the moral concepts of autonomy and beneficence, and justifications for paternalism.

Autonomy

Roughly, what gives a human being (or a porpoise, or Mr. Spock) moral standing is the capacities that comprise the ability to be moral. Persons can think in terms of moral rules, and they can consider their own actions in terms of those rules, and they can constrain their action to conform with the rules that they accept as action guiding. These capacities amount to the ability to be autonomous and mark an individual's choices as worthy of respect.

Respect for autonomy requires us to allow others to make their own choices and to live by their own lights. Respect for autonomy tells us to leave others alone and to tolerate their choices. It also tells us that morality requires us to presume that others are autonomous and to treat them accordingly.

In respecting autonomy we should regard an individual's demonstration of self-motivated action or voluntary behavior as sufficient reason for requiring respect as an autonomous agent. Stated negatively, and more to the point, only reasons for concluding that the other is incapable of making an autonomous choice (the particular one in question) or that the other belongs to a class of individuals that are typically incapable of autonomous choice (e.g., children) could justify intervention.

This standard presents a strong presumption in favor of regarding other humans as autonomous beings, capable of making rational choices relative to their own goals. Even when another's choice strikes us as a bad idea, foolhardy, or dangerous, for the most part we must respect the decision and leave that person alone to take whatever risks he or she may choose.

Beneficence

Beneficence, however, is also an important principle of ethics. It is derived from the understanding that anyone needing help would want others to provide it, and requires that we act for the good of others. Since morality demands that we treat others as we would wish to be treated ourselves, we are obliged to treat others with beneficence, the principle of mutual love.

Paternalism

The simultaneous commitments to beneficence and to the moral standing of persons (i.e., respect for autonomy) create the problem of paternalism. Rational beings who are governed by both the principle of mutual love and the principle of respect find that in some situations they are directed by beneficence to interfere with another's choice, while respect directs them to leave the other alone. The duty of beneficence seems to require involvement in the lives of others; respect seems to require that we allow others to do their own thing. The problem for anyone who governs action according to both of these principles is to determine when paternalistic interference can be justified.

In his 1972 paper, "Paternalism," and in a follow-up entitled "Paternalism: some second thoughts," Gerald Dworkin (1983a, 1983b, 1998) articulated one of the most influential frameworks for approaching justified paternalism. In those papers, he discusses paternalism in terms of parents' restrictions on the choices of their children. With respect to parental paternalism, he suggests that such interventions "may be thought of as a wager by parents on children's subsequent recognition of the wisdom of the restrictions" (Dworkin 1983a). Dworkin recommends that we think of paternalistic interference as "being a kind of insurance policy that we take out against making decisions that are far-reaching, potentially dangerous, and irreversible" (Dworkin 1983a). Hence, Dworkin concludes that the concept of "future-oriented consent" justifies paternalistic intervention.

Using Dworkin's model, however, is not very helpful in situations where we cannot know what the adolescent would be happy with tomorrow, or the day after. Future-oriented consent as a test for autonomy turns on what the future holds. When the outcome is obvious or when the one who agrees would be satisfied with the decision even in the worst-case scenario (e.g., think of a Jehovah's Witness who prefers death to the eternal damnation expected after a blood transfusion), we can be sure that the choice is autonomous. But in cases of genuine uncertainty, Dworkin's construct is not informative. When weighing probabilities is a significant issue, we know that there are features of the alternative foreseeable outcomes that are desirable and others that are not. We know that there are aspects of the different alternatives that are appealing, others that are unappealing, and that a great many consequences of the choice are unknown and unknowable. In such cases, future-oriented consent cannot produce a judgment until the future occurs. Because so many of our choices are fraught with uncertainties, we are frequently uncertain about what to choose and no one can honestly say that tomorrow we would be happy with having chosen one alternative or another. In that light, future-oriented consent becomes useless as a mechanism for determining when paternalistic interference would be appropriate since the constraints would have to be put in place before the fact.

Examples and intuitions

The method of bioethics suggests starting with examples in order to shed some light on an enigmatic problem (Brody 1991).[1] So, for guidance with questions of justified paternalism and to inform our position on adolescent decisions about transplantation, let us consider some hypothetical examples.

---

[1] Baruch Brody has called this the "downwards-up model."

If I wanted to cut off my healthy hand, or even just a healthy finger, I imagine that most people would feel justified in paternalistically interfering and stopping me. I also imagine that I would not be able to find a surgeon who would be willing to perform the amputation for me, even if I were willing to sign all of the necessary consent forms.

Imagine that my child was involved in an accident and because of tremendous blood loss now needed a blood transfusion (i.e., a life-preserving transplant with low likelihood of serious harmful side effects). If it was likely that the child would die without the transfusion and likely that the transfusion would help her to live, I imagine that most people would not accept her refusal of the blood, regardless of her reasons. Similarly, few people would accept my refusal of blood products on her behalf, regardless of my reasons.

Imagine that I delivered a baby and after examination the child's kidneys were found not to function and several additional serious congenital anomalies were also identified. Because a cadaveric kidney transplant in a newborn is likely to be rejected, it is unlikely that one would be offered, regardless of my wishes, because it would be more just to allocate the organ to someone with a better chance of long-term benefit and because the foreseeable horrifying ordeal for the infant might not be worth the small chance of benefit. And because initiating a plan for a living related transplant after the child was sufficiently large and well nourished would require tremendous parental cooperation, providing peritoneal dialysis in the interim and willingness to donate a kidney later on, my decision would rule, regardless of my reasons. The justification for the invasive treatment would be the long-term success of a living related-donor transplant, but no one could compel me to be an organ donor for my child.

On the other hand, if I wanted to donate one of my healthy kidneys to my seven-year-old child who had kidney failure and needed one, people would support my choice and the kidney transplant team would be eager to cooperate. Nevertheless, pressure from other family members and society at large (which raises eyebrows whenever parents survive a fire unscathed while their offspring perish) could be so coercive as to make a parent feel unable to withhold consent.

If, however, I wanted to donate my heart to save my child, I am sure the heart transplant team would refuse to cooperate. And if I wanted to donate one kidney to each of my two children who each needed one to avoid dialysis, I imagine that the kidney transplant team would either not accept my consent as valid or simply refuse to act on it.[2]

---

[2] Or consider the recent headline case of a father who wanted to donate his second kidney to his adolescent daughter after she lost his first donated kidney to rejection subsequent to non-compliance with her anti-rejection regimen.

If I was willing to be a bone marrow donor for a total stranger, my consent would be accepted and I would be seen as a hero. On the other hand, if I volunteered my three-year-old child who, when asked, said "yes," or presented my seven-year-old who clearly articulated her willingness to donate marrow to save the dying stranger, it is not obvious whether people would accept their agreement as consent. If these children were agreeing to donate a kidney instead, it would be even more likely that people would refuse to count their consent. Yet we might be inclined to accept the consent of a large child (or child-like older individual) to donate blood for the stranger or the consent of one sibling to donate a kidney to the other and we might even determine that the child's consent was not necessary for the moral acceptability of that donation.[3]

I suspect that this survey of responses produces a clear and uniform set of intuitions. When the risk of death without treatment is great and when treatment offers a high likelihood of preserving life with low likelihood of causing physical harm, neither a child's nor a parent's refusal of blood transfusion is respected. When death is a certainty for the heart donation, people reject my consent. When death is only a remote possibility, my consent to a non-medically indicated amputation is refused while my consent to kidney or marrow donation, which may involve no less of a risk, or even a greater risk, is accepted. So, risk itself could not be the crucial consideration.

When it comes to a child's consent, because their decisional capacity is questionable, our acceptance of their donation is uncertain. But when the risk is small or when the need is urgent, the quality of the consent and even the need for consent seem irrelevant. So consent, in itself, could not be the sole criterion for our decisions.

And when the anephric infant's situation is urgent, we do not compel a parent to provide labor-intensive care and we do not forcibly remove a parent's kidney for transplant to the child. We sometimes accept limits on resources (no cadaveric kidney for the anephric infant) and beneficence (no sacrifice of my heart for my child), perhaps because the chance for a good outcome seems so remote or because the sacrifice seems too great. So urgency, alone, does not dictate the answer.

In the case of one child donating for another sibling, the children's familial relation is significant. But personal relationship is unnecessary for the acceptability of my marrow donation for the dying stranger. So familial bonds do not supply a sufficient account either.

Risk, consent, likelihood of success, wherewithal, and relationship all seem to be considerations in deciding when to perform a transplant or to accept an organ

---

[3] Recent legal cases have reached just such conclusions (e.g., *Strunk* v. *Strunk* [445 S.W.2d 145 (1969 Ky.)]; *Hart* v. *Brown* [29 Conn. Supp. 368; 289 A.2d 386 (1972 Conn. Supr. Ct.)]; *Little* v. *Little* [576 S.W.2d 493 (1979 Tex. App.)]).

donation, but how they fit together and why is not clear. Why does agreement sometimes have to be respected? When can consent be set aside? If we accept the consent of recipients and prospective donors, we respect their autonomy. If we refuse to accept their consent out of concern for their good we are treating them paternalistically. Is such paternalism ever morally acceptable?

A Kantian answer

While it is common to see paternalistic action in conflict with respect for autonomy, there is a way of reconciling the two as the good parent does. Immanuel Kant, the nineteenth-century philosopher who focused our attention on the primacy of autonomy, wrestled with the problem of justifiable paternalism. In what follows I will adopt a Kantian approach to the issue as it presents itself in modern transplant practice.

In Kant's framework, we are bound to "cast a veil of philanthropy over the faults of others" (Kant 1983: 466). Respect for the other as an end in himself requires us to presume, whenever possible, that his action is autonomous. We have

a duty to respect man even in the logical use of his reason: not to censure someone's errors under the name of absurdity, inept judgment, and the like, but rather to suppose that in such an inept judgment there must be something true, and to seek it out. (Kant 1983: 463)

In other words, as far as possible, Kant demands that we try to consider another's actions *as if* they were freely done, autonomously. Respect requires us to try to think of what another does as something we too would find reasonable if only we knew the facts of the situation as we should imagine the other does. The standard suggests, however, that when another's act cannot be comprehended as something reasonable, in spite of a sincere effort to imagine a context in which it might be reasonable, we have grounds for paternalistic intervention.

Obviously, since paternalistic interference is ideally applied before another's autonomy-threatening act could be performed, in some cases an assessment of the other's capacity for autonomy is the paramount consideration: a person might be either incapable of making the decision in question or incapable of reason. In some cases the other's choice could be the salient consideration. We could decide that although there was no independent reason (e.g., known intoxication or psychosis) to suppose that the person lacked the capacity for autonomy, if this particular choice were enacted the person's future autonomy would undoubtedly be compromised. In each situation, after finding the other's choice inappropriate or capacity inadequate, the paternalistic agent must ascertain whether or not failing to interfere would make the other's future autonomous action impossible. If it would, because autonomy is such a significant good in the Kantian scheme, the agent would be morally bound to perform the paternalistic act of beneficence. On the other hand, when there would be no irremediable effect on the other's autonomy, regardless of how foolish or undesirable one might think the action, "[w]hat they count as belonging to their happiness is left up to them to decide" (Kant 1983: 388).

The end of the other's continued existence as an autonomous being, therefore, serves as the limiting conception for paternalism. (1) When autonomy can only be preserved by paternalistic action (e.g., stopping me when I want to cut off my own hand), because it preserves autonomy, the only thing which has absolute worth, we must interfere. (2) When a person's capacity for autonomous action is not jeopardized by their choice (e.g., when I want to donate marrow to a stranger) paternalistic interference would not be justified. (3) If, however, there is no possibility of preserving autonomy (e.g., the requisite mental status can never be restored) no duties *qua* "end in itself" can be owed to the other.

Physical welfare as well as psychological well-being (Kant 1983: 393–4) count as needs which must be met for continuing agency. Seriously compromising either (but not merely making oneself somewhat worse-off or somewhat diminishing one's chance for continued agency) would make future autonomous action impossible. These autonomy-preserving justifications for paternalistic interference explain why Kant sees "minors and the mentally deranged" as broad classes of people who are generally exempted from the autonomy-respecting rule (Kant 1983: 454). Without autonomy-preserving paternalistic interference the future autonomy of minors can be jeopardized. Without such interference the temporarily deranged might never have their autonomy restored.

Besides referring to needs as a test in determining the appropriate domain for paternalistic interference with another, we can also rely upon a Kantian recast version of hypothetical consent. An act of paternalism is justified by hypothetical consent when I could not imagine how another could possibly assent to it. Paternalistic interference would be justified if a paternalistic agent were to find that he could not "contain the end of this action in himself" (Kant 1983: 430). To illustrate, consider some of the previous examples. Paternalism would be justified when I wanted to cut off my healthy hand. Because an agent could not imagine any end which another might adopt that would motivate such an action (i.e., hypothetically, s/he could not conceive of herself consenting to the self-amputation), s/he must paternalistically act to preserve autonomy and stop me from severing my hand. Paternalism would not be justified for the adult stranger's bone marrow donation because an agent could imagine a rational person consenting to accept some pain, scarring, and inconvenience to save another's life.

This autonomy-preserving hypothetical-consent test differs from other models for delimiting paternalism which rely upon hypothetical consent (VanDeVeer 1980, Dworkin 1983a, 1983b) in that it does not ask the paternalistic agent to conceive what s/he could not know – whether the beneficiary would or would not consent, which is the test invoked in "substituted judgment." Kantian hypothetical consent is assessed straightforwardly, on this view, according to one's own conception of what would gain the consent of any rational agent.[4]

This test for the appropriateness of paternalism, in a typical Kantian fashion, relates to the form of the agent's willing rather than to external criteria of the beneficiary's condition. Instead of requiring proof of the other's lack of rationality or competence, the moral standard demands only a sincere effort to test one's judgment by the autonomy-preserving principle of paternalism.

Surrogate decision making

When healthcare decisions have to be made and the patient cannot make decisions or lacks the capacity to make the particular decisions at issue, a surrogate is called upon to make decisions on the patient's behalf. Competent adults are allowed to designate a specific person as a proxy to make decisions for them about health matters when they are unable to do so for themselves. Adults can also make their wishes about health care known through an advance directive. These mechanisms are not available for children because in most cases it is appropriate to assume that they lack the capacity to make such decisions. Instead, we presume that parents are the appropriate surrogates for making decisions on behalf of their children, unless they are making decisions by an inappropriate standard or they show themselves to lack capacity for making the decisions.

Standards for surrogate decision making

In adult medicine we accept three alternative standards for surrogate decision making: substituted judgment, best interest, and reasonableness. Substituted judgment involves the surrogate deciding about treatment based on an assessment of what the patient would have chosen in the situation at hand. Best interest involves the surrogate choosing between alternatives with a view to achieving what is best for the patient all things considered. The reasonable-person standard allows the surrogate to take account of a wider array of considerations in making a decision about what is a reasonable course of action under the circumstances, including the impact on other family members, and the costs and burdens of prolonged treatment.

---

[4] Concern about the patient's idiosyncratic views, personal history, previous statements, etc. have limited relevance according to the rational-agent perspective, while they would count a great deal for those who base hypothetical consent on a determination of what the particular beneficiary would have wanted. Furthermore, healthcare workers must always be alert to the possibility that their own personal history may influence their view of rationality. It is the view of rationality rather than the view of the patient's or healthcare provider's idiosyncrasies which may justify and direct paternalistic interference.

Substituted judgment and best interest arise as standards in some state law that relates to end-of-life decisions. The reasonable-person standard is a far more common legal standard for decision making.

Assessing a surrogate's decisions

When the healthcare team can accept the view that the surrogate is relying upon any one of the three acceptable standards in making decisions on behalf of the patient, the surrogate's decisions should be allowed to govern the patient's care. However, "the veil of philanthropy" that we appropriately extend to decisions that people make for themselves does not cover surrogate decisions. Because health professionals have a moral duty to act for their patient's good, they have a responsibility to scrutinize surrogate decisions for their patients and to be ready to challenge their authority when the decisions seem to violate all of the appropriate decision-making standards. In other words, one should be allowed far greater discretion in healthcare decisions for oneself than in those that one makes on behalf of another. Surrogate decisions are subject to far greater inspection and interrogation than decisions that one makes about one's own care. For example, an adult patient may refuse some particular life-preserving treatment because it would involve a breech of his or her religious convictions. That person could not refuse the same treatment for his or her child on those grounds.

And just as patients may lack the capacity to make decisions about their health care, surrogates may also lack capacity. In fact, because of their responsibility to the patient, health professionals should be alert to the possibility of surrogate lack of capacity and be prepared to challenge inappropriate surrogate decisions, especially when the decisions are likely to have a serious and harmful impact on the patient (Rhodes and Holzman 2004).

Case discussion

With some understanding of the problem of just allocation of scarce transplant organs, with the autonomy-preserving criterion for paternalistic interference in mind, and with some guidelines for assessing surrogate decisions, let us examine the complicated case of this 16-year-old who needs a transplant of liver and small bowel. The moral acceptability of providing her with the transplant is certainly not obvious.

Just allocation in this case

Triage allocation of transplant organs requires us to consider the likelihood of success of the transplant. That other recipients would have a significantly greater chance of surviving with the organ could justify withholding an organ from someone who would surely die without one. Intestinal transplantation is a relatively new therapy and it has not yet achieved the level of success that we find in the transplantation of some other organs. At this point in the intestinal transplant experience with children, overall patient and graft survival is about 70% at one year and 50% at five years. The surgery is only offered to those who live with intravenous nutrition, and primarily to those who are not likely to survive long without the transplant because of complications or other indications for a poor prognosis. In this environment of offering a transplant in relatively few circumstances, there is still a shortage of transplant organs. About 30% to 60% of intestinal transplant candidates die while waiting for an organ. Yet, given the population who would be candidates for intestinal transplantation, there is no reason to expect a worse outcome for our patient than any other. Hence, there is no reason for her not to be listed for an organ (OPTN 2003, Table 1.14).

The allocation problem in our patient's case, however, is complicated by her need for a liver as well as small bowel. Properly selected patients who receive liver transplants now can be expected to have an 80% to 95% chance to survive at least five years. Clearly, that prediction cannot be made for our patient. Patients who need only liver transplantation but who have a significantly lower likelihood for success (e.g., only 60% to 70%) could be ruled out for getting a liver transplant from the national organ pool on triage criteria. Even after triage excludes patients with a less favorable chance for success from liver transplant listing, and even after innovative techniques, such as reduced, split, and living related transplant, have increased the supply of organs available, about 10% of listed children die waiting for liver transplantation (OPTN 2003, Chapter 5). Our patient certainly would not meet the liver transplant standard for likely survival. However, additional considerations could incline us to list her for a liver transplant.

It is certainly a matter of chance that some people's illness afflicts the bowel while for others it afflicts the liver. Technology has provided a successful therapy to rescue those with liver failure. The procedure to save those with small-bowel failure is not as well perfected. Perhaps this inequality in available therapy justifies some license in allocating some liver transplants to patients who also need small-intestine transplants. To the extent that the disparity in success is merely the result of developing expertise in one area before adequately exploring the other, fairness is certainly an issue. To the extent that the disparity of results is an unavoidable difference related to the special physiological problems of different organs and our current technology, holding the line at triage would be appropriate.

Presently, a transplanted liver is believed to protect the intestines from rejection after transplantation. That could improve the chance for success of a combined organ transplant enough to allow combined liver/small-bowel transplantation patients to be considered for liver transplantation along with the rest. Using animal models aggressively to develop a better understanding of the particular physiological problems of these transplants and to further refine the technology should be the first path to improving their success. Yet, when that route takes us to its limits, fairness, in this case an effort to equalize success, could at least justify the allocation of some transplant livers in an attempt to improve the odds of success with combined liver/small-bowel transplantation. That reasoning would allow allocation of some transplant livers to patients who need small-bowel/liver transplantation until we knew that the disparity in success could not be reconciled.

Patient autonomy and justified paternalism in this case

Using the autonomy-preserving principle of paternalism, should this 16-year-old's choice about transplantation be respected or should her refusal be overridden? The answer is determined by the assessment of whether her choice reflects autonomy. If it is an autonomous decision it must be respected. On the other hand, if we view her choice as a non-autonomous act, we would have to consider how refusing transplantation might affect her future autonomy.

While morality usually requires us to presume that the decisions others make are autonomous, the choices of children are the classic exception to that rule. We always feel duty-bound to evaluate our children's acts, to teach them how to think,[5] and to protect them from the predictable harms of their choices (e.g., disability, loss of freedom, death). We do this so that when our children become autonomous, they will be free of handicaps and able to do what they choose. Adolescents fall into a gray zone where it is unclear whether to assume that they need paternalistic protection or that they are fully autonomous. Often the justifiable presumption is that the adolescent's autonomy status is somewhere between childhood and maturity. In these cases, choices with the most serious consequences should be examined; some of their choices should be respected and others constrained. The autonomy-preserving principle of paternalism informs us that the likelihood, extent, and degree to which predictable harms might restrict future autonomy determine whether an adolescent's choice should be restricted or respected.

The psychiatric consultants involved in this case found our adolescent patient to lack the capacity to make decisions about her transplantation. Even though her unique perspective could give her the greatest insight for making a decision, the account of her experience and her comments support the psychiatrists' conclusion. Taken together, these considerations provide good reason for doubting that she has the capacity to make decisions about transplantation and for not accepting

---

[5] This is a particularly Kantian example. See, for example, "The didactic of ethics" (Kant 1983).

her transient refusal of transplantation. The alternative is to involve surrogates for decision making.

Also, based on our patient's previous history of taking responsibility for her daily care, the psychiatrists concluded that she would adhere to her post-transplant medical treatment. So, in spite of the problems that many adolescents have with adhering to their post-transplant care regimens, the assessment of our patient's future compliance with post-transplant therapy should allow the team to proceed with a transplant if that accorded with the surrogates' decision.

Furthermore, considerations of risk, likelihood of success, and the wherewithal required for success, should all be taken into account. Because an optimal outcome is unlikely, because the risks of prolonged suffering are significant, and because a tremendous amount of physical, emotional, and financial resources are needed for success, it is not hard to imagine that reasonable people of good will could come to different conclusions about whether or not to go ahead with transplantation in this complex case. For these reasons, a good deal of discretion should be allowed to the surrogates.

Surrogate decision making in this case

Because of their relationship and clear commitment to the well-being of their daughter, our patient's mother and stepfather are the obvious surrogates for making decisions about her transplant. Yet, because surrogates should not be accorded the same presumption of respect for their decisions as should be allowed for a person who makes decisions for herself, the transplant team is appropriately somewhat skeptical about their choices. In particular, the stepfather's guilt about having previously been willing to let her die when she was gravely ill raises questions about the reasonableness of their decision to proceed with transplantation.

Three questions should be asked about the surrogate's decision. Are they using an appropriate standard for considering what to do? Are they choosing to compromise future autonomy? Are they choosing something that cannot be comprehended as reasonable? Because they seem to be trying to decide what will be best for the patient, the team can have confidence that they are using an appropriate standard for surrogate decision making. Furthermore, because proceeding with transplantation is more likely to enhance the patient's autonomy than to compromise it, and because the decision can be seen as reasonable, the transplant team can feel secure that the decision is acceptable. These considerations make it clear that it is important to evaluate the approach of the surrogates in determining whether they should be making decisions on behalf of a patient who lacks the capacity to decide for herself. Then it is important to examine the decision of the surrogates, rather than their state of mind, in deciding whether to go along with their choice.

Summing up

This case of intestinal transplantation for an adolescent is complex for many reasons. None of the issues it raises has a simple answer. This discussion has touched on three central ethical issues. Others raised by Drs. Garcia-Careaga, Castillo, and Kerner are also compelling. Taken together they illustrate that transplantation in the pediatric setting is challenging, not only for the many technical problems it presents, but also because of the difficult moral terrain that has to be negotiated. Successful organ transplantation requires a tremendous team effort. Some of that energy has to be directed to the moral concerns.

9.3 Topical discussion

Innovation and risk

The more novel a treatment, whether in the medical community at large or in a particular treatment center, the higher the risks for a patient considering a treatment, as the discussion by the physicians in this case reveals. Not only does the technology associated with a novel procedure improve, the statistics improve for a given center as the associated surgeons gain experience, so the risk for the first patient in a procedure or in a center is much higher than for later candidates. The last three decades of organ transplantation offer a case study in the costs and benefits of innovation in surgical techniques, and have been extensively commented upon by scholars in many disciplines. Our authors raise questions not only about the feasibility of this particular procedure for this particular disease, but also about the justice of the distribution of the healthcare dollar between expensive procedures that benefit a few and less expensive treatments for other diseases that may benefit more – much discussed questions of utilitarian ethics and public health. The open and decentralized US system of health care and reimbursement renders many such considerations moot, since there is no designated "healthcare dollar" in that society that cannot be allocated in other ways.

Adolescence and decision making

Both this case and the next represent difficult healthcare decisions about high-risk medical treatments involving adolescents. Fluctuation between independence and dependence normally characterizes this stage of human development, and caregivers must acknowledge both the adolescent patient's wishes and the ultimate decision-making right of the parent or surrogate. Professional societies address decision making by adolescent minors by distinguishing between "consent" and

Ethical Dilemmas in Pediatrics: Cases and Commentaries, ed. Lorry R. Frankel, Amnon Goldworth, Mary V. Rorty, and William A. Silverman. Published by Cambridge University Press. © Cambridge University Press 2005.

"assent." The distinction acknowledges the formal status as minor of a child until the legal age of majority, but is designed to encourage the greatest possible exchange of information and elicitation of values between parents, caregivers, and the adolescent patient. Discussion in the literature acknowledges that both the likelihood of success and the consequences of refusal need to be taken into consideration in weighing the preferences of adolescents and their parents in treatment choices. If the stakes are low, refusals are more likely to be accepted than if the treatment being offered is life-sustaining or offers a high likelihood of serious improvement.

The adolescent patient in this case is described as being passive about the decision to transplant and incurious about – perhaps even unwilling to hear about – the complex procedure, its demands, and consequences. At an age where many adolescents are developing their independence and separate identities, this young woman had few contacts outside the family and a long history of medical dependence. Rhodes notes that the decisional capacity of adolescents in general is ambiguous but concludes that in this case, because of the seriousness of the consequences of refusing a transplant and the patient's disinterest (or inability) in acquiring relevant information, the candidate should not be considered capable of refusing and the parents' decision to proceed should be accepted. Granowetter, commenting on the next case (Chapter 10), wishes she had heard more discussion in the case about what was known about the values and interests of the patients before they became incapable of expressing their wishes.

Informed consent

Informed consent is a professional issue with ethical implications and legal teeth. It is a *global* issue: it arises in virtually every clinical encounter. And it is a *central* professional issue: it is crucial for physician–patient relationships, a litmus-paper test for the adequacy of communication between the caregiver and the patient. Lying behind the paired issues of consent and refusal is the ethical issue of *autonomy*: both negative (the right of non-interference; freedom from restraint or coercion) and positive (the right of self-determination; the control of my body and life). It has legal teeth because, in law, unconsented touching is a tort.

The legal implications of informed consent in the clinical setting have been developed through a series of court cases in which judges have suggested what ought to have been done instead of what was done. The standards are discussed at length in Rhodes' commentary, and are evolving in the direction of greater patient participation. Consent for research, though not explicitly at stake in the cases presented here, is also a controversial and much-discussed issue.

Capacity and voluntariness are preconditions for valid informed consent, conditions which are typically unavailable in pediatric patients, for whom parents or other surrogates decide. The "information" elements which need to be disclosed include the nature of the therapy, its purpose, risks, and predictable consequences, benefits, and probability of success, as well as discussion of feasible alternatives and prognosis if the therapy is not given. If the patient or surrogate understands the physician's recommendation, a decision can be made and authorized by signing a consent form. The literature on informed consent emphasizes that it is a process of communication and comprehension, not simply a signature on a form, that validates the consent process.

Problems with the ideal of informed consent

It's impossible. Not every individual is the ideal communicator – or the ideal listener. The context of clinical practice provides institutional limits on both the hearer and the speaker. Individual thresholds for information differ. And communicability itself is a limit: even if you talk forever about what I should expect, I will never know what something is like for me until I experience it. That is why clinicians have to try so hard even to asymptotically approach the ideal of informed consent, and why a personal relationship between physician and patient, on which trust can be based, is so important.

It may be undesirable, or undesired. In some cultures there are explicit conventions governing disclosure of bad news that may run counter to those mandated by current medical expectations. Indeed, ancient Hippocratic practice recommended against disclosure of bad news. Some clinicians express concern about the therapeutic effects of some kinds of disclosure, and what few empirical studies have been done suggest that patients not only rely heavily on the clinical expertise of their physicians, they tend to follow physician recommendations and in some cases may explicitly request the doctor to decide. (Any such requests should be witnessed and documented.)

It's a theoretical nightmare. It is justified by both the value of autonomy and by the value of beneficence – it's my right, and it is in my best interest. But while the two should reinforce each other, in some situations they may contradict. So practitioners need to develop a delicate ethical sense.

In practice, it is the rock on which every failure of professional clinical practice founders. If anyone does not like the results of an intervention or decision, they can always argue failure of informed consent (since it is, after all, impossible), and sue.

FURTHER READING

Applebaum, P. S., Lidz, C. W., and Meisel, A. *Informed Consent: Legal Theory and Clinical Practice* (New York, NY: Oxford University Press, 1987).

Arnold, R. M., Shaw, B. W., and Purtilo, R. Acute, high-risk patients: the case of transplantation. In *Surgical Ethics*, ed. L. B. McCullough, J. W. Jones, and B. A. Brody (New York, NY: Oxford University Press, 1998), pp. 97–115.

Faden, R. R. and Beauchamp, T. L. *A History and Theory of Informed Consent* (New York, NY: Oxford University Press, 1986).

Ghanekar, A. and Grant, D. Small bowel transplantation. *Current Opinion in Critical Care* **7** (2001), 133–137.

Ghobrial, R., Farmer, D., Amersi, F., *et al.* Advances in pediatric liver and intestinal transplantation. *American Journal of Surgery* **180** (2000), 328–334.

Goldworth, A. Standards of disclosure in informed consent. *In Ethics and Perinatology*, ed. A. Goldworth, W. Silverman, D. K. Stevenson, and E. W. D. Young (Oxford: Oxford University Press, 1995), pp. 263–278.

Ross, L. F. Health care decision making by children: is it in their best interest? *Hastings Center Report* **27** (6) (1997), 41–45.

Part IV

Institutional impediments to ethical action

Institutional arrangements can impede or facilitate ethically excellent medical care. As clinical ethics matures, increasing attention is being paid to the institutional contexts in which health care is provided, and the ethical impact of recent changes in methods of care delivery. The growth of this new area of bioethical focus is adumbrated in the third of the articles in this section. Thinking about ethics in organizations, as well as in the interactions between individuals, can take various forms. Clinical ethics problems can be caused or exacerbated by structural arrangements within institutions. Recurrence of similar clinical ethics problems can sometimes be prevented by institutional changes in staffing, accountability, or interventions. Further, many clinical ethics issues, such as confidentiality, informed consent, or disclosure and truth telling, have institutional analogues which must be addressed by different strategies than their individual-level counterparts. Institutional structures or routines can cause ethical problems in particular cases, and sources of ethical distress which are out of the control of individual caregivers can sometimes be ameliorated by scrupulous attention to institutional processes. Heightened sensitivity to ethical issues in clinical practice opens the door to considering ways in which the organizations within which clinicians practice can improve their ethical climate.

The three cases in this part call attention, in different ways, to structural sources of ethical perplexities. In one case, the structure of medical practice causes difficulties that thoughtful structural interventions can ameliorate; in another an institutional component, the ethics committee, carries out its function in a way that impedes, rather than facilitates, the ethical climate of an institutional unit. The final contribution explicitly addresses the ethical impact on traditional medical practice of changes in the structure of healthcare reimbursement.

In Chapter 10, Lorry Frankel and Joseph DiCarlo describe two end-stage cancer cases where increasing complexity of medical management led to multiple failures – both of organ systems and of communication systems. When several medical specialties or divisions are involved in the care of one seriously ill patient, concurrent decisions are constantly being made about treatment options. Any of them in isolation might have predictable outcomes, but it can also happen that in combination they fail to arrest the decline of a dying patient. Frankel and DiCarlo's first case illustrates the difficulty of coordinating care with one family and two professional decision makers, and underlines the importance of coordination between caregiving teams. Their second case adds another complicating factor: assuring adequate communication with the family when rapidly changing conditions necessitate changes in the care plan. In this age of specialty medicine, few individual doctors can be both intensivists and oncologists, or oversee all aspects of a complex case involving several disease processes. But when medical management is distributed among various specialties, it is easy to lose track of the important question of who is talking for – and to – whom. An institution with complex patterns of responsibility in critical units needs to open an explicit discussion about what structures or mechanisms will facilitate communication between care teams, and how to maintain what the respondent calls "clear and ongoing communication" with the family.

The physician respondent, Linda Granowetter, returns the discussion to the question of futility, which when defined narrowly as true physiological futility, she suggests, can open discussions among family and professional caregivers. The absence of such discussions, as the two cases illustrate and the commentator emphasizes, is itself an ethical failing. Dr. Granowetter's lucid commentary points to another way in which these two cases differ from the other cases in this part: the two patients are old enough to have considered preferences which need to be factored into decision making. She laments, "in no part of these case histories do I see anyone specifically speaking about the child's perspective." As Rosamond Rhodes suggests in her commentary on a transplantation case in Chapter 9, when pediatric medicine has to deal with adolescents, the tentative and volatile nature of their decisional capacity can further complicate complex cases.

If the first chapter in this part represents a problem for which there may be an institutional solution, the second represents an ethical problem which has an institutional cause. In Chapter 11, nurse educator Joy Penticuff presents the case of an infant with necrotizing enterocolitis for whom intravenous feedings were becoming increasingly painful. While there was family and caregiver consensus that the number of venopunctures to restart hyperalimentation should be limited, the way that decision was reached and the misrepresentation about who initiated the discussion caused great damage to unit morale. Policies and procedures surrounding the operation of the ethics committee failed the practitioners in this case, and represent an ethical failure on an institutional level.

Dr. Penticuff takes the occasion of this troubling case to expand on a particularistic and case-sensitive "ethics at arm's length" that represents a powerful and immediate version of clinical ethical sensitivity. Penticuff contrasts bioethics, which often approaches cases from the standpoint of principles, with nursing ethics, arising out of the particularities of nursing practice. She echoes the concern of Dr. Silvers in Chapter 5 for attention to relationships and the particular details of specific cases. The psychological impact of clinical decisions on the caregivers most intimately involved in the care of the patients is also specifically invoked as an ethically relevant consideration in ethically troubling cases.

The respondent, philosopher Mary Rorty, calls attention to the fact that although there is general agreement that it is equally appropriate, ethically and professionally, to either withhold or withdraw inappropriate medical treatment, including artificially provided nutrition and hydration, the formulation of the decision in this case was to limit the number of venopunctures for restarting hyperalimentation. She explores psychological issues and differing approaches to ethical deliberation as possible reasons for this formulation of the decision, and criticizes the institutional ethics committee for their role, suggesting that the perception within the institution of the kind of decisions the committee makes can damage their standing and usefulness. Her thoughtful critique of the impact of the ethics committee process on the hospital as a whole is a contribution to the literature on ethics consultation, as well as a move toward an organizational ethics.

Chapter 12, by Douglas Diekema, departs from the format of the rest of the book. Explicitly asking what effect the shift in healthcare delivery from fee-for-service medicine to managed care will have on the ethical practice of medicine, a physician who also has a Master's degree in public health presents four cases illustrating ways in which managed care poses a challenge to the physician–patient relationship. Cost-containment strategies explicitly adopted by some managed care organizations restrict the access of patients to referrals to specialists, limit the range of treatment options physicians can offer, offer incentives to physicians to limit care, and can even limit the access of patients to the health system. The new model of healthcare financing which managed care represents casts traditional clinical ethics issues such as disclosure and truth telling, informed consent, and fiduciary responsibility in a new light, and can introduce conflicts of interest into physician–patient relationships which physicians must guard against.

Respondent Nancy Jecker continues Dr. Diekema's examination of managed care strategies by discussing rationing within managed care organizations. She spells out clearly several methods of rationing adopted by MCOs for cost containment, including limits on providers, refusal of treatment to non-subscribers, practice guidelines which limit physician discretion, and various financial incentives which can encourage undertreatment, reduce time spent with patients, limit specialist referrals, reduce hospital admissions and lengths of stay, and substitute cost for quality in treatment decisions. Dr. Jecker raises the question of whether physician–patient relationships as we know them can survive in this new environment, or whether, as one commentator suggests, medicine needs a new ethics to go along with its new economics. Resisting the notion that physicians can ignore rationing decisions, she suggests that they might respond by explicitly paying attention to issues of justice and making the rationing process publicly accountable, consistent, and less arbitrary and unfair.

In discussing managed care strategies the contributors are discussing systemic, rather than merely institutional, constraints on ethical care. The move from ethical consideration of cases to ethical consideration of institutions, organizations, and structures represents the next stage of evolution of healthcare ethics.

10.1 Ethical problems encountered with oncology and bone marrow transplant patients

Lorry R. Frankel and Joseph V. DiCarlo

Introduction

In an attempt to inform the reader of the ethical problems encountered in the pediatric intensive care unit with the care of oncology and bone marrow transplant patients, we present two cases, one of leukemia and the other of Hodgkin's lymphoma. The issues which these cases raise are complex, as they involve medical input from multiple services, concerns about communication and informed consent, the initiation of aggressive therapies with limited benefit, and decision-making power.

The first case involves a nine-year-old girl with acute lymphoblastic leukemia (ALL) who developed respiratory failure and *Candida* sepsis. The second case involves a 16-year-old female with Hodgkin's disease who underwent a bone marrow transplant (BMT) and then sustained complications in the post-transplant period.

The two cases

Multisystem organ failure and acute lymphoblastic leukemia

AD was a nine-year-old Latina who developed respiratory failure soon after her chemotherapy for relapsed lymphoblastic leukemia. She was first diagnosed with leukemia in Central America at the age of four. After the girl received an incomplete course of therapy, her mother brought her to the United States in hopes of receiving adequate treatment. She was treated into remission within a few months, but two years later the recurrence of her cancer was discovered on routine screening examination of her cerebrospinal fluid.

Re-induction therapy was begun, consisting of four intravenous chemotherapeutic agents as well as three medications delivered into the cerebrospinal fluid. She had great difficulty this time around, with mouth and throat pain and protracted

Ethical Dilemmas in Pediatrics: Cases and Commentaries, ed. Lorry R. Frankel, Amnon Goldworth, Mary V. Rorty, and William A. Silverman. Published by Cambridge University Press. © Cambridge University Press 2005.

vomiting resulting in hospitalization for extreme dehydration. Her chemotherapy was continued at reduced doses. Cell counts dropped as expected from therapy, leaving her with temporary reductions in platelets, white blood cells, and red blood cells. She received nutrition intravenously. After ten days of hospitalization, her respiratory status became labored, even though her white blood cell count had recovered and there were signs of remission from her leukemia. She began to show signs of sepsis as indicated by an elevated temperature to 40.9 °C. Blood cultures were obtained on successive days and eventually grew fungus, *Candida albicans*. Antifungal and antibacterial treatment were begun, but her respiratory distress worsened, and she became hypotensive. She was transferred from the oncology ward to the pediatric intensive care unit for further stabilization and management.

Intravenous fluids and dopamine were used to treat her hypotension, and increasing concentrations of oxygen were needed to support her through her pneumonia. A fiberoptic bronchoscopy was performed to obtain culture material from the lungs. *Candida albicans* was again isolated. Over the next two days her respiratory status further deteriorated, and her clinical picture was consistent with acute respiratory distress syndrome (ARDS). This syndrome carries a 38% mortality rate in previously healthy patients; in the severely immunodepressed bone marrow transplant population, mortality approaches 100%. This child's prognosis was somewhere in between. Her mother remained at the bedside as much as possible throughout this period, but was struggling to continue breast-feeding her one-year-old son. Through an interpreter, she was informed that her daughter's lungs had failed, and that intubation and mechanical ventilation would be necessary in order to support respiration. She consented.

Respiratory function declined further, necessitating treatment with very high (70–100%) concentrations of oxygen to yield marginally adequate serum oxygen levels (50–60 torr). High ventilator pressures were needed as well. Strategies were adopted to limit the exposure of the lungs to high pressures, with only modest success. Eventually suboptimal blood gas parameters were accepted, in order to limit complications from the ventilator.

The child's cardiovascular function improved after several days of therapy, and liver and kidney function remained intact, but lung function continued to worsen. The arterial pH hovered for days between 7.15 and 7.24, along with a greatly elevated carbon dioxide level (65–80 torr). Physicians counseled the mother that survival was unlikely, and that perhaps interventions should be limited and that a do not resuscitate (DNR) order should be placed on the chart. The child's mother disagreed. One week later, pulmonary function worsened and the child developed a pneumothorax which required chest tube placement. At this juncture the mother again refused to agree to a DNR status.

After a month of treatment, antifungal therapy was discontinued. After five weeks of mechanical ventilation, a hospital-acquired infection complicated her management. Dopamine was again started, antibiotics were added, and intravenous sites were changed. Pulmonary function declined further. Experimental therapy with inhaled nitric oxide was then instituted after obtaining informed consent from the child's mother. The nitric oxide seemed to improve oxygenation, but lung function plateaued at the very dysfunctional level described in the previous paragraph. She continued in this hopeless state for another two weeks.

The child's oncologists remained actively involved in her care and supported the mother's decisions at all times. This created a number of conflicts regarding realistic goals of treatment between the oncologists and the intensivists. The intensivists were impressed with the deterioration of her pulmonary status: refractory hypoxemia and hypercarbia unresponsive to conventional intervention with little hope of improvement. On the other hand the oncologists felt that since her oncologic process appeared to be in check, aggressive ICU support (including experimental therapies) was indicated. Finally, her prolonged struggle with ARDS and sepsis resulted in her demise. It is important to note that her leukemia, due to her relapse and phenotype, carried a very poor prognosis.

Bone marrow transplant with respiratory failure

The second patient was DC, a 16-year-old female with Hodgkin's disease who failed conventional therapy and was referred from a tertiary medical center to our facility for BMT. She received a peripheral stem cell transplant. On day 6 following her transplant she began to develop multisystem organ failure and was transferred to the PICU, where she was treated for respiratory failure, necessitating mechanical ventilation, renal failure requiring a form of dialysis, and cardiovascular insufficiency which initially responded to inotropic support. She was placed on multiple antibiotics as part of our prophylaxis against infection. Perhaps because they failed to recognize these problems as transplant-related, and had been encouraged about the success of the BMT while DC was still in the transplant unit, her parents remained very optimistic and encouraged not only continuation but an escalation of support.

Numerous conferences were held with the family. Both intensivists and oncologists were present, and the unlikelihood of DC's survival was discussed in realistic terms. Despite cautionary input from the medical team, the family was supported by the oncologists in continuing to ask for multiple interventions and increased support. An adult intensivist/pulmonologist was consulted and concurred with our pessimistic outlook for the patient. Although the family did not want to discontinue aggressive support, and were not being asked to do so, they did agree to a DNR order. The next day, the attending physician decided to discontinue inotropes because it was felt that the child's hemodynamic condition was stable and that she would be less predisposed to the adverse effects of these agents. This was done without the parents' knowledge. When the parents discovered that their child was no longer on medication to support her blood pressure, they became very angry and demanded that the agents be restarted. After lengthy discussions the family agreed with the medical decision. Over the next four days, the family was permitted uninterrupted visits with their child. Finally, the child developed a series of dysrythmias and died.

A year after her death, the parents requested a meeting with the medical staff. They were still very angry over a number of issues including the unilateral medical decision to discontinue inotropic support, the communication between the nurses and their daughter, and the decision to have the bone marrow transplant done. Following the meeting, many of the parents' questions were answered, but they were left with other concerns. Most notably, they were still confused about the transfer of their child from the bone marrow unit to the ICU, which had resulted in different physicians and nurses caring for their child. Finally, they indicated that they were led to believe that her mortality risk even with a BMT was minimal. They never really understood the complexities of BMT and issues surrounding critical care interventions, including the non-beneficial character of the treatment in the ICU.

Ethical issues

The first child described here had leukemia with a poor prognosis, while the second, with Hodgkin's lymphoma, had failed conventional therapy and required a bone marrow transplant. Both patients presented to the ICU with severe respiratory failure (commonly called ARDS), and thus with very poor prognoses. Should the families have been offered invasive therapy (i.e., mechanical ventilation) or, as occurred in both cases, should the patients have been placed on life support? Could the children's physicians withhold these options?

Clearly, these two cases presented significant ethical problems to the physicians, families, and patients. The introduction of mechanical ventilation in patients similar to ours has not been shown to provide beneficial treatment. In a large series of adult and pediatric BMT recipients who developed respiratory failure and required mechanical ventilation, survival rates were virtually zero. Hence the unwillingness of the intensivists to offer ventilatory assistance to BMT patients, contrasting with the desire of the parents and the willingness of the oncologists to escalate support. Furthermore, as care was escalated, discussions regarding the possibility of limiting the duration or extent of therapy met with significant resistance on the part of the parents and oncologists. This situation created many difficulties among the various

ICU attendings when they were asked to provide a higher level of support for these complicated patients.

A number of ethical questions will be discussed as the basis for our conclusion.

(1) Can invasive therapies be withheld if the caregiving team is divided in opinion, as they were in both cases, or must they proceed with treatment?

As intensivists, we cannot hope to detail the beliefs and values surrounding the material facts of each individual caregiver. But their judgments were framed by two important considerations: the probability that a particular treatment or set of treatments would be of benefit to the patient; and the value of the outcome, if the given treatments were of benefit.

Although the intensivists were pessimistic about the benefit of treatment to a degree that outweighed whatever value could be placed on a possible outcome, the oncologists viewed the value of producing a beneficial outcome as overriding considerations concerning the possibility of producing this result. The parents, who wanted their child to live, either ignored or denied the non-beneficial nature of the treatments. They sided with the oncologists.

It goes without saying that complete concurrence by the caregivers concerning the goals and associated treatment strategies was needed, and that such unanimity was required prior to communications with the parents about these matters. But what is the correct thing to do when such concurrence is not achieved?

Several considerations weigh in at this point. First, when caregivers are divided over which invasive therapies are to be provided, the patient can become the possible victim of ineffective treatment. Second, to limit invasive therapies without unanimity of opinion can easily create a distrust of the caregivers by the parents and create disharmony among all of the concerned parties. Third, if invasive therapies are, in fact, non-beneficial, this will become evident in due course, as it ultimately did for the caregivers and parents in the two cases – as will be discussed more fully in answering question 3. Given these circumstances, it is right to provide an array of medical care rather than to attempt to be selective.

Since complete concurrence had not been achieved in the two cases described, the physicians proceeded to provide full care for the children, which in one case included not only mechanical ventilation but also renal replacement therapy in the form of dialysis or hemofiltration in order to assist in fluid and electrolyte management, medication to support blood pressure and heart rate, and finally, broad-spectrum antibiotics and antifungal agents in order to treat suspected or proven infections. Of course, the family needed to be made fully aware of the impact of the decision to continue support in this manner.

We have found the use of multidisciplinary conferences helpful to all the caregivers involved with the patient. They provide the family with an opportunity to meet with all the physicians at one time to obtain their input regarding medical management. This is seen as an attempt by the treating physicians to cooperate and to do what is best for the child. By this means, it is hoped that the family and treating physicians will reach a shared understanding of how far to go.

(2) If the caregivers favor invasive therapy but the family insists on "comfort care only," should the family's wishes be honored?

Family wishes are very important in instituting any form of aggressive therapy since the family is in the best position to understand their child's wishes and the impact that the disease process has on their child and themselves. Only if it is clear that the disease process which has produced the need for life support is reversible (e.g., airway obstruction secondary to mucositis), and is not severe pulmonary disease (such as ARDS), should one attempt to convince the family that a short trial of mechanical ventilation is reasonable.

In our two cases, both patients sustained severe acute lung injury compatible with ARDS, hence the concern demonstrated by the intensivists regarding the initiation and continued support required for these patients. As a general rule, the less confidence there is for a successful outcome of treatment (whatever this is understood to mean), the more the caregivers should defer to the parents' wishes.

(3) Once invasive care has been instituted, should the medical team recommend or insist on its discontinuation when the patient fails to improve?

Throughout the course of ICU care, the option to discontinue aggressive treatments needs to be revisited with the healthcare team, and with the parent(s) and/or family, on a periodic basis. Once it has been made clear that the patient is no longer receiving any benefit from the further use of life support, judgments have to be made concerning quality of life and futility of care. The treating physicians must clearly articulate this to the family with the strong recommendation to discontinue support when it is virtually certain that the outcome will be death. If the family insists upon continuing care in hopes of having their child survive with the continued use of the ventilator, then this has to be accompanied by a tracheostomy in order to transition the patient to home ventilator care. However, this is seriously complicated by the fact that the child most likely will require a level of support more sophisticated than can typically be offered at home. Most families do not have the medical, physical, financial, and psychological resources to make this happen. But, once it is clear that the pulmonary system, cardiovascular system, or other body functions are not responding, then limiting or discontinuing support is indicated.

Given the important moral value of parental autonomy, recommending is morally more justified than overriding parental wishes. However, physicians are morally justified in insisting on cessation of treatment when it is clear, as it was in both cases, that treatment was non-beneficial. Reaching consensus between the contending parties is clearly superior to coercion. But to achieve this requires time and careful negotiations with the family.

However, there is no guarantee that such negotiation will lead to a resolution of the conflict. When conflict is irresolvable, the physicians are left in the difficult position of having to decide whether medical expertise outweighs parental preference or the converse. The physicians must then work with the other care providers to develop a plan which sets limits, is consistent, and deters further escalation of care. This permits the parents to continue to actively participate and advocate for their position, yet allows the medical decision making to remain with the physicians.

Conclusion

In both of these cases it was clear that overriding the parents' wishes would be inappropriate. However, we failed as care providers by not enabling the parents to clearly understand the various scenarios for their children. In the first case, the reluctance on the part of the oncologist to accept the very poor prognosis reinforced the mother's belief that her child's pulmonary deterioration was transient and that supportive care was clearly indicated. Thus, providing newer therapies such as nitric oxide and high-frequency ventilation, which had no clear benefit, only reinforced the mother's perception that more could be done and should be provided to her daughter, despite the fact that these were not medically indicated.

The second case provided the care provider with the issue of the removal of a pharmacologic agent without the family's authorization and/or concurrence. The family perceived this drug as essential to support their child's cardiovascular status. Although this act by the attending physician did not lead to an immediate change in hemodynamics, it raised the question of parental involvement in bedside decision making. The family's insistence that it should not only be informed but must also concur with the medical management led to significant friction over who was in charge between the family and the care providers. This confrontation could have been avoided if the parents had been informed about the medical decision before it was implemented. However, because it was done in a unilateral manner, the parents' perception that the physicians were not working in their child's best interests was reinforced.

Obviously, there was frustration encountered in caring for these complicated patients. However, it is the care providers' obligation to work with the various physician groups and the family to reach a common goal. When conflict arises between family and medical personnel, and our aggressive efforts are unsuccessful, we need to reconsider our management plan and inform the family that limiting support, making the child a DNR, or withdrawing support are reasonable options.

Clarifying what these three involve for the family requires effective communication and the development of appropriate expectations. At the outset, the family must be aware that whatever is done, high-quality and compassionate care will continue. If the decision is to withdraw life support then the family must be made aware that the child's comfort is of most importance. The family must also understand that withdrawal of life support may not result in the child's immediate demise. It is incumbent for us to work with the family in coming to conclusions which are in the patient's best interest.

FURTHER READING

Bojko, T., Notterman, D. A., Greenwald, B. M., De Bruin, W. J., Magid, M. S., and Godwin, T. Acute hypoxemic respiratory failure in children following bone marrow transplantation: an outcome and pathologic study. *Critical Care Medicine* 23 (1995), 755–759.

Butt, W., Barker, G., Walker, C., Gillis, J., Kilham, H., and Stevens, M. Outcome of children with hematologic malignancy who are admitted to an intensive care unit. *Critical Care Medicine* 16 (1988), 761–764.

Keenan, H. T., Bratton, S. L., Martin, L. D., Crawford, S. W., and Weiss, N. S. Outcome of children who require mechanical ventilatory support after bone marrow transplantation. *Critical Care Medicine* 28 (2000), 830–835.

Randle, C. J. Jr., Frankel, L. R., and Amylon, M. D. Identifying early predictors of mortality in pediatric patients with acute leukemia and pneumonia. *Chest* 109 (1996), 457–461.

Shorr, A. F., Moores, L. K., Edenfield W. J., Christie, R. J., and Fitzpatrick, T. M. Mechanical ventilation in hematopoietic stem cell transplantation: can we effectively predict outcomes? *Chest* 116 (1999), 1012–1018.

Todd, K., Wiley, F., Landaw, E., *et al.* Survival outcome among 54 intubated pediatric bone marrow transplant patients. *Critical Care Medicine* 22 (1994), 171–176.

van Veen, A., Karstens, A., van der Hoek, A. C., Tibboel, D., Hahlen, K., and van der Voort, E. The prognosis of oncologic patients in the pediatric intensive care unit. *Intensive Care Medicine* 22 (1996), 237–241.

10.2 Ethics in the pediatric intensive care unit: oncology and bone marrow transplant patients

Linda Granowetter

Introduction

Doctors Frankel and DiCarlo present summaries of the course of two pediatric oncology patients who suffered severe ARDS and multisystem organ failure in the course of aggressive therapy. The first child was a nine-year-old who had previously received inadequate care for acute lymphoblastic leukemia (ALL), subsequently achieved remission, and suffered respiratory failure while undergoing therapy for a central nervous system relapse. Isolated central nervous system relapse of ALL which occurs between 18 and 35 months after diagnosis may have a six-year survival rate as high as 59% ± 5% (Gaynon *et al.* 1998). The second child, a 16-year-old who was either refractory to therapy or relapsed, had Hodgkin's disease. Survival rates reported for such patients treated with stem cell transplantation vary from study to study, but a recent report cites a four-year survival of 52% (Horning *et al.* 1997.)

The central ethical conundrums cited by Drs. Frankel and DiCarlo focus on the appropriate limits of heroic care, and revolve around the resolution of conflicting opinions: there are conflicts between the two sets of medical caregivers, and conflicts between the parents and the caregivers. I believe that a discussion of these important questions must be preceded by a question. Ultimately, in choosing to limit heroic care for a patient with a poor prognosis, whose decision is it anyway? Even if the physicians were unanimous in the view that further aggressive care would be futile, do physicians have a right to withdraw such care in the face of parental opposition? What about the patient in all this? I would like to address this question first, and then consider the complicating issues of conflict between caregivers, and conflict between caregivers and parents.

Ethical Dilemmas in Pediatrics: Cases and Commentaries, ed. Lorry R. Frankel, Amnon Goldworth, Mary V. Rorty, and William A. Silverman. Published by Cambridge University Press. © Cambridge University Press 2005.

Whose decision?

I believe that the perspective in the United States regarding the question of who is the ultimate decision maker is that patient autonomy should be upheld, unless there are very compelling reasons to do otherwise. In most states, there are provisions for mature adults with capacity to state their views, for example by appointing a healthcare proxy, or by describing their wishes specifically. The do not resuscitate (DNR) order is to be placed on the patient's chart to protect the patient's autonomy. This autonomy is to be respected if the patient requests aggressive therapy or if the patient refuses heroic treatment. In New York State, where I practice, it is very clear that the patient or designated proxy is the decision maker. Futility is defined very narrowly as true physiologic futility, meaning death would be imminent even with an attempt at resuscitation; a broader definition of futility, meaning general lack of benefit, is not accepted. My first response to this law was negative; it seemed to make futile care an option for all patients. However, after years of working under this law, I have come to believe that it can be used to facilitate open discussions about death and end-of-life care, and to prevent parents from believing that their child was denied a chance at life.

It is the ethical responsibility of the physician to make sure the patient, or appropriate proxy, has the opportunity to state his or her wishes. It is also imperative that the risks of heroic care and resuscitation and the chances for a good outcome are described fully, honestly, and with minimal bias. The medical evidence that exists should be presented. The subjective view of the medical caregiver should be avoided, as much as is feasible. When the medical literature is clear that a patient has no or very little chance of meaningful recovery, the physician is obligated to clearly explain the futility of the situation to the patient or proxy. The discussions must be sensitive and supportive, yet factual. Ideally, there is not one "DNR discussion," but ongoing conversations, reflecting the developments in the patient's condition. In other words, it is not the role of the physician to "get a DNR." It is the role of the physician to facilitate decision making by offering clear information. The way we medical practitioners speak of DNR – "getting it" or "the parents refused DNR" – demonstrates our biases against giving the patient and parent choices. We need to develop respect for a process which gives the patient or proxy genuine voice.

Decision making regarding the institution of heroic care and resuscitation of a child raises special issues. In this culture, the death of a child is viewed as profoundly abnormal. In addition, it is often assumed that a child lacks capacity, and no further thought is given to the child's wishes. There are studies that speak to young children's capacity in regard to research (King and Cross 1989, Susman et al. 1992) and the ability to choose between experimental research treatment and palliative care (Nitschke *et al.* 1982). In order to protect the autonomy of a child, we must understand the child's level of cognitive, moral, and emotional development (Susman *et al.* 1987). There is less known about children's capacity to forgo heroic life-sustaining treatment; however, the concept that children should be given voice has been addressed (Leikin 1989). Employing what is known about children's development, we must attempt to determine the capacity of each minor patient, child or adolescent.

The child's perspective

When a child lacks capacity, it is generally agreed that the parent(s) speak for the child. A child may lack capacity because of devastating illness which renders them incapable of communicating their views, as in these cases. Alternatively, a child may lack capacity because of developmental age. I must wonder if there was any thought to determining the wishes of the young patients in the two cases under discussion before they became medically incapacitated. In the first case, the child was nine: old enough to have opinions, perhaps young enough to lack full capacity. In the second case, the child in question was 16: mature enough in the minds of most to have full capacity. Both patients may have expressed some opinions about their care prior to becoming incapable of communicating. In no part of these case histories do I see anyone specifically speaking about the child's perspective. The parents were considered to speak directly for the patients, and, as the patients were rendered without capacity due to their medical conditions, this is both reasonable and legal. However, it is highly likely that these patients did leave clues as to their beliefs, and it is the ethical obligation of all involved to at least consider the wishes of the patient.

All pediatricians have seen children with devastating illness clearly state that they will do "anything" to get well, and suffer significant medical intrusions without complaint. Other children make it clear that they hate the hospital, hate needles, and want no part of invasive care. When a child or young adolescent has an illness with a high likelihood of cure, they are generally not given the option to refuse medical care inasmuch as it assumed that their moral reasoning and abstract thinking are too immature to make decisions which would obviously jeopardize their life. However, when the course of the disease has taken a profoundly negative turn and cure is no longer possible, the decision now affects primarily quality of life, and not the maintenance of life itself; different standards should apply. In a study in which children as young as seven who had relapsed disease and a very poor prognosis were asked in a family conference whether they wanted experimental medicine or comfort care (Nitshcke *et al.* 1982), the children generally expressed the same choices as the parents. However, this report reflects data on a small number of patients.

I am inclined to believe that most parents speak for their children, although this may not always be true, and we should not presume it is always the case.

When the choices are profoundly difficult, I would ask the parent "What do you think [the child's name] would want?" To me, this is an ethical imperative. Further, it is an excellent clinical tool, since it helps parents move from their own paralyzing fear of loss and grief, in order to consider the child's perspective. No loving parent wants to lose a child, and thus they might choose to subject a child to treatments that they would themselves decline. In asking them to consider the child's perspective, a parent may be able to understand the futility issue more clearly, and they may move towards preventing needless intervention out of respect for the child's wishes, beliefs, and desires. We professionals must remember that the parents are supposed to speak for their child, not only for themselves. In the case reports under discussion, we do not learn much about the patient's wishes, so I must assume that the parents speak for the children.

Conflicting opinions

In order for any parent to speak for a child regarding escalating, continuing, or discontinuing aggressive care in the face of a poor prognosis, he or she must be offered the facts that are known. The question framed earlier was "Can invasive therapies be withheld if the caregiving team is divided in opinion, as they were in both cases, or must they proceed with treatment?" I would say that the central issue is how the teams of physicians can present their views to the parents, in order to give the parents unbiased information. It is the responsibility of the physicians to prevent their own biases from intruding upon the decision making, if at all possible. In the first case, the oncologists were presented as "siding with the mother," and the intensivists as "impressed with the deterioration of her pulmonary status." It is stated that there were many conferences with the parents and both the oncology team and the intensive care team. The inference is that the conflict between the teams, pitting the hope of the oncologists against the pessimism of the intensive care team, confused the parents. I believe that the intensivists and the oncologists were obliged to review the relevant literature, to understand what the best prognosis could be, given published data and experience, and to develop a plan to relate this information to the parent in the least biased way. It seems that the intensivists had doubts about the validity of re-induction therapy for ALL and Hodgkin's disease altogether, when the literature supports the idea that this treatment is valid. The oncologists seemed not to be fully aware of the intensive care literature regarding the poor prognosis of respiratory failure in the setting of bone marrow transplantation and/or intensive chemotherapy. It was imperative that the practitioners understand the literature, speak with and teach one another. If there was insufficient data to prognosticate for a patient, the physicians were obligated to inform the parents as to what might be expected on the basis of clinical experience. If the difference in outlook between the teams could not be resolved, the parents should have been told that this was an area in which there was no absolute answer, and the experiences of the teams differed. In these two cases, the conflict between the teams seemed quite dramatic. At one point the intensivists posited the viewpoint that "survival rates were virtually zero" for respiratory failure in this setting. Yet older studies exist that suggest that some patients do survive, perhaps in the range of 5–9% (Nichols *et al.* 1994). Newer studies report 16–25% survival for oncology patients who required inotropes or ventilators during intensive care admissions (Keengwe *et al.* 2000), and in a review restricted to pediatric stem cell transplant patients survival was reported as 50–70% when intervention was limited to inotropes and 15% if a ventilator was required (Tomaske 2003). Although these data demonstrate a relatively poor chance for survival, there is a precedent for cure. A parent might well be justified in wanting further therapy when there is a possibility, albeit a small one, of a cure.

My personal view, hearing these cases and knowing the literature, is that I would agree with the intensivists that the medical evidence predicts that these two children would almost certainly die because of severe respiratory failure and other complications. Yet I would acknowledge that it would not have been completely unprecedented for such a child to survive. My perspective is that it was the ethical obligation of both the oncology and intensive care staff to inform the parents that the outlook for survival was extremely poor. However, for me, the rule of patient autonomy ultimately puts the final choice in the parents' hands. The parents are then given the awesome responsibility to sift through the information presented in order to make a choice for the child. My experience does bias me. I have been involved with more than one patient for whom the expected chance of recovery after heroic intervention was essentially nil. I have, with medical facts in hand, presented profoundly pessimistic viewpoints to the parents, and I have indicated that I believed that a DNR order would be appropriate and most kind. In more than one such instance, I have been humbled to see the child survive, and survive well. Thus, I will continue to present the facts, as I know them. I will advocate a DNR order when the prognosis is truly grim, and I will fully support patients and parents who choose palliative or otherwise limited care in such a situation. However, at the same time, I am committed to supporting the parents' (and patient's) right to choose.

Futility

Does this mean that physicians are required to provide care, even if they believe it is absolutely futile? Is it unethical to compel physicians to deliver care in which they have no faith? After all, a physician who does not believe in abortion is not required to perform abortions. At the other end of life, should a physician do what he or she believes is entirely futile? I would suggest that, for the most part, they should respect patient/parent autonomy. This does not mean that a child with highly resistant metastatic cancer and heart failure should be eligible for a heart transplant. It does not mean that a patient must be given a third marrow transplant just because the parents want to try again. When the physician knows that there is absolutely no known reason to believe that interventions of these kinds would eventuate in meaningful survival, they should not be offered. However, once a heroic treatment has been offered, the physician can not suddenly refuse to give further care without clear evidence and patient/parent involvement in decision making.

To pursue the question of futile care more fully, I think it is useful to ask why a physician would not want to provide care he or she deems futile. If the physician feels that the patient is suffering, it is his or her duty to make sure that the patient receives adequate analgesia. If the physician wants to limit care because "it is horrible to see the parent with false hope, day after day," I would say that such reasoning is profoundly paternalistic and inappropriate. Although I have known that feeling myself, I believe it is unethical to allow our perception of the parents' suffering to limit their child's access to care. If the physician wants to limit care because "it is a poor use of resources," I would argue the physician should not make social policy at the bedside. The physician might instead join a social or political campaign to educate the public about the appropriate limits of medical care, or become involved in research regarding medical outcomes and futility, or participate in panels attempting to develop guidelines on the issue of heroic care. In my view, it is not ethical to refuse care to an individual because the state's or hospital's resources are limited, unless this is part of a clear, consistent, and non-discriminatory policy. Another possible reason physicians might want to limit "futile" care is their own anguish in being powerless to heal: they do not want the patient to linger because each moment of the patient's time on life support is evidence of medicine's limitations. To physicians who feel "futile" care must be limited, I must remind them that our goal is to do no harm. If the patient is not suffering, and the parents want to continue care, is anyone harmed? Although there may be economic and resource utilization issues raised by continuing care in such a case, these issues must be addressed politically and socially. These broader issues should not inform the argument for individual patients.

Communication and informed decision making

The issue of clear communication and informed decision making is critical in these cases. The parents of the child with resistant Hodgkin's disease were said to be angry a year after the child's death because of the doctor's "unilateral decision to discontinue inotropic support." As a physician, I agree with the caregivers in this case that each medical order need not be co-signed by the parent. However, when heroic life-saving interventions have begun, and the parents have made it clear that they want "everything done" except, as in this case, full resuscitation, the physician is ethically obligated to discuss changes in the level of care with the parent. The physician should change care because of the patient's medical condition, not as a surreptitious attempt to limit care. If indeed the decision to limit inotropic support was medically appropriate, it should have been explained to the parents, thus developing rather than interfering with trust. We must remember that after the child has died, it is the parents who live with the grief. We have the potential for harming the parents, if they feel that the physicians were dishonest or ignored their wishes. It is also said that these parents had understood that the "mortality risk even with a BMT was minimal." It is obvious that the informed consent process for the BMT must address all risks, and especially that of mortality. To be fair to the oncology physicians involved, many parents hear very selectively. The medical literature supports the idea that despite an attempt to inform parents of the real risk of procedures such as marrow transplantation, as many as 50% of parents and patients do not absorb all the information about risks (Lesko *et al.* 1989). This again underscores the need for clear and ongoing communication.

Conclusion

In summary, I believe that the autonomy of the patient must be respected. For children and adolescents this means that the child's perspective must be considered, but in most cases it is the parent who must ultimately decide. It is the responsibility of the physicians involved to impart the facts, compassionately and without bias. My personal perspective is that it is tragic that too often parents opt for interventions that are destined to be futile, and these choices result in a prolonged dying process for the patient. Nonetheless, I believe we must ultimately accept the fact that the patient or parent must have the right to choose. In order to minimize the excessive use of inappropriate care, I exhort physicians to continue to study and examine the facts pertaining to the results of heroic interventions, and not initiate clearly futile care. In addition, I exhort physicians to talk with parents and patients before a crisis occurs, so there is a basis for decision making, based on a prior understanding of the patient's and parents' general perspectives about heroic care. I urge physicians troubled by the inappropriate use of high-cost futile interventions to develop care plans and decision trees based on evidence, so that their limitation of care is not arbitrary, but based on coherent medical standards.

10.3 Topical discussion

Coordination between services

The structural organization of the contemporary hospital can constitute an obstacle in its own right to effective communication with patients and their parents about the plan of care in complex medical cases. Intensive care units providing technically sophisticated support are typically staffed with specialists in critical care, but the patients whose illnesses have reached a critical point can be referred to those services from a variety of different specialties – transplant, cardiology, pulmonary medicine, oncology. When the attending physician on the referring service and the ICU attending have different priorities, opinions, or treatments for the same patient, whose opinion governs care? This is not a question that should be determined by power within the institution or hierarchy of medical specialties, but realistically, there are few areas of human interaction in which relative power does not play a role. Coordination, communication, and cooperation between services is a problem of organizational structure, too important to be left prey to the personalities and varying skills of individuals.

The problem of coordination and communication arises on many levels. In many hospitals, the physicians in training, the residents, have more contact with individual patients than their supervisors, the physicians who are training them in their specialty, but quite rationally might fear to challenge their decisions. The various professional groups among clinicians, united by a Hippocratic commitment to the well-being of their patients, nonetheless may have differing priorities, reflecting their different professional ethics. Three shifts of nurses have intimate and continuing contact with patients and their families, and their perspective on patient and family needs to be included in care conferences. Scholars of organizational structure in other industries have noted a tendency for more horizontal and egalitarian

Ethical Dilemmas in Pediatrics: Cases and Commentaries, ed. Lorry R. Frankel, Amnon Goldworth, Mary V. Rorty, and William A. Silverman. Published by Cambridge University Press. © Cambridge University Press 2005.

managerial structures to improve efficiency and effectiveness, but many of these innovations have not been carried over into health care. ·

Rationing at the bedside

After a brief plateau, the percentage of the gross national product of the USA devoted to health care is once again on the rise. The central role of the physician in containing medical costs is universally acknowledged, but Hippocratic ethics requires the physician to give primacy to the interests of his patient. Acting as rationers can create in physicians a conflict between the needs of their own patients and the needs of other patients. On the other hand, in any given case, there is arguably no one better able to decide whether a treatment is appropriate or not than the patient's physician. While there is some question about whether physicians are the ideal agents for rationing decisions, there is little agreement about who would be better. It is worth considering the role of the physician as gatekeeper in the larger context of distributive justice. Attempts to limit or override physician discretion in decision making, particularly in the form manifested in the early years of managed care, have proven unworkable or widely unacceptable.

DNR

All the literature on "do not rescuscitate" orders emphasizes that such an order does not mean that all care should be withdrawn from the patient. But the psychological difficulties that parents confront in allowing such orders to be written are complicated, as in this case, by fears that other treatments will be withdrawn as well, "abandoning" their child. Although the discontinuation of inotropic support was related to its adverse effects and had nothing to do with the DNR, inadequate communication allowed the parents to torture themselves with that possibility.

Empirical evidence is accumulating about the morbidity and mortality of patients who have been resuscitated. On the basis of such information, physicians are often in the position of being unable in good faith to recommend treatments that surrogates may nevertheless desire for their loved ones, thus creating ethical problems for practitioners.

The Janus-face of medicine: an art or a science?

Since the beginning of the twentieth century it has been understood that medicine is not only an art but a human science. In reports on the medical condition of patients the tension between the two approaches has been visible in many ways. In morning rounds on the units, the residents and medical students often report to the attending physician on the current status of their patients with a potentially bewildering numerology: blood pressure, temperature, blood chemistry, oxygen saturation, ventilator settings, followed by examination of the lung X-ray, the printouts of MRI or CT-scan readings.

In ethics committees as well, sometimes the details of the patient being discussed – name, sex, age – are changed, not only to protect the privacy of the patient, but to isolate for specific consideration the ethical issues involved in difficult cases. But the scientists are also passionate participants in personal interactions, intensely involved in the sufferings of their patients and compassionate supporters of their families, and ethics committees know well that it is the particular situation of that individual that determines what the ethical issues might be. This tension between the two faces of medicine plays out in interesting ways in the various cases presented in this book, as the scientist and the caregiver wrestle with the choice of the voice in which to tell their stories. The apparent impersonality of a case report is a thin veneer over the recollected anguish of a painful encounter. To choose to be a practicing physician is to choose to accept the challenge of balancing both of the Janus-faces of medicine.

FURTHER READING

Chambliss, D. F. *Beyond Caring: Hospitals, Nurses and the Social Organization of Ethics* (Chicago, IL: University of Chicago Press, 1996), especially Chapter 4.

Orentlicher, D. *Matters of Life and Death: Making Moral Theory Work in Medical Ethics and the Law* (Princeton, NJ: Princeton University Press, 2001), especially Chapter 9.

Penson, R. T., Rauch, P. K., McAfee, S. L. *et al.* Between parent and child: negotiating cancer treatment in adolescents. *The Oncologist* 7 (2002), 154–162.

Rowe, M. The structure of the situation. *Hastings Center Report* 33(6) (2003), 37–44.

11.1 Nursing perspectives on withholding food and fluids in pediatrics

Joy Penticuff

Introduction

There are few ethical dilemmas in the care of sick children more difficult than the dilemma of deciding to withhold food and fluids. This chapter presents such a case and discusses the ethical, psychological, and organizational issues it raised. In addition, the experiences and perspectives of the nurses in the case are discussed.

The case

Latasha was 18 months old when her medical condition necessitated the decision of whether to withhold artificial food and fluids. She had been born prematurely, at 30 weeks gestational age, and in the second week of life had developed necrotizing enterocolitis. Surgery to remove affected bowel left Latasha with a minimal amount of bowel function and she required continuous hyperalimentation (intravenous fluid that does not require digestion) to sustain life. It was estimated that less than 10% of her nutritional needs could be met through oral nutrition. A central hyperalimentation line was surgically placed and Latasha was discharged home.

Over the next year Latasha developed multiple infections of the central line and was repeatedly hospitalized for line replacement and treatment of sepsis. Over time, her liver function deteriorated and she became jaundiced. In the month prior to her case being brought to the pediatric ethics committee, Latasha developed total lower-body paralysis in association with central nervous system changes resembling multiple infarcts.

At the time that her case was brought to the ethics committee, Latasha had been hospitalized for about two months. All central line placement sites had been exhausted and only peripheral vessels were available as routes for continuous

Ethical Dilemmas in Pediatrics: Cases and Commentaries, ed. Lorry R. Frankel, Amnon Goldworth, Mary V. Rorty, and William A. Silverman. Published by Cambridge University Press. © Cambridge University Press 2005.

hyperalimentation. Latasha was undergoing venopunctures about every 24–48 hours because of repeated infiltration at peripheral IV sites. Latasha's parents, and the nurses and physicians caring for her, realized that she was terminally ill, and believed that she was suffering, in part because of her general condition, but also because of the painful venopunctures required to maintain continuous hyperalimentation.

Latasha's parents did not want her to undergo further suffering and they requested an ethics committee meeting to explore options. They requested that, should the hyperalimentation IV infiltrate, not more than three attempts be made to restart it. The ethics committee agreed that it was ethically justifiable to support this request. The family knew that not to restart hyperalimentation would eventually result in Latasha's death, but they understood also that her liver failure was untreatable.

For several days the nursing staff were able to maintain adequate hyperalimentation, although several times they reached the limit of three attempts to restart the IV. Ultimately, however, there came a point at which the IV could not be restarted in three attempts, and artificial nutrition was no longer administered. Oral nutrition was provided, but everyone involved in the case understood that Latasha could not survive without hyperalimentation. Latasha died ten days after cessation of hyperalimentation, experiencing some seizure activity and finally lapsing into a coma a few hours prior to her death.

Ethical issues

The major points of the ethics committee discussion of this case were as follows:
- Latasha's liver failure was a terminal medical condition;
- The frequent venopunctures required to maintain hyperalimentation constituted burdensome therapy;
- The burden of repeated venopunctures was not offset by benefit to the child.

It is noteworthy that the request put to the committee by Latasha's family was not that her hyperalimentation be withdrawn, but that there be a limit to the number of venopunctures performed in each instance of restarting hyperalimentation. In essence, the parents' focus was on limiting the amount of pain their child might endure. They realized that even if hyperalimentation could be maintained indefinitely, Latasha ultimately would succumb to liver failure because her liver was unable to metabolize the nutritional elements in the hyperalimentation fluids.

The strategy elemental to the family's request, and to the committee's discussion, was that of deciding the proportionality of harms and benefits. The decision to allow only three attempts to restart the IV was a means of limiting the burden of therapy, and this limitation reflected the reality that there was no effective treatment to reverse Latasha's deteriorating liver function. On the other hand, this rather indirect approach to cessation of hyperalimentation reflected also the parents' and committee members' deep reluctance to withhold life-sustaining nutrition from a child. The decision forced all involved to confront both the reality and the symbolism of a child's death by starvation, and it engendered a deep sense of violating a basic ethical obligation. Nonetheless, there was committee consensus that the decision was ethically justified, based on the principle of non-maleficence. Not to limit the number of venopunctures would be to prolong a painful process of dying. There was agreement about the ethical decision across all the disciplines represented on the committee: hospital chaplaincy, medicine, nursing, and social work.

Nursing perspectives

The multidisciplinary ethics committee concluded that it was ethically justifiable to limit pain-producing attempts to restart life-sustaining hyperalimentation in this case. In further describing this case, I wish to explore what in it was unique to nursing ethics. In doing so, I move from general bioethical concepts to those perspectives that are derived from the particularity of the experience of providing nursing care 24 hours a day to sick children.

Nurses have traditionally been and continue to be the professional group in closest proximity to hospitalized children and their families. This proximity produces interactions between the child and his or her nurses, and between the child's family and the nurses, that are qualitatively different from the interactions of children and families with physicians, social workers, and other professionals. I contend that what is unique about nursing ethics is derived from what is unique in nurses' interactions, relationships, and obligations to child patients and their families.

The element of proximity – care within arm's length – generates an *ethics within arm's length* (Penticuff 1997) that is in essence more particularistic, personal, and affective than what is found in general bioethical concepts. In giving nursing care to children, each nurse must look, must touch, must listen, to a child – an innocent – who is in some way vulnerable and needy. The element of proximity makes the reality of the child's pain, anxiety, and bewilderment inescapable. Thus, pediatric nurses confront, within arm's length, the unanswerable question: How can God be good and children suffer?

The nurses who cared for Latasha, both before and after the final IV was discontinued, generously gave their time to talk with me about their experience of the case a few months after Latasha's death. I wanted to find out how her nurses were affected by the decision to limit attempts to restart hyperalimentation and how they experienced caring for Latasha and her family during the long interval between the ethics committee decision and Latasha's death. Three core elements of nursing ethics within arm's length – particularity, personal involvement, and affect – were apparent in their descriptions of how they cared for Latasha and her parents in the last weeks of her life.

Particularity

The experience of giving nursing care to Latasha during this final phase of her life demonstrated an inability to generalize from that experience. It was a singular experience, not comparable with other instances or situations of caring for other child patients. Granted, the circumstances of Latasha's case were unique. But it may be a characteristic of nursing ethics that our comprehensive view of the patient, and our sense that many facets have moral relevance and must be taken into account in ethical decision making, give rise to an ethics that eschews generalization and application of distant or formal theories and categories.

Personal involvement

Proximity also makes inescapable the immediacy of a sense of obligation to alleviate a child's pain, fear, and bewilderment. After the ethics committee decision, Latasha's nursing care required that a fundamental nursing obligation – to feed the patient – be broken. The nurses were the ones to check Latasha's IV site and discern that the hyperalimentation fluid had infiltrated. The nurses were the ones to remove the malfunctioning IV. It was the nurses who experienced the personal responsibility of not being able to restart the IV within three attempts. The nurses were the ones who continued to provide hour-to-hour comfort, knowing all the while that Latasha could not survive the withholding of intravenous feeding. In this case, a basic notion of what it is to be a pediatric nurse was challenged. Indeed, the adage "to nurse is to nurture" was violated.

Affect

A recent addition to the bioethics literature is the concept of *ethical anguish*. Again, nurses' care of patients within arm's length engenders emotional responses that professionals who do not interact with patients over prolonged time and through intimate contact are not likely to experience.

Psychological and organizational issues

A number of significant psychological and organizational issues were raised in the implementation of the family's request to limit attempts to restart Latasha's hyperalimentation. The primary psychological issue was that of the guilt of those nurses who could not restart Latasha's final IV.

A concomitant psychological factor was their anxiety about the procedure. The most skilled nurses in the hospital were called upon to attempt the venopuncture each time Latasha's IV infiltrated, and the pressure on these nurses was intense. With each attempt the number of possible IV sites diminished. The child's peripheral veins had been used for so long and had been so traumatized from the local tissue damage caused by infiltration of concentrated hyperalimentation fluid that the odds of achieving a successful venopuncture were very slim.

Another difficult emotional situation was the nurses' close experience of seeing Latasha's responses to the repeated painful attempts to restart her IV. The nurses caring for her also witnessed her family's anguish through a period of weeks of uncertainty and finally through the ten days in which hyperalimentation was forgone.

Latasha was conscious until about 12 hours before her death; she recognized her nurses; they had cared for her through her many previous hospitalizations. To watch her slowly die was an agony for all involved.

Organizational factors

Probably the most consequential organizational factor in this case was the nurses' lack of input into the decision to withhold further IV fluids after the third attempt to restart the IV was unsuccessful. In discussing the case later with the nursing staff, it became apparent that the nurses at the bedside did not have a clear understanding of the function of the pediatric ethics committee of the hospital. This lack of bedside nurses' input into hospital ethics committee discussions is not unusual. Based on my research and informal conversations with bedside nurses and nurse administrators, I would estimate that only about half the nurses providing direct patient care in hospitals today are aware of the functions of their institutions' ethics committees. They have little knowledge of the role of nursing on these committees and rarely do they overcome their sense of intimidation and actually request that a case be brought to the committee.

In this case, even though the nursing staff were unclear about how the ethics committee decision had been arrived at, there was a great deal of unit-based nursing administrative support for the nurses providing bedside care. Although there was wide agreement that limiting Latasha's suffering was the morally correct thing to do, all of the nurses providing care had real emotional struggles in implementing this decision.

Another interesting aspect of how the decision was presented to the nurses at the bedside was that Latasha's parents were reluctant to portray themselves as having initiated the request that IV attempts be limited. It may be that the parents had had such close relationships with the nurses over time that they did not want the nurses to believe that any move that would hasten Latasha's dying could originate with her parents. This stance by her parents certainly increased the nurses' confusion about the role of the ethics committee in the decision to limit venopuncture attempts.

The bedside nurses' lack of clarity about how the hospital's pediatric ethics committee functioned and who had the moral authority to decide to withhold life-sustaining therapy were issues that needed to be addressed at an institutional level. In this case, two nurses closely involved in Latasha's care were unaware that the request to limit IV attempts originated with the parents. Some nurses were under the impression that the pediatric ethics committee had initiated this treatment plan and had recommended this plan to the family.

This misimpression may have come about partly because of the family's need to place responsibility for the decision on the ethics committee when they discussed the decision with staff nurses close to Latasha. The lack of communication between the pediatric ethics committee and bedside nurses also played a role in the misunderstanding.

The impact on the nursing staff of the ethics committee's decision to support Latasha's parents' request was quite serious. But all the nurses interviewed felt several months after her death that the decisions made to limit further suffering for Latasha were ethically correct. Those nurses closest to Latasha felt that her death was inevitable due to liver failure, and they did not want her to have to experience multiple, painful, desperate attempts to find IV hyperalimentation routes. The pressure on nurses "not to be the first to fail" had been ongoing and severe. Nurses called upon to restart the IV felt highly anxious. They also felt, toward the end of Latasha's life, that the situation had become futile. Everyone knew that death would come inevitably, even if the current IV insertion were successful. As IV sites became more and more scarce, the nurses began to face the reality that Latasha would not live much longer. Efforts were turned to making her last days as comfortable as possible and to supporting her family.

The fact that Latasha did not die within the 48–72 hours predicted after her final IV infiltrated was a source of much anxiety and emotional turmoil for staff and family alike. As mentioned previously, Latasha knew and trusted the nurses caring for her. She was old enough to talk, she recognized the staff, she smiled and laughed and played in those months before liver deterioration, sepsis, paralysis, and repeated venopunctures took their toll on her mood and endurance.

This group of nurses were extraordinary in their ability to continue to care sensitively for Latasha, to support her parents, and to support each other. Although an employee assistance program was available to the nursing staff, they chose instead to talk about the situation among themselves rather than to go to strangers outside their work group. It is fortunate that this staff felt a strong sense of cohesion and mutual support, because it is not unusual for ethical dilemmas and difficult resolution processes to be destructive to work-group relationships.

The head nurse of this unit had done a commendable job of developing a staff that could rise to meet the challenge presented by Latasha's family's request and the affirmation of that request by the ethics committee. In my judgment, many other staffs would not have been able to carry out such a request without significant deterioration of staff–family and staff–staff relationships. The key role played in this case by the head nurse is a good example of the fundamental importance of organizational factors to the resolution of ethical dilemmas in pediatrics.

The limited understanding and sense of lack of input into the ethics committee's deliberations about this case are also examples of why it is necessary for the workings of such committees to be highly visible to nurses caught up in intense ethical dilemmas. While this staff was able to overcome their sense of having no say in the resolution of the dilemma of withholding artificial nutrition in this case, in a less cohesive or less well-supported staff, high rates of disillusionment and turnover may have occurred.

Toward the end of her life, the nursing staff and others involved in her care said goodbyes to Latasha. When she died, her room was left intact for a while so that staff could accustom themselves to the fact that she was no longer there. In the last few days, the nurses took care to allow Latasha's parents and family privacy and time alone with their child. Latasha's nurses demonstrated caring, courage, and discipline in remaining committed to her and to her family, and in supporting each other through the entire process.

It is obvious that it would have increased the nurses' understanding of how this resolution process was put into place if several nurses most closely involved in Latasha's care had been included in the meeting of the pediatric ethics committee. Although nursing was represented in the meetings, the views of nurses at the bedside could have been informative and their participation would have helped them to feel that their views were important to the committee. One would hope that ethics committees would seek the participation of those nurses (perhaps one or two) most involved in the daily care of the children for whom ethical decisions are being deliberated.

It also seems valuable for a series of in-service education programs and written materials to be developed to describe the role of ethics committees to all nursing and medical staff, to prevent misunderstanding and to disseminate information about the committee's role as a resource when staff and families confront ethical dilemmas in the care of children.

11.2 Ethics and clinical decision making: withholding food and information

Mary V. Rorty

Introduction

The moving story of Latasha's death and the care she received in the course of her dying brings home the poignancy of death in the pediatric unit. The conflation of the beginning of life and its end runs deeply contrary to our normal expectations and fondest hopes for children, and, as in this case, involves in its course people who are deeply committed to giving every possible support to vulnerable patients and their families.

I will comment on three aspects of the case Dr. Penticuff presents: the withdrawal of nutrition and hydration in infants; the relation of nursing ethics and clinical ethics; and the operation of the hospital ethics committee.

Withholding and withdrawing nutrition and hydration in infants

There are many reasons why it is difficult to deprive young children of the nutrition and hydration needed to sustain their lives. One often mentioned reason is the symbolic importance of nourishment; another is the extent to which not nourishing children goes in the face of our strongest instincts and inclinations. The relative unpredictability of the course of illness in the young makes it harder to take a decisive position which might seem to determine what that course will be.

It is interesting that, as Dr. Penticuff emphasizes, in Latasha's case the decision made was not directly one to withdraw nutrition and hydration, but specifically to limit the number of venopunctures for restarting hyperalimentation after infiltration of a site. On the one hand, framing the decision in terms of limiting venopunctures was economical: it directly addressed the issue creating the problem, which was the suffering caused by repeated attempts to restart the IV. To that extent it

Ethical Dilemmas in Pediatrics: Cases and Commentaries, ed. Lorry R. Frankel, Amnon Goldworth, Mary V. Rorty, and William A. Silverman. Published by Cambridge University Press. © Cambridge University Press 2005.

was a decision to limit a painful therapy, not a decision to withdraw nutrition and hydration per se. On the other hand, one can speculate whether some of the moral distress surrounding this case was caused by exactly this refusal to address directly the momentous consequences of the decision. It may have been a desire for precision that led the decision makers to frame it as they did; but did a desire to evade the responsibility contribute as well?

If the decision had been explicitly rather than indirectly one to withdraw nutrition and hydration, would there have been less pressure on the nurse responsible for finding a viable site for the next attempt? In the situation described, it seems unlikely that there was anyone unclear about what the consequences would be. However, a more explicit decision to withdraw, for which the pain of restarting the treatment was the proximate justification, might have depersonalized the decision for the nurses carrying it out, and made it less traumatic, not only for the individual who failed at the third attempt, but even for the nurses who successfully restarted, knowing what the consequences of failure would have been.

The decision to limit the number of venopuctures to restart hyperalimentation in Latasha's case is equivalent to the decision to withdraw nutrition and hydration. A decision to withdraw nutrition and hydration is one that is generally considered both ethically and legally possible, and a case of necrotic bowel in infants is one of the paradigmatic situations in which it may be considered appropriate (Nelson *et al.* 1995). Nutrition and hydration are generally agreed to be medical treatments on a par with mechanical ventilation and other life-sustaining technologies. In cases when the treatment is medically futile, or continuing to provide such treatments is inhumane, decisions to withdraw treatment are allowed even by the relatively strict child abuse regulations. A more frequently applied standard of the patient's best interest could also allow for withdrawal of treatments in cases such as that described by Dr. Penticuff (Weir 1995). In Latasha's case, the patient was suffering multiple system failures, including the central nervous system and the liver, as well as her alimentary system. Latasha's life expectancy was severely limited, and no curative or corrective treatment was available that could reverse the course of her deterioration. The degree of suffering experienced by the child from continuing hyperalimentation could in such circumstances outweigh the benefits that could accrue to her. It seems there was no legal or ethical reason not to make the more explicit decision to withdraw the treatment.

If there was no legal or ethical reason not to decide to withdraw treatment, perhaps pyschological reluctance can explain the way the decision was framed. It is clear from many surveys that there is a considerable reluctance to make the decision to withdraw hydration and nutrition. In a survey cited by Ashwal and colleagues (1992), members of the Child Neurology Society found that 75% "never" withheld fluid and nutrition from infants and children, even those in a permanent vegetative state. Dr. Penticuff mentions the deep reluctance of the parents and committee members to withhold life-sustaining nutrition from a child, and the symbolic weight of nourishment in our understanding of our responsibilities to infants. The decision to limit the number of tries to re-start, however, had the same effect as a more explicit decision.

In a case where neither law nor morality stand in the way of a decision to withdraw treatment, the question might still arise of who has the authority to make that decision. The physician bears the ultimate responsibility for making such decisions, and the preferences of the parents must count as one of the major factors to be taken into consideration. Should there be any disagreement about the appropriate plan of care, the availability of an ethics committee in the institution can be a source of advice, judgment, or help (Stahlman 1995). In the case described, there seems to have been an enviable unanimity of decision makers, although insufficient attention was paid to communication. Parents and physicians agreed; the case was submitted to the advisory judgment of the institution's ethics committee; and despite the confusion engendered by the way the decision was reached, the nursing staff seemed to agree that the decision to limit Latasha's suffering was correct.

One might speculate that had there been any disagreement between the caregivers, the physicians, and the parents, or between the parents, a quite different case would have been taken to the ethics committee. Such decisions are difficult and painful; it seems to one observing from outside the institution that considerable care was taken to cover some of the most important bases in reaching the decision. Although providing "appropriate" nutrition and hydration is often advantageous to infants, the decision of when such provision is appropriate can require complex discretionary decision making on the part of the caregivers, and it seems that considerable attention was paid to making that decision. In light of that attention, the failure to involve the nursing staff in the decision is a surprising – and inappropriate – oversight.

Nursing ethics and clinical ethics

There has been considerable discussion in the literature about whether nursing ethics is a subset of medical ethics or of bioethics, or whether it is as specifically different as the professions themselves. The answer to that question may depend upon the larger ethical theory that is held by the participants in the debate. Nursing ethics has often been described as more contextual or situational, less theory-driven, as particularistic, or more focused upon relationships than bioethics generally (Cooper 1990). One of the most interesting developments in recent philosophical ethics has been a proliferation of attempts to develop an ethics of care, and a number of contributions have come from nursing. There are several themes common to most versions of an ethics of care. First, they acknowledge that human beings are to varying degrees constituted by, defined by, the relationships in which they stand to others (Benner 2004). Not only contractual ones, but such natural relationships as parent, neighbor, or colleague are integral to the ethical self and have moral status. Second, such emotions as love, care, sympathy, empathy, or compassion are not distractions, irrelevant to the essentially rational work of ethical decision making, but are rather clues to our deepest-held values and the stuff of which morality is made (Tong 1998). Third, there is a general humility about the capacity of ethics to be turned into a science, and a skepticism about the desirability of doing so. Ethical principles have the status of empirical generalizations or thumb-rules for action, rather than premises for deductive conclusions (Cooper 1991). Fourth, care ethicists tend to give great weight to context or situation. The importance laid on experience suggests that the perspective so important to ethics of care is a function of that experience (Tronto 1999).

A definitive formulation of an ethic of care has not yet emerged, but feminists, bioethicists, and nurse ethicists are working to develop alternatives to universalizable and impartial ethical theorizing. Patricia Benner (Benner and Wrubel 1989), Sally Gadow (1983), and Jean Watson (1988), among nursing theorists, have made important contributions to the growing literature. In suggesting that nursing ethics tends to be characterized by particularity, personal involvement, and affect, Dr. Penticuff contributes to this increasingly popular direction for ethical theorizing. A very similar description of clinical pediatric ethics by a physician contrasts "close-up" with "distance" ethics (Duff 1987). Dr. Penticuff's description of "ethics within arm's length" as more particularistic, personal, and affective than bioethics in general seems quite right, and may serve to distinguish both nursing ethics and clinical ethics in general as a subset or outgrowth of bioethics.

Insofar as the activities associated with a specific profession are different from those of another profession, it is to be expected that there will be some differences in the ethical perspectives of the two. Both medicine and nursing are dedicated to the best interests of the patient, and so operate under a common and unifying paradigm which provides a stable basis for agreement. But the ordering or priority given to values shared in common may differ depending upon the experiences of different individuals in the same situation. The professional responsibility of nursing for a broad range of patient needs in addition to the patient's specifically medical care, and a strong emphasis on responsibility to the family, especially in pediatric nursing, may call into prominence, in a given case, different values than those emphasized by attention to the medical situation alone. Certainly the knowledge about the patient and the family which is available to the nurse because of the intensive contact required by bedside nursing makes the input of the nurses *essential* in any approach to ethical issues which arise in clinical contexts.

While the expertise required by one profession may differ from the skills and competencies required by another, one of the important presuppositions of clinical ethics is that there is no profession that has a monopoly on ethical expertise. Clinical ethics presupposes that all individuals with a moral stake in a given clinical case need to be heard when ethical decisions have to be made.

The role of the ethics committee in the life of the institution

Not all the distress caused by this case was avoidable. But one of the avoidable contributing factors was the mystery surrounding the decision to limit venopuncture. There are several important issues raised by the process in Latasha's case. One is the role of the ethics committee in the institution, as perceived by the rest of the hospital staff. Another is the protocol of the committee itself. Is it typical for the operation of this ethics committee that the immediate caregivers are not included in the processes of the committee, either at the information-gathering or at the information-dissemination stage of the committee's consultations?

Who was seen to have made the decision in Latasha's case? From the description given, it sounds as though the decision appeared as a decision of the ethics committee rather than as a decision of the care team and family in consultation with the ethics committee. Does this ethics committee wish to be perceived by the people in the institution as the legislator of such decisions, rather than as a support system for the people responsible for making those decisions? Their failure to involve the bedside nurses in the deliberations can contribute to such an understanding of the role of the committee. Their lack of participation in the decision, and lack of information about how the decision was made, strongly impacted the morale not only of the individual bedside nurses most involved in the care of Latasha, but of the whole unit. In this case Dr. Penticuff describes a cohesive and well-supported staff able to survive the threat to unit morale. But it is worrying that the role of the ethics committee in this case was to constitute such a threat. No one could deny that the people most involved in Latasha's care have a moral, as well as emotional and professional, stake in decisions that impact her care. Ignoring that moral stake is demeaning to their professional and personal contribution to the function of the hospital. Limited understanding of and lack of input into the decisions made in this case led to moral distress; in other circumstances they could have had consequences for the treatment itself or have led to litigation for the institution.

Dr. Penticuff, along with the nurses in the unit, is very generous to attribute some of the communication failures to the parents' unwillingness to hurt their relationship with the nursing staff. The committee may have been explicitly asked to withhold information about who initiated the request for limiting IVs, in which case it would face a conflict between communication and confidentiality as competing ethical imperatives. The suggestion that the parents were reluctant to portray themselves as having initiated the request is probably correct, but perhaps short-sighted on their part, as well. The nurses were committed to their support, as well as to the support of Latasha, and would in the case described have been better able to support them had they had more adequate information about what was going on. Anyone who has been involved in ethics consultation in hospitals has quickly learned that the single most important contributor to ethical problems in institutions is communication: failures of communication, inadequate communication, inappropriate communication, miscommunication. Insofar as any committee can hope to contribute positively to the ethical climate within the hospital, it needs to pay serious attention in its protocols and procedures to issues of communication, and there is some reason to wonder if the committee in this institution has done so. Even if communication and confidentiality, competing obligations of the ethics committee, were at odds in this case, the conflict does not seem to have been explicitly addressed by the committee. Both prudence and common courtesy suggest that the workings of the ethics committee need to be highly visible to all those who have a moral stake in the resolution of ethical issues at the bedside. This case could have served as a clarion call to the ethics committee to address communication issues explicitly in their protocol.

Ethics committees function differently in different institutions. Their composition is ideally multidisciplinary; and apparently this committee appropriately included representatives from nursing. One wonders how those representatives were expected to function, however. Was it only the nurse representatives who had the responsibility for communicating with the nursing staff? Compartmentalizing the responsibilities in that way would complicate the operation of the committee. Did the committee consider its responsibility to include the effects of its operation on the ethical climate of the institution, or only to approve or veto suggestions brought to it?

Dr. Penticuff's conclusions about the number of nurses in hospitals who understand the functions of their institution's ethics committee are discouraging, and represent a serious problem for committees. The problem is exacerbated by the fact that the role of such committees is different in each institution, and is changing as the expectations of such committees expand to include organizational ethics issues. It is the obligation of any such committee to be very clear and explicit about its role, structure, and procedures; to disseminate that information widely within the institution by various educational strategies; and to periodically re-examine its role and procedures in light of changing situations. Older and well-established committees are no less likely than newly formed committees to require regular self-scrutiny as well as continuing institution-wide education of the sort recommended by Dr. Penticuff.

Ethics committees have in the past been primarily concerned with clinical issues. But no profession is more aware than nursing of the extent to which organizational constraints impact clinical ethics. Recent changes in the accreditation process recommended by the Joint Commission for the Accreditation of Healthcare Organizations mandate an expanded role for ethics in hospitals to encompass organizational issues as well (JCAHO 1997). This mandate represents an opportunity for ethics committees to expand their focus from consultation on specific clinical cases to a broader consideration of the ethical climate of the healthcare organization as a whole. Many clinical ethics cases have organizational implications. The case presented is an excellent example. The role of the ethics committee in this case in fact contributed to distress and demoralization of a crucial clinical unit. A successful clinical ethics process would examine why this happened and what structural changes in the protocol of the ethics committee, in the method of communication between different services in the unit, or in hospital policies, might prevent similar incidents in the future, and help the institution as a whole to run more smoothly. Many clinical ethical issues – disclosure, privacy, confidentiality, communication – have organizational analogues which specific cases can introduce into discussion so as to broaden the concerns of the ethics committee. Some ethics consultations, as we have learned to our dismay, arise because of organizational constraints that create conflicts of interest or conflicts of commitment in the individuals who function in various roles within the institution. An effective ethics process in an institution must prepare itself to address these broader issues of organization ethics.

Conclusion

Latasha's case represents a sorry example of good intentions gone awry and hard decisions made harder by thoughtlessness. For whatever reason, perhaps even with good intentions of protecting them, the people involved in making decisions for Latasha's care failed to respect the bedside nurses, and failed to acknowledge their agency as caregivers for the seriously ill child. They were not mere means to the child's care, but active participants in what should have been a collaborative joint enterprise. The ethics committee's failure to recognize and acknowledge the injustice done to them by withholding information about the decisions being made speaks ill of the role that the committee is playing in the life of the institution.

11.3 Topical discussion

Ethics committees and case consultation

The nation's experience with "Baby Doe" laws in the 1980s led to a reaction against deciding problematic ethical cases through the courts. Institutional ethics committees established to deal with particular clinical areas such as dialysis allocation or treatment of newborns served as a model for clinical ethics committees, intended to serve as an intermediary between individual physician decisions and extramural judicial interventions in ethically troubling cases. By 1993, the Joint Commission for the Accreditation of Healthcare Organizations (JCAHO) began to require all hospitals of more than 200 beds to have ethics committees with responsibility for education, policy formation, and case consultation. No specific procedures are required, but the multidisciplinary committee described in this case has become widely accepted as standard. Not all committees are equally effective within their institutions, and attention to supporting the role and processes of those committees is an important organizational concern.

The Society for Bioethics Consultation (now the American Society of Bioethics and Humanities) has developed guidelines for clinical ethics consultation. They emphasize the importance of working to ensure that all involved parties with a moral stake in the outcome of a given case have a chance to have their voices heard, and recommend documentation of the results of all consults.

Authority and responsibility

The traditional and legal authority of physicians to determine medical care has long been mediated by nurses and other allied health professionals who are given the responsibility of carrying out their decisions. This hierarchical structure of medicine

Ethical Dilemmas in Pediatrics: Cases and Commentaries, ed. Lorry R. Frankel, Amnon Goldworth, Mary V. Rorty, and William A. Silverman. Published by Cambridge University Press. © Cambridge University Press 2005.

has to some extent been ameliorated by the contemporary "team" approach to hospital care, but collaborative practice requires information sharing and discussion of options.

The unit nurses in this case were the proximate agents for a care plan apparently formulated outside of the unit, and because of inadequate communication they found themselves carrying out orders they had no voice in determining. Indeed, no attempt was made to clarify the source or rationale of the plan, leading to confusion and exacerbating stress. Were the parents and physicians thoughtless, or did they misunderstand what appropriate respect for the role of the nurses required?

Moral distress

Conceptualized in the mid-1980s, moral distress has spread from its origin in nursing ethics to apply in many realms of health care. If moral *dilemmas* arise when a caregiver must choose between incompatible courses of action, each of which has ethical justification, moral *distress* arises when the agent is clear about the ethically appropriate course of action but institutional constraints make it difficult to do it. Much of the literature on moral distress focuses on the psychological consequences of frustrated ethical agency: loss of self-esteem, demoralization, and guilt.

Working conditions that impede, rather than support, actions required by the professional ethics of healthcare providers can be a source of moral distress. Among the factors reported in the literature as contributing to moral distress are inadequate staffing, with its concomitant lack of time and resources; lack of supervisory support; hierarchical structure and its associated power differential; legal constraints; and badly implemented institutional policies. Virtually every cause of distress in the literature cites failures of communication, and every strategy for reducing impediments recommends ways of improving it.

It is simplistic to think that conflicts between physicians and nurses or between caregivers and surrogates about appropriate care are the only sources of moral distress. More recent explorations focus on conflicts of commitment, noting that all caregivers, physicians as well as nurses, are increasingly torn between their accountability to their patients and their accountability to the institutions in which they practice. Of particular concern to both individuals and organizations throughout the healthcare system is the current pressure for cost containment, as well as continuing pressure for quality improvement. The moral dilemma of balancing cost and care is the most salient cause of moral distress in nurses at all levels and in all roles in healthcare organizations, and can usefully be seen as causing an organizational analogue to moral distress, a misalignment of values, to the organizations them-selves. An organization committed to excellent care for reasonable cost may insti-tute policies oriented toward cost containment that are perceived by internal con-stituents as constraints upon the quality of care required by their professional clinical judgment.

In this case, the belief of the bedside nurses that the ethics committee, rather than the caregivers, had been responsible for the care plan may have led them to see that committee as an inappropriate third-party intervention in already complex hospital hierarchies and roles – not an institutional facilitator but an impediment to agreement among those with an immediate stake in the case.

Nursing ethics

Socialization into a profession is a process of impressing its intrinsic values upon its members. Nursing, like medicine, is a Hippocratic profession, insofar as it has as its central focus the well-being of the patient. But the activities associated with that profession may lead to a different understanding or prioritization of those common values. One of the most frequently drawn contrasts in priorities is the parodic contrast of "care" versus "cure" – as though any clinician were not committed to both.

The American Nursing Association has a code that is a professional analogue to that of the American Medical Association. In addition there has been con-siderable work in the nursing literature on the theoretical foundation of nursing practice, including elaboration of the ethical values associated with that practice. Dr. Penticuff characterizes nursing ethics as essentially "particular" and relational. Because nursing care includes primary responsibility for the life functions of medi-cal patients, some nurse theorists have developed sophisticated versions of an "ethics of [nursing] care" that draws on feminist, phenomenological, and pragmatic ethi-cal theory. It is fair to say that there is more interesting theoretical work on ethics being done in nursing than in any other health profession, although the insights developed are inappropriately neglected outside that profession.

In the clinical setting, among those who have a moral stake in the treatment of each patient are physicians and nurses, social workers and chaplains, administrators and regulators, as well as family members. Clinical ethics as a practice, as exempli-fied in the operation of clinical ethics committees, encourages the expression and acknowledgment of these different perspectives. Organizational and professional structures decree that the attending physician has the final authority, but profes-sional (or personal) differences need to be expressed and heard, whether or not they are determinative of the resolution of ethically problematic cases.

FURTHER READING

American Nurses Association. *Code of Ethics for Nurses with Interpretive Statements* (Washington, DC: ANA, 2001).

American Society for Bioethics and Humanities. *Core Competencies for Health Care Ethics Consultation* (Glenview, ILL: ASBH, 1998).

DeRenzo, E. G. and Strauss, M. A feminist model for clinical ethics consultation: increasing context and narrative. *HEC Forum* **9** (1997), 212–217.

Drane, J. F. *Clinical Bioethics: Theory and Practice in Medical–Ethical Decision Making* (Kansas City, MO: Sheed and Ward, 1994), Chapters 1 and 11.

Erlan, J. A. Moral distress: a pervasive problem. *Orthopedic Nursing* **20** (2001), 76–80.

Levi, B. Withdrawing nutrition and hydration from children: legal, ethical and professional issues. *Clinical Pediatrics* **42** (2003), 139–145.

Liaschenko, J. and Davis, A. J. Nurses and physicians on nutritional support: a comparison. *Journal of Medicine and Philosophy* **16** (1991), 259–283.

Lynn, J. and Childress, J. F. Must patients always be given food and water? *Hastings Center Report* **13** (5) (1983), 17–21.

Raines, M. L. Ethical decision making in nurses: relationships among moral reasoning, coping style and stress. *JONA's Healthcare Law, Ethics and Regulation* **2** (2000), 29–41.

Wilkinson, J. M. Moral distress in nursing practice: experience and effect. *Nursing Forum* **23** (1987–8), 17–29.

12.1 Ethics and managed care

Douglas S. Diekema

Introduction

In recent years, insurance organizations in the United States have increasingly adopted managed care strategies in an effort to control the steadily rising costs of health care. The strategies employed by these managed care organizations (MCOs) have in many cases challenged the ethical integrity of physicians caring for patients enrolled in them (Kassirer 1993).

Most healthcare delivery systems pose some challenge to the physician's primary obligation to seek the good of the patient. Payment methods – fee for service, salary, per-capita prepayment – can and do affect how medical professionals pursue the delivery of health care (Hillman 1987, Hillman *et al.* 1989, Hemenway *et al.* 1990). Traditional healthcare delivery with physician reimbursement on a fee-for-service basis provides an incentive for physicians to utilize unnecessary or marginally beneficial diagnostic and therapeutic interventions, sometimes to the point of causing harm. Managed care changes the nature of the incentives. Both fee-for-service and managed care challenge physician integrity by creating a potential conflict of interest. In fee-for-service, providing overtreatment has the potential to increase physician income. Under managed care, physician financial welfare is often tied to reducing utilization of consultation, diagnostic, and therapeutic modalities.

Managed care does not inherently lead physicians to put their own welfare above that of their patients any more than fee-for-service systems. However, the challenge to the physician's primary obligation to his or her patient changes form. In this chapter I will explore four ways that managed care poses a challenge to the physician's primary obligation to seek the good of the patient.

Ethical Dilemmas in Pediatrics: Cases and Commentaries, ed. Lorry R. Frankel, Amnon Goldworth, Mary V. Rorty, and William A. Silverman. Published by Cambridge University Press. © Cambridge University Press 2005.

Cases

(1) Duties of disclosure and managed care

> Dr. Jones is seeing 13-year-old Katie for a laceration she suffered when a friend's large dog lunged at her and bit her cheek. The cut on Katie's face is quite large, deep, and somewhat complicated. Though Dr. Jones possesses very good suturing skills, she would feel most comfortable having a plastic surgeon do the repair. However, Katie belongs to an MCO that requires pre-authorization for any plastic-surgery referral. When Dr. Jones discusses the laceration with the MCO's authorizing physician, she admits that she could do an adequate job on the repair, but believes a plastic surgeon could do better. He refuses to authorize the referral.

Dr. Jones finds herself in a difficult position that has become increasingly common in managed care environments. MCOs may seek to control the costs of medical care directly by limiting the services available to their subscribers or requiring pre-authorization before certain expensive interventions are utilized. One common form of direct control is to limit the drugs that are available on an MCO's formulary. The MCO will then refuse to pay for any non-formulary drugs that a physician might prescribe. In this case, Katie's MCO is directly controlling the use of an expensive consultation service by requiring pre-authorization for referrals to a plastic surgeon. Direct controls such as pre-authorization or limitation of certain diagnostic or treatment options seek to reduce costs by eliminating non-beneficial or marginally beneficial medical treatments. In this case, the MCO has decided that the marginal benefit associated with the use of a plastic surgeon instead of a primary care physician to suture a laceration does not justify the increased cost to the MCO (or to the patient – or patient's employer – in the form of increased premiums).

Dr. Jones finds herself in an awkward position because the therapeutic intervention she believes to be in the patient's best interest has not been approved by the MCO paying for Katie's care. How can she fulfill her obligation as Katie's physician and operate within the constraints posed by the MCO?

The physician's primary duty must remain patient-centered (Pellegrino and Thomasma 1988; Churchill 1997). In other words, Dr. Jones must recognize that despite the multiple constraints she faces each day, her role as a physician calls her first to attend to the best interests of her patients. The physician's role is grounded in the principle of beneficence – the obligation to seek the good of the patient. In situations where the "best" care may not be covered, Dr. Jones can meet her obligation in two important ways.

First, Dr. Jones has an obligation to all of her patients to deliver competent care. If she believes that she does not possess the skills necessary to competently suture Katie's laceration, she should refuse to do so, and pressure the MCO to authorize someone with those skills to perform the procedure. The essential feature here is the question of competence. It can be argued in almost every case of patient care that there exists a physician or specialist somewhere who is perhaps more adept at performing the evaluation or procedure in question than the patient's own physician. However, it is neither possible nor desirable for all patients to receive the "best" medical care. The fact that a plastic surgeon could possibly achieve a better cosmetic result does not in and of itself make it wrong for Dr. Jones to do the procedure. Nor is it wrong for the MCO to refuse authorization – as long as another physician can competently perform the procedure. Therefore, Dr. Jones must first make an honest assessment of her own abilities in this situation. If she has the skills to suture this laceration, then the simple presence of another physician whose skills exceed hers does not oblige her to refuse to perform the procedure.

Dr. Jones must couple an honest assessment of her competence in this situation with another duty, however. In its simplest form, the dilemma facing Dr. Jones arises from the trade-off between the marginal benefit of a plastic surgeon and the cost of that service. What Dr. Jones must realize, however, is that the trade-off must ultimately be weighed by the person who will bear the burdens or benefits of whatever decision is eventually made. The decision involves personal values as much as medical considerations. Is a plastic surgery closure worth the added cost? Since the benefits and costs are born by Katie and her family, the decision belongs to them, not Dr. Jones. Katie and her parents should be given the option of paying out of pocket (or appealing to the MCO later) for a plastic surgeon if they feel it is worth the cost for the possibility of a better cosmetic outcome.

If any duty becomes essential in a managed care environment, it is the physician's duty to be honest in disclosing these trade-offs to the patient and the family. The principle of informed consent continues to apply in the managed care setting. Simply because a family has chosen a healthcare insurance plan that excludes coverage of certain services does not exempt the physician from disclosing those services as alternatives in the therapeutic plan. In this case, Dr. Jones should discuss her conversation with the MCO representative. She should disclose her own competence and comfort level with doing the procedure, the fact that a reasonable alternative exists (the plastic surgeon), her assessment of the likelihood and extent to which the outcome might differ if performed by a plastic surgeon, and the cost to the family of a plastic surgery referral. Dr. Jones has an obligation to deliver quality medical care to Katie. While she does not have an obligation to deliver the *highest* level of care to each of her patients, she does have an obligation to disclose the various alternatives available and help them in understanding the trade-offs of each choice. In that way she fulfills her obligation as a caring physician who seeks the best for her patient as determined by the patient.

(2) Incentives to limit care

Mr. and Mrs. Miller have brought their six-week-old son, Zach, to the clinic today because he has been fussy and had a fever at home. Dr. Smith, who also cares for the other three Miller children, notices that Zach does indeed have a fever and a runny nose, but is unable to find any other source for the fever on his examination. Up until recently, Dr. Smith's approach to all children under two months of age with fever has been to fully evaluate them with a spinal tap, blood culture, and urine culture followed by a two-day admission for antibiotics until the cultures proved negative for bacterial infection. However, Dr. Smith's practice patterns have recently come under scrutiny by the MCOs to which many of his patients belong. Several MCOs, including the one to which the Millers belong, have threatened to drop Dr. Smith from the plan if his costs don't drop. As a result, Dr. Smith has changed his practice. He explains to the Millers that Zach appears to have a cold and that he would prefer to do no further evaluation at this time, but to see Zach back in the morning for another examination. Mrs. Miller tells Dr. Smith that she trusts his judgment but is curious why he is managing Zach differently than he had managed Zach's older sister when she presented with a fever at seven weeks of age.

Managed care organizations often seek to control costs by utilizing incentives to influence physician behavior. These incentives can take many forms. Some MCOs may refuse payment after the fact for what they perceive to be wasteful care. Others use capitation payments to shift the risk of over-utilization from the MCO to the physician. Many utilize payment mechanisms which include bonuses that reward productivity or frugality, tying income either directly or indirectly to performance. Others withhold portions of the physician's income that may or may not be returned based upon either the financial status of the MCO or the physician's individual performance. In most cases, the physician stands to benefit financially by decreasing the utilization of medical services among his or her patients. The positive aspect of these schemes is that they provide an incentive for physicians to eliminate wasteful or marginally beneficial practice patterns. The danger, however, is that the same incentives apply when physicians decrease the utilization of services that would clearly or potentially benefit a patient.

Dr. Smith faces another kind of incentive. Through review of utilization patterns and cost profiles of individual physicians, MCOs may decide to drop certain physicians from their plan. In certain markets, the loss of patients that results from such a decision could be devastating to the physician. Therefore, the threatened loss of participation in the plan can be a powerful incentive for a physician like Dr. Smith to change his practice patterns.

What all of these incentive mechanisms share is that they create a conflict of interest for the physician. They pit the financial self-interest of the physician against the welfare of his or her patients by making at least a portion of the physician's income or financial welfare dependent on decreasing utilization of medical services. The conflict of interest this represents can pose a serious challenge to the physician's ethical integrity, especially when the physician's interests conflict with his or her obligation to seek the good of the patient (Pellegrino 1995b).

As physicians come under the control and direction of managed care corporations – entities for which maximizing shareholder earnings may take priority over patient good – their professional integrity must remain steadfast. The integrity of healthcare providers requires that they reject a pure buyer–seller characterization of medical practice in order to advocate for the good of their patients (Yarmolinsky 1995). Physicians must insist that arrangements with business-owned managed care companies not undermine their ability to deliver medically appropriate care to their patients. At a minimum, the physician concerned primarily about fidelity to his or her patient must assure that arrangements with economic entities be carefully considered. Connections between physician incentives and individual patient care decisions should be as remote as possible and as small as possible (Morreim 1995). Incentives spread over the performance of groups of physicians, for example, pose less of a conflict than those that apply to an individual physician (Emanuel 1995). These arrangements need not entirely disrupt the connection between medical care and cost-consciousness on the part of the physician, but they must not interfere with the physician's ability to function as a trusted caretaker for the individual patient (Hillman 1987). The American Medical Association has reminded physicians that "medicine is a profession, a calling, and not a business . . ." (American Medical Association Council on Ethical and Judicial Affairs 1995b). It may be – as some have suggested – that paying physicians salaries is the only way to eliminate completely the concerns raised by financial motivation of physician behavior so that there is no financial incentive to either over-provide or under-provide medical treatment (Johnson 1990).

The financial pressures faced by Dr. Smith do not change his moral obligation to seek the best interests of his patients. Even if he feels pressured to limit what he delivers, the fiduciary nature of his role as physician demands that he deliver reasonable and appropriate medical care. If his recommended course of action places Zach at risk, Dr. Smith should reconsider his recommendation. On the other hand, if Dr. Smith believes that his recommended plan of action is a reasonable one that does not pose a significant risk to Zach, he still owes Zach's family an honest assessment of alternatives, the risks and benefits of each alternative and the management strategy he is recommending, and those financial arrangements which may bias the recommendation he is making to the family.

In some cases, the economic arrangements made between MCOs and the physicians they employ may represent a threat to informed consent. Physicians may face incentives that encourage them not simply to withhold care, but also to withhold information from their patients about the very care they are withholding (Morreim 1995). When economic incentives "gag" physicians, patients may not be made aware of important alternatives in the management of their illnesses. In most cases, the incentive to remain silent arises from the conflict between the physician's financial self-interest and the welfare of the patient. In a fee-for-service system, the physician had an incentive to over-utilize diagnostic and therapeutic modalities, but because these things were being done to the patient, the patient in most cases was aware of the services being utilized. With incentives to under-utilize, however, many patients remain ignorant of what is being withheld. They may have no way of knowing that a valuable service has not been discussed.

In a few cases, this silence can be coerced in the form of contracts between physician and MCO. Physician David Himmelstein was terminated from his corporate employer after publishing and criticizing the details of his contract, a contract that included significant economic incentives to restrict care to patients: "Physician shall agree not to take any action or make any communication which undermines or could undermine the confidence of enrollees, potential enrollees, their employers, their unions, or the public in US Healthcare or the quality of US Healthcare coverage," and "Physician shall keep the Proprietary Information [payment rates, utilization-review procedures, etc.] and this Agreement strictly confidential" (Woolhandler and Himmelstein 1995). MCO policies which restrict the physician's ability to communicate openly with the patient about potentially beneficial alternatives (including those not covered by the patient's MCO), to make honest recommendations, and to disclose conflicts of interest, are morally inappropriate and legally questionable (American Medical Association Council on Ethical and Judicial Affairs 1995, Martin and Bjerknes 1996). Informed consent and fidelity to patient interests remain essential components of moral duty in the role of physician. Any MCO policy that interferes with those duties should be vigorously opposed. Woolhandler and Himmelstein (1995) comment, "It is hard to be a good doctor. The ways we are paid often distort our clinical and moral judgment and seldom improve it. Extreme financial incentives invite extreme distortions . . . many physicians scrambling to preserve their careers will be tempted or forced into the corporate embrace. But if we shun the sick or withhold information to benefit ourselves, we conspire in the demise of our profession." Patients trust that physicians will act as their agents and have their best interests as a primary concern. That trust is important to the healing relationship. The conflicts of interest built into existing financial and organizational arrangements between physicians and corporate payers threaten to destroy that trust (Rodwin 1995). At a minimum, these financial incentives must be revealed to the patient (Morreim 1997). Likewise, the duty of informed consent requires that physicians continue to discuss reasonable alternatives with their patients, even if some of those alternatives are not covered by the patient's insurance plan.

(3) Beyond disclosure to patient advocacy

Dr. Jones has seen four-year-old Daniel repeatedly over the past several weeks for persistent fevers. She initially diagnosed Daniel with a urinary tract infection, but further evaluation has resulted in the discovery of a Wilms' tumor, a rare tumor of the kidney that occurs only in children.

Dr. Jones has explained to Daniel's parents that the primary treatment involves surgical removal of the abdominal mass. Depending on the stage of the tumor, radiation therapy and chemotherapy may also be necessary. Daniel's MCO has authorized a referral to a urologist, Dr. Hall. As Dr. Jones discusses the case with Dr. Hall, Dr. Hall admits some mild discomfort. Until recently his practice has included only adult patients, and he has never seen or operated on a child with a Wilms' tumor. Nonetheless, he accepts the referral. Dr. Jones, uncomfortable with Dr. Hall's revelation, once again discusses the case with an MCO representative. Despite her arguments that standard of care would require referral to a pediatric surgeon with experience in the management of Wilms' tumor, the MCO will only authorize a referral to a physician within their plan. Since they have no pediatric surgeons, Dr. Hall will have to suffice.

Most MCOs utilize a panel of physicians who have contracted with the MCO to provide services to MCO subscribers. Since an MCO usually contracts for discounted rates with its panel of physicians, costs are controlled by limiting referrals to physicians belonging to the MCO. Referrals to physicians outside of the plan can be expensive for the MCO, and the MCO has more difficulty monitoring and restraining the costs of services provided by a non-plan provider. In some cases, the panel of physicians who have contracted with an MCO may not include a full complement of subspecialty providers. The MCO to which Daniel belongs does not have a pediatric surgeon as part of the plan. It is less expensive for the MCO to use non-pediatric surgeons.

There may be times when a physician owes more to his or her patient than simple disclosure. Dr. Jones owes Daniel's family an honest assessment of her recommendations. She should inform them of the MCO's decision, but she must also share her own judgment that Daniel should be seen by a pediatric surgeon for this procedure. Yet having informed Daniel's family of her recommendation does not necessarily give them the ability to make other choices (Zoloth-Dorfman and Rubin 1995). To go outside of the plan without authorization to see a pediatric surgeon may be what is best from the perspective of Daniel's health care, but Daniel's family could be devastated by the resulting unreimbursed costs of that care.

Dr. Jones must decide when more than honest disclosure is required of her. Honest disclosure seems sufficient when the gains offered by an uncovered service or procedure would be marginal. When Dr. Jones evaluated Katie's laceration, the net gain offered by a plastic surgeon in repairing a simple laceration was marginal. In that case, honest disclosure of the alternatives was an adequate response on the part of Dr. Jones, leaving the family to decide whether the services of a plastic surgeon would be worth the additional cost to themselves.

However, when a service that has been denied MCO authorization would likely prevent substantial harms or offer substantial benefits, Dr. Jones owes a duty to advocate on behalf of her patient with the MCO. This duty certainly begins with a formal appeal to the MCO by the physician on behalf of the patient (Howe 1995).

Dr. Jones is capable of bringing forward a more powerful argument for the necessity of a pediatric surgeon than Daniel's family. She must recognize that the diagnosis alone can be overwhelming, and that simply to inform Daniel's family of the option to appeal to their MCO would be unfair and cruel. The appeals process within many MCOs can be formidable, and Daniel's family should not have to find their way through it without the help of their physician.

If, despite her best efforts, Dr. Jones is unable to convince the MCO to pay for a pediatric surgeon, she should again honestly provide her assessment to Daniel's family. If she truly believes that inferior or dangerous care is being provided to Daniel, she should convey that to his parents, along with a discussion of their options. If Daniel's care is truly being jeopardized, it might be appropriate to recommend consultation with a lawyer. Such recommendations are extreme and should represent only a last resort in situations where the decision of an MCO clearly places the health of one's patient at risk and where all less intrusive alternatives have been explored without a satisfactory resolution. Of course, such a recommendation might also place the welfare of Dr. Jones at risk. Being dropped from the MCO's physician panel is a real risk for physicians who undermine the confidence of patients belonging to that MCO. Nonetheless, if she is to take her role as a physician seriously in seeking the good of her patient, she will recognize a duty to help her patient seek necessary care, even at some risk to her own welfare.

(4) The non-plan patient

Dr. Green is a pediatrician who works in the emergency department of a hospital owned by a health maintenance organization (HMO). At 10 o'clock one evening, as Dr. Green is about to evaluate a six-month-old child with a fever, the registration clerk informs him that the patient is uninsured. The HMO policy is not to offer services to non-plan patients who cannot provide either insurance or proof of ability to pay for care. Dr. Green has been informed previously that these patients should be transferred to the public hospital across town.

As we have discussed in the previous cases, Dr. Green has a primary duty to his patient. The medical needs of the patient must be addressed before the financial desires of the HMO within which the physician practices. Not only is Dr. Green under a moral obligation in this case to assure that this six-month-old child with a fever would not be endangered by a transfer to another institution, but he is constrained by federal statutes and regulations. The federal Emergency Medical Treatment and Active Labor Act (EMTALA) requires that a hospital with an emergency room provide an "appropriate medical screening examination within the capability of the hospital's emergency department, including ancillary services routinely available to the emergency department," to *any* individual who comes to that emergency room and on whose behalf a request is made for an examination or treatment of a medical condition (42 USC 1395dd). The purpose of this medical screening examination is to determine whether an "emergency medical condition" exists. If no emergency condition is discovered, the hospital's duty under EMTALA ends. The patient may be refused further care or transferred to another institution. However, if an emergency medical condition is discovered during the screening examination an additional duty arises. The hospital must either provide further medical examination and treatment (within the capacity of the hospital's staff and facilities) necessary to stabilize the individual's medical condition, or provide for an appropriate transfer to another facility. EMTALA defines "to stabilize" with respect to the emergency condition to mean "to provide such medical treatment of the condition as may be necessary to assure, within reasonable medical probability, that no material deterioration of the condition is likely to result from or occur during the transfer of the individual from a facility."

Thus, before Dr. Green can consider sending this family to the public hospital across town, he has a moral and legal duty to assure that the child does not have a serious medical condition that might pose a danger to the child during the transfer. If there is any question, Dr. Green should take steps to assure adequate stabilization of the child's condition and only then consider whether a safe transport is both appropriate (from the perspective of the child's interests) and legal (from the perspective of EMTALA and any relevant state transfer laws) (Diekema 1995).

This final case hints at another concern raised by the increasing presence of for-profit corporations as the owners of MCOs. For-profit MCOs have increasingly characterized the practice of medicine as a business. This market model of medicine threatens to change the primary focus of those who practice medicine. Emanuel and Steiner (1995) argue that healthcare institutions have three primary missions that benefit the public: patient care, teaching, and biomedical research. Raising funds and maximizing profit have historically been a means to support and further those primary missions. It is possible that medicine can become so commercialized that securing financial resources for the profit of stockholders may become its *primary* mission. We are increasingly encouraged to think about medicine in terms of efficiency, profit maximization, ability to pay, and competition of providers. The values of the marketplace (the maximization of profit or income) threaten to overwhelm the primary values of medicine (to seek to benefit the patient). "Let the buyer beware" replaces trust in this model (Lundberg 1995). Changes in the language people use to describe medical relationships reflect more significant changes in the relationships themselves. When customers and clients replace patients, we also risk losing the ethical tradition in which the term patient was embedded. Healthcare providers cannot become primarily business-persons or corporate employees without losing touch with their moral tradition (Relman 1992). The metaphors of business and industry imply different moral expectations of providers than the moral expectations required of physicians as professionals (Pellegrino 1994,

Pellegrino and Thomasma 1994). Furthermore, as the case above illustrates and as George Annas (1995) has recently pointed out, "There is no place for the poor and uninsured in the metaphor of the market."

In this setting, healthcare providers must heed the warning of Edmund Pellegrino (1995a) that "corruption inevitably afflicts any health care system not designed with care of the patient as its primary driving force." Physicians must bring integrity to their roles as patient caretakers:

> The role of gatekeeper entails an erosion and a violation of the commitment to the patient's welfare that must be the primary moral imperative in medical care. This commitment flows from the nature of illness and the promise of service made by individual physicians and the profession as a whole. That commitment has a basis in the empirical nature of the healing relationship in which a sick person – dependent, vulnerable, exploitable – must seek out the help of another who has the knowledge, skill, and facilities needed to effect cure. It is inevitably a relationship of inequality in freedom and power in which the stronger is obliged to protect the interest of the weaker. (Pellegrino 1986)

This role of gatekeeper becomes especially problematic when it goes beyond a "sense of responsible stewardship over communal resources and a concern for problems of distributive justice" to an interest in expanding the profit margins of companies, the dividend and portfolio values of shareholders, and the salary and benefit packages of highly paid MCO executives (Zoloth-Dorfman and Rubin 1995).

As physicians struggle to maintain their integrity in this increasingly corporate culture, they should celebrate what is good about managed care. At the same time, however, they must actively resist those elements that threaten to weaken their advocacy of what is best for their patients, including and especially those patients who are economically or socially disadvantaged (Winkenwerder and Ball 1988).

12.2 Challenging fidelity: the physician's role in rationing

Nancy S. Jecker

Introduction

Dr. Douglas Diekema has set forth a series of cases illustrating ethical concerns that arise for pediatricians practicing medicine in managed care settings. This chapter explores how the environments of managed care alter the physician's ethical role as patient advocate. The approach to this topic will be twofold. I begin by exploring rationing within managed care organizations (MCOs), using the cases set forth in the previous chapter to illustrate distinct rationing methods and criteria. Then I identify the limits these forms of rationing impose on patient advocacy, with an eye to clarifying the pediatrician's ethical role in healthcare rationing.

Possible methods of rationing within MCOs

Rationing occurs whenever physicians, hospitals, MCOs, purchasers, or others deny beneficial health care to patients under conditions of scarcity. But what is scarcity? In some instances, the raw materials from which healthcare services are made are themselves limited and there is not enough to provide them to everyone who stands to benefit. This first kind of scarcity is referred to as "resource scarcity" to emphasize the finite nature of the resources required to produce healthcare services (Morreim 1995). One example of resource scarcity is organ transplantation. The supply of hearts, lungs, kidneys, and other organs required for transplantation is currently insufficient to meet demand. Another example of resource scarcity is specialty care. In rural areas of the United States, medical specialists may be unavailable to patients who need them.

In other situations the raw materials required to provide health care are at hand, but the means to pay for services is limited. This second kind of scarcity, called "fiscal

Ethical Dilemmas in Pediatrics: Cases and Commentaries, ed. Lorry R. Frankel, Amnon Goldworth, Mary V. Rorty, and William A. Silverman. Published by Cambridge University Press. © Cambridge University Press 2005.

scarcity," underscores that the dollars needed to pay for health care are often in short supply (Morreim 1991). Fiscal scarcity can occur, for example, when patients lack healthcare coverage altogether and lack the means to pay out of pocket for the care they need. It also can occur when MCOs exert pressure on providers to reduce the cost of health care through financial penalties and rewards, resulting in patients being denied beneficial services.

Is rationing occurring in MCOs? If so, by what methods, and according to what criteria? Let us address these questions by briefly reviewing the cases of Katie, Zach, Daniel, and the six-month-old child (I will call her Julie), presented in the previous chapter. With respect to each case, we shall ask the following: Was health care rationed? If health care was rationed, what were the conditions of scarcity leading to rationing? Who was responsible for carrying out rationing? What ethical criteria might be invoked to justify rationing?

In the first case, 13-year-old Katie belonged to an MCO that denied her access to a plastic surgeon to repair a large facial laceration. The MCO's authorizing physician reasoned that an adequate suturing job could be done by Katie's primary care physician; hence the additional cost of specialty care was not justified. In this situation, financial considerations were the primary factor affecting the MCO's refusal to pay for referral to a plastic surgeon. No one disputed that (1) Katie could benefit from the care of a plastic surgeon and (2) this benefit was denied due to the cost of providing it. In other words medical care was rationed under conditions of fiscal scarcity. The MCO's policy was not to authorize payment for all services subscribers could benefit from. Nor was it to allow patients or their families to make informed medical choices in consultation with their physician after reviewing all medical options. Instead, the MCO policy was to deny care if it determined that less expensive care was "adequate."

Although the MCO set the policy for approval or denial of services, this policy was carried out by physicians. The MCO's authorizing physician was the person who said "no" to the primary care physician's request for a specialty referral. The primary care physician was, in turn, responsible for telling the patient and her parents that the request for a plastic surgeon to repair the laceration was denied.

An appeal to ethical criteria may not have figured at all in the actual deliberations at any stage; nonetheless, it is essential to consider possible ethical rationales for this decision. One ethical criterion that might be called upon to justify rationing in this situation is medical need. According to this line of thinking, referral to a plastic surgeon to repair the laceration on Katie's cheek would presumably result in a better cosmetic result; however, Katie does not medically need the best possible cosmetic result. Rather, what she needs is a repair of the laceration.

A second line of ethical reasoning might appeal to the criterion of benefiting the greatest number. According to this way of thinking, in order to produce the greatest good for the greatest number of patients, the MCO must deny referrals for procedures that can be performed safely and adequately by the primary physician. The MCO could argue that reducing costly specialty referrals enables it to provide better primary care to benefit a larger number of its subscribers.

A final way of thinking about the denial of specialty care to Katie holds that plastic surgery should be offered first to patients who would receive the greatest benefit. Arguably the benefit Katie would receive is marginal, since the primary care provider could do an adequate, albeit imperfect, job.

A second possible illustration of healthcare rationing is seen in the case of the six-week-old who presented at a pediatric clinic with fever and runny nose. Zach stood to benefit from a work-up to rule out bacterial infection as a source of fever; this benefit was denied because the MCO to which Zach belonged had informed Zach's pediatrician that he would be dropped from the health plan if he did not reduce the cost of caring for patients. This resulted in the physician changing his previous practice pattern by ordering fewer costly diagnostic services and hospital admissions, and replacing these with less expensive services, such as monitoring patients in the clinic over time to see if complications developed. As with the previous case, the expertise and resources required to provide services were not in short supply, but the dollars to pay for these were limited. Rationing occurred if the work-up that Zach was denied had a reasonable chance of offering him a significant medical benefit. If there was not a reasonable prospect of benefiting Zach, then rationing did not occur. For instance, rationing did not take place if the diagnostic work-up would serve only to provide psychological benefits, such as reassuring Zach's mother, or legal benefits, such as minimizing legal liability for the physician if complications developed and Zach's parents sued.

Let us assume that rationing occurred, and that Zach had a reasonable chance of benefiting from diagnostic procedures such as spinal tap, urine culture, and hospital admission for antibiotic treatment until cultures proved negative for bacterial infection. Who would we hold responsible for actually carrying out rationing? At one level, it was the physician who signed on with the MCO and thereby agreed to conform his conduct to its policies. When various health plans threatened to drop the physician for practicing expensive care, he apparently did not protest, but instead altered his practice patterns to align them with the MCO's fiscal constraints. The physician also carried out rationing in the sense that he made a decision about how to alter his practice in order to cut costs. He might have chosen instead to continue working up infants under two months of age who presented with fever, and cutting back expenses in other ways. Finally, the physician carried out rationing in the sense that he was the one who said "no" to the patient and parents. He sent them home without further testing. He had to answer Zach's mother when she asked why her son was being treated differently than her daughter had been when she was an infant. In short, the physician was expected to offer a plausible defense or explanation of rationing to patients and/or families.

Seen from a different vantage point, however, it is the MCO, not the physician, who bore the brunt of rationing. After all, the MCO had much more to do with creating the conditions of fiscal scarcity that led to rationing than the physician did. It was the MCO that sought to reduce its costs through a policy of dropping, or threatening to drop, from its plan physicians who provided relatively more expensive care. In the absence of this decision, Zach's physician would not have altered his practice pattern and Zach would have been worked up to rule out bacterial infection. In short, the MCO establishes limits on how much providers can spend in the course of caring for their patients, and enforces these limits by creating incentives for providers to reduce the cost of care.

Yet, looked at differently, the MCO is simply responding to market forces, doing its best to compete with other health plans for the business of purchasers (usually employers) in an environment of intense competition. MCOs that successfully reduce costs are able to offer better rates to purchasers, expand their businesses, and ultimately increase profits (or, in the case of not-for-profit MCOs, increase the funds available to invest in their product).

According to what underlying ethical criteria were healthcare services distributed in Zach's case? From the perspective of the physician, the central consideration appeared to be his own financial wherewithal. Zach's physician was reasonably concerned about his own livelihood because a number of MCOs had threatened to drop him. More generally stated, this criterion calls for allocating scarce resources in order to reduce financial risk to providers, hospitals, or health plans. Another possible rationing criterion was likelihood of medical success. Zach's physician might have reasoned that a practice of monitoring infants whose fever was below a certain level over a fixed period of time, and thereby delaying a decision about antibiotic treatment and diagnostic procedures, would be just as successful as working up infants when they first presented. Yet, in the absence of research demonstrating this, the physician had only his own clinical impressions to go on. Presumably these were quite limited, since the physician had only recently begun to delay treatment decisions in this kind of case.

The third case was that of Daniel, a four-year-old diagnosed with Wilms' tumor. Daniel's pediatrician recommended surgical removal of the tumor and was uncomfortable when the MCO to which Daniel's parents belonged referred Daniel to a urologist who had neither seen nor operated before on a child with a Wilms' tumor. The rationale the MCO gave was that there were no pediatric surgeons in the plan; therefore the urologist, who had until recently treated only adults, would suffice. Yet let us assume that pediatric surgeons were available in some capacity, either to join this MCO's plan, or to contract their services to the MCO. Assuming this, financial considerations would most likely be the driving factor leading the MCO to exclude pediatric surgeons from its list of available specialists. Understood in this way, fiscal scarcity was once again a driving force behind rationing. In other words, the patient was denied substantial benefits due to financial pressures to reduce healthcare costs.

The party who bears the burden of facing the patient and family most directly is, once again, the pediatrician. Depending on the knowledge level of the patient's parents, the physician may have some degree of choice about how much to disclose to the parents about the urologist referral. For example, if Daniel's parents lack medical sophistication about the disease and tend to accept the physician's recommendations at face value, then the physician may be in a position to choose whether or not to disclose rationing. In such situations, some ethicists argue that physicians have a strong legal and ethical duty to discuss the economic factors affecting care (Morreim 1991). Others hold that the legal, and perhaps the ethical, duties of economic disclosure can be fully discharged by MCOs at the time patients enroll in a health plan (Hall 1994). If rationing is disclosed and the parents protest and enlist the physician's help, the physician would be in the position of choosing whether to assist them in appealing to the MCO to reconsider its decision. Even if the pediatrician decides to do this, however, she may not be successful. Yet she would have at least forced the decision back to the MCO, conveying that the rationing choices the MCO had made did not meet professional standards of care. Ultimately, the pediatrician may lack the time, energy, or ability to provide this degree of advocacy for every patient who needs it. Or she may fear that continued protests would result in the MCO dropping her from the plan. Alternatively, the physician might judge that the MCO's policies were unlikely to change, and she should therefore terminate her contract with the MCO.

As with the previous case, the MCO in this third case might have reasoned that in order to compete against other MCOs for the business of purchasers, it must reduce costs. The question is not whether to ration care, but how to ration. What kinds of services will the MCO deny? The problem with blaming "market forces" is that this approach holds no identifiable individual accountable. If the physician passes the buck to the MCO, which in turn passes the buck to "market forces," then no one steps up and assumes the responsibility for rationing choices, and no one is considering whether these choices meet justice standards (Reiser 1994). Alternatively, if pediatricians and other physicians do what they can, both individually and as a profession, to define and ensure competent care for their patients, then others will be more likely to follow suit. MCOs may find it more difficult to impose arbitrary cost restrictions, and purchasers may be less likely to expect cut-rate deals from health plans. To the extent that government can be made aware of physicians' and patients' concerns about healthcare rationing, it is better able to develop appropriate regulations to guide the rationing practices of MCOs.

One criterion that might be used to support the practice of excluding pediatric surgeons or other medical specialists from the list of providers a health plan offers is the criterion of benefiting the greatest number of patients. As described previously, this criterion holds that limiting the number of specialists available to serve subscribers is justified by showing that the MCO uses this money to provide more primary care services to benefit a larger number of patients. Of course, this assumes that the MCO will actually devote the money saved through limitations on specialty care to the provision of primary care. If the money is spent on executive salaries, shareholder dividends, advertising campaigns to increase market penetration, or in other ways, then this argument is no longer sound.

Another option the MCO might have considered would be to include pediatric surgeons among its list of providers, but restrict access to them for certain patient groups. For example, if the criterion of benefiting the largest number of patients was used, the MCO might refuse Daniel access on the ground that since Wilms' tumor accounts for about 7% of all cancers in children, and childhood cancers are themselves relatively rare, it could benefit more patients by providing pediatric surgeons first to groups with more common ailments.

Alternatively, the MCO might invoke the standard of maximizing life years saved, reasoning that dollars should be spent first on treatments likely to prolong life for the greatest number of years. Applied to Daniel, this criterion would justify rationing care if Daniel's chance of survival was relatively low. Ordinarily, when treatment is started early, there is a fairly good survival rate (50–80%) for children diagnosed with Wilms' tumor. Yet we could imagine a situation where Daniel's individual prognosis was poor. His parents might have delayed bringing him to the pediatrician when he complained of abdominal pain. His treatment was further delayed when the pediatrician initially diagnosed a urinary tract infection, rather than Wilms' tumor. It might have taken several weeks to schedule another appointment with the pediatrician when symptoms persisted following antibiotic treatment. Since this form of kidney cancer spreads rapidly, it might have reached other organs by the time a correct diagnosis was given, thereby diminishing Daniel's chance of survival.

The final case under consideration involves six-month-old Julie. Julie's parents lacked healthcare coverage when she presented with fever to the emergency department of a hospital owned by a health maintenance organization (HMO). The HMO policy was to deny Julie an obvious benefit, namely, a preliminary evaluation to determine if she was stable enough to transfer to another hospital. Quite clearly, the emergency department possessed the material resources and professional expertise to provide this. As with the previous cases, fiscal scarcity, rather than resource scarcity, gave rise to rationing.

Who did it? Seen from one perspective, the HMO rationed care by setting a policy of denying beneficial treatment to patients like Julie. Seen from a different perspective, the registration clerk and the physician signed employment contracts agreeing to carry out the HMO's policies. It was therefore they who rationed care, assuming that they carried out the HMO's policy and told Julie's parents to go elsewhere.

According to what criteria was care rationed? The most obvious criterion is ability to pay. Julie's parents lacked insurance and proof of the ability to pay out of pocket for emergency services. The HMO might have applied this same criterion differently. For example, it might have chosen to devote sufficient resources to comply with the law by agreeing to evaluate uninsured patients and treat those who were not stable enough to transfer. This minimal responsibility would ensure that patients who arrived on their doorstep were not injured by the delay resulting from going elsewhere. Or the HMO might have chosen to assume a positive responsibility to serve the community by caring for a limited number of uninsured patients even if they were stable enough to transfer (Jecker 1995). This approach enables the HMO to ration health care while simultaneously limiting the effects of rationing on disenfranchised and vulnerable groups (Thomasma 1995).

Methods and criteria for rationing within MCOs

The cases discussed above illustrate distinct methods and criteria for rationing within MCOs. These methods and criteria are summarized below.

Methods

(1) Limits on providers: Daniel's plan did not include pediatric surgeons.
(2) Refusal of treatment to non-subscribers: Julie did not belong to the HMO.
(3) Financial incentives leading to rationing: in the cases discussed, financial incentives led providers to:
  (a) undertreat patients (all four cases show financial pressures resulting in patients receiving less treatment)
  (b) reduce time spent with patients (Zach was seen for a follow-up clinic visit, rather than a full diagnostic work-up)
  (c) limit specialist referrals (Katie was not referred to a plastic surgeon; Daniel was not referred to a pediatric surgeon)
  (d) substitute less costly treatment with greater risks/fewer benefits (Katie, Zach, and Daniel were offered less costly treatments with fewer benefits and/or greater risks)

(e) reduce hospital admissions and lengths of stay (Zach was not admitted to the hospital at the time he presented at the clinic; the HMO's policy was to refuse all care, including hospital admission, to Julie).

(4) Practice guidelines limiting physician discretion: Katie's pediatrician was not given a choice about whether she or a plastic surgeon would perform Katie's surgery; Daniel's urologist was not given a choice about whether he or a pediatric surgeon would remove Daniel's tumor.

Criteria

(1) Benefit the greatest number of patients
(2) Patient's ability to pay
(3) Risk of legal or financial liability to providers, hospitals or health plans
(4) Medical need
(5) Likelihood of medical success
(6) Life years saved

These methods and criteria for rationing restrict pediatricians' ability to advocate on behalf of patients. Should these restrictions be accepted? Or would accepting these forms of rationing erode the integrity of physicians' medical judgments (Callahan 1998), arouse the suspicions of patients (Jecker and Jonsen 1997), and raise concerns about diminished quality of care (Milstein 1997)? Some ethicists argue that physicians can no longer sustain a single-minded and unequivocal commitment to patients (Morreim 1995). Instead, they must acknowledge a "new medical ethics" that goes hand-in-hand with medicine's new economics. A quite different view holds that the pediatrician is ethically required to protest rationing at every turn, seeking to ensure the very best care possible for every patient. According to this position, the doctor cannot ethically serve as a "double agent," weighing allegiance to individual patients against monetary costs to health plans and society (Angell 1991; see also Purtillo 1995 and Stone 1997).

Is there a middle ground? Some have suggested that financial restrictions and the rationing practices they give rise to should be monitored and regulated, rather than outlawed (Orentlicher 1995, 1996b). But what role should physicians have in monitoring rationing? Dr. Diekema suggests that physicians can ethically deny beneficial treatments to patients, so long as they ensure patients receive competent care. Yet this approach can take us only so far. It assumes that fiscal scarcity does not require harder choices, choices involving the denial of medically necessary services. But the current healthcare system in the USA does not pay for all patients to receive a level of care that physicians consider "adequate." Medically necessary services, such as home health care for the disabled, drug treatment for patients with AIDS, mental health care for the chronically mentally ill, birth control for women of reproductive age, and other services are routinely excluded from health care coverage. This shows that even if a more robust healthcare system was in the offing, medically necessary care is currently rationed and will continue to be rationed in the immediate future. How should these hard choices be made? Consider the following example. Suppose health care is rationed in accordance with the criterion of benefiting the largest number of patients. This might result in rationing costly but medically necessary services, such as organ transplantation, that benefit a small number of patients. If physicians are obligated to provide all competent care to patients, it is difficult to see how they could ethically abide by this approach, even if it were sanctioned by society or its representatives.

What more viable approaches to rationing exist for the physician? To begin with, physicians should acknowledge a role in healthcare rationing. As long as the conditions of fiscal scarcity persist, rationing of one form or another will occur and physicians will be party to it, as the examples discussed above attest. Those who refuse to participate in rationing decisions, insisting that their own patients should always receive the very best care, should be asked to consider their obligations to the larger population of patients. While fidelity to one's own patients, and to the bond between patient and physician, is an important value, it is not an ethical absolute. Instead fidelity to patients must be considered in tandem with other important values, such as social justice (Jecker 1990). The refusal by some physicians to have a hand in rationing may spring from resentment toward MCOs, rather than fidelity to patients. Thus, physicians may resent intrusions into the doctor–patient relationship by third-party payers, and may feel general distress about a perceived loss of physician autonomy in clinical decision making (Ellsbury *et al.* 1987, 1990, Ellsbury and Montano 1990). The antidote here is to encourage physicians to exert an influence at various levels (e.g., MCOs, hospitals, physician groups, professional organizations, and at all levels of government) in designing the restrictions to which they and their patients will be subject.

Becoming more self-conscious about rationing and choosing to make more deliberate decisions leaves many questions unanswered. According to what methods and criteria should health care be rationed? This chapter has not set forth a conception of what a just healthcare system would look like. But even without such a conception in hand, improvements in justice can be made. Thus, the phenomenon of rationing can be defined and identified, the parties involved in rationing can be pointed out, and the methods and criteria for rationing can be talked about and assessed. Such efforts can help to ensure that rationing processes will be more publicly accountable, more consistently applied, and less vulnerable to manipulation by unfair and arbitrary influences. Such efforts can also make it more difficult to sustain glaringly unjust practices. By becoming more aware and forthright about their role in rationing, physicians help with the tasks of envisioning justice and evolving toward a more just healthcare system.

ACKNOWLEDGMENTS

This chapter was first drafted during a sabbatical year devoted to the study of ethical issues in managed care. The author acknowledges generous financial support from the Sierra Health Foundation (grant #95MOOI).

12.3 Topical discussion

Information and decision making

In an ideal world, in which each patient can assess the quality of medical care and the MCO can determine what maximum profit is, one could determine the Pareto optimal point, i.e., the point of compromise achieved between the competing aims of the patient and MCO in which each can veto the other.

In the real world, quality assessments of medical care by the patient (and for that matter by other individuals or groups of individuals, whether they be part of the healthcare system or not) are fragmented and distorted by economic concerns ("can I afford it?" or "can I reduce costs?"). In addition, it is not at all clear whether the concept of maximum profit has a determinate meaning, or an appropriate application, in the healthcare arena. Furthermore, the patient does not have decision-making powers that are equal to that of the MCO. He or she may opt out of a particular MCO but cannot directly bargain with the MCO for better terms, however these are understood. Indeed, the marketplace itself places powerful constraints on the competing demands of both the patient and the MCO. Thus, the point of compromise is not likely to be the Pareto optimal point.

Conflicts of interest and conflicts of commitment

A complex and difficult feature of professionalism is the level of autonomy of the practitioner. Professionals are expected to exercise their expert judgment in their practice, and to abide by their professional code of ethics, which should override other considerations if a conflict should arise. Yet most professionals today are also employees, partners in practice, or in contractual relationships, and, as a result, organizational or partnership interests sometimes conflict with professional

Ethical Dilemmas in Pediatrics: Cases and Commentaries, ed. Lorry R. Frankel, Amnon Goldworth, Mary V. Rorty, and William A. Silverman. Published by Cambridge University Press. © Cambridge University Press 2005.

judgment or the demands of a professional code. Such conflicts are ordinarily labeled conflicts of interest. While countries with a national health service may be better able to control financial conflicts of interest for physicians, in the USA fee-for-service medicine has in the main been replaced by managed care, and both models offer opportunity for conflict of interest. Fee-for-service medicine can provide an incentive for over-treatment, and managed care risks providing incentives to under-treat. One of the major criticisms directed toward the risk-sharing financial incentives to reduce utilization introduced by some managed care contracts is that they create a conflict of interest for the contracting providers, between their professional concern for the patient's best interest and their own financial advantage. Conflicts of interest need to be recognized, disclosed to all affected parties, and in some cases may even lead to the need to withdraw from the situation.

Conflicts of interest are usually distinguished from conflicts of commitment, although they overlap. Conflicts of commitment are those sets of role expectations where competing obligations prevent someone from honoring both commitments, or honoring them both adequately. Professionals with obligations to a group of patients cannot always serve each patient equally well. Even without considerations of financial conflict of interest, a physician may be professionally committed both to clinical care and to advancing medical science. Clinicians may also occupy administrative roles in their institutions, as well as roles as parents or children, as citizens or volunteers.

Organizations too face conflicts of interest and conflicts of commitment. One of the criticisms most frequently made of for-profit managed care is that the obligation to serve the patient, constitutive and definatory of the social institution of health care, is in possible conflict with the need to make profits for shareholders.

Current legal structure in the USA creates an additional complication. Managed care organizations have appropriate commitments both to their own financial survival and to the care of the patients of the providers with whom they contract. But unlike individual physicians, most plans are sheltered through provisions of a 1974 law, the Employee Retirement Income Security Act (ERISA), from being sued for malpractice, despite the fact that health plans are increasingly dictating treatment decisions through their contractual arrangements, and are thus seen, by both providers and patients, as co-responsible for treatment damages.

HMOs and MCOs

The idiosyncratic history of medicine in the United States illustrates problems faced by few other nations in determining how best to meet the health needs of its citizens. Unlike many nations, the United States early established private practice, fee-for-service medicine as the model of healthcare delivery, rather than a centrally controlled national health service. Only a few organizations (for instance, the non-profit Kaiser Permanente group) adopted an alternative model: pre-paid direct service medical plans, where membership in a health maintenance organization (HMO) with salaried doctors and proprietary hospitals provided participants with comprehensive care for a fixed annual membership fee. This early corporate model spread after World War II, but was strongly resisted by organized medicine.

Until the mid-1970s the medical system was almost entirely made up of independent practitioners and local non-profit hospitals. Increasing linkages between doctors, hospitals, medical schools, and health insurance companies paved the way for what some observers have called the "corporatization of medicine." This involves several tendencies: greater horizontal integration, as hospitals and other healthcare institutions combine into larger regional and sometimes national systems; greater vertical integration, as organizations dealing with a single level of care join with organizations that handle other types and levels of care; and increasing consolidation, both regionally and nationally. Finally, the greatest difference from earlier models of care delivery is the eclipse of non-profit health care by for-profit health plans, whose success in enrollment in the last 20 years has made them the de facto health policy of contemporary medicine in the USA, despite the salient conflict of interest between the social mission of healthcare provision and the business model of profit seeking.

Health insurance in the USA has been predominantly employer-based, with government taking an increasing role as payer after the introduction of Medicare and Medicaid. As healthcare costs in the USA began to assume a greater and greater share of the gross domestic product, both government and employers began to encourage the growth of managed care organizations (MCOs), characterized by contractual relationships with selected physicians and hospitals, who agree to furnish a specified set of services to enrolled members, either in exchange for a fixed monthly premium or for reduced rates on a fee-for-service basis. The institutional and individual providers typically must accept utilization and quality controls as part of their contract. Those enrolled in an MCO are given financial incentives to use these providers, with "out of network" services either not covered at all or available only at higher out-of-pocket costs. The growth of the managed care organization as a socially sanctioned third-party intermediary between the provider of services and the governmental or employer payer has many ethical implications for physicians, some of which are illustrated in the cases discussed in this chapter.

Who should be the gatekeeper?

Rationing is someone's or some institution's deliberate decision about how to distribute a scarce good among competing persons. Seen in this light, rationing is unavoidable, since there is no healthcare resource that is infinite – be it the time or skill of physicians, the availability of beds or of nursing care, or the financial resources of the patient, the institution, or the society. But the language of "rationing" remains unpopular, at least partly because of its inherent ambiguity and the various polemical uses of the term. Distribution decisions we object to we call "rationing" in the polemical sense, while distribution decisions we agree with we call "appropriate priority setting."

The important question in discussing rationing of healthcare resources is not *whether* to ration – for in that matter there is little choice – but *how* and *where* to ration. It is essential to determine how decisions of distribution are made, and by whom. While cost should not be the only consideration in determining care, ignoring cost is irresponsible in the current healthcare environment, when government, third-party payers, and the general public are exerting pressures to contain rising healthcare costs. Cost-constraint mechanisms are being exerted on the governmental (macro) level, with certificate-of-need laws or state plans for the distribution of (shrinking) Medicaid funds, and on the institutional (meso) level, with utilization reviews or pharmaceutical formulary committees in hospitals, and with financial incentives and quality controls contractually negotiated by managed care organizations and insurance companies. In countries with national health services, a pooled budget limits the cost of health care and provides some guidance for priorities in distribution. This option is not available in the USA.

Some of the resistance to the idea of rationing on the micro or "bedside" level relates to a Hippocratic assumption that it is inappropriate for a physician to refuse to offer a potentially beneficial service to a patient because of its expense alone. Taken literally and without qualification, this may be both impossible and undesirable. But rules or procedures externally imposed upon physicians which constrain their capacity to exercise professional judgment in determining appropriate treatment cannot control costs without seriously damaging the quality of care. Physicians trained in the economics of medical decision making are in the best position to evaluate the benefits of available options, to communicate honestly with their patients about both costs and benefits, and to advocate for their conscientious judgments with decision makers on other levels.

An issue not discussed in this volume is the mechanism of cost control that consists of limiting access to health care altogether. The number of people in the USA who are not insured is large and rising. Healthcare providers who daily confront the human costs of these social policy choices are among those most active in working for change in the current fragmented and inconsistent system. Finding an appropriate balance between cost and quality is a problem that health systems in every nation face. No single "gatekeeper" suffices. The appropriate balance will be found when providers at all levels, from individual physicians to managed care organizations, are equally conscious of and equally responsible for cost, quality, and access. It is toward this balance that the healthcare system is evolving.

FURTHER READING

Robinson, J. C. *The Corporate Practice of Medicine* (Berkeley, CA: University of California Press, 1999).

Rodwin, M. A. Conflicts of interest and accountability in managed care: the aging of medical ethics. *Journal of the American Geriatrics Society* **46** (1998), 338–341.

Russell, B. J. Health-care rationing: critical features, ordinary language and meaning. *Journal of Law, Medicine and Ethics* **30** (2002), 82–87.

Starr, P. *The Social Transformation of American Medicine* (New York, NY: Basic Books, 1982), Chapter 5.

Ubel, P. A. "Rationing" health care: not all definitions are created equal. *Archives of Internal Medicine* **158** (1998), 209–214.

Ubel, P. A. and Arnold, R. The unbearable rightness of bedside rationing: physician duties in a climate of cost containment. *Archives of Internal Medicine* **155** (1995), 1837–1842.

Werhane, P. and Doering, J. Conflicts of interest and conflicts of commitment. *Professional Ethics* **4** (1995), 47–82.

Wong, K. L. *Medicine and the Marketplace: Moral Dimensions of Managed Care* (Notre Dame, IN: University of Notre Dame Press, 1998).

References

Abu-Elmagd, K. and Bond, G. (2003). Gut failure and abdominal visceral transplantation. *Proceedings of the Nutrition Society* **62**, 727–737.

Ad Hoc Committee of the Harvard Medical School (1968). A definition of irreversible coma. *JAMA* **205**, 337–340.

Alecson, D. G. (1995). *Lost Lullaby*. Berkeley, CA: University of California Press.

Allen, M. C., Donohue, P. K., and Dusman A. E. (1993). The limit of viability: neonatal outcome of infants born at 22 to 25 weeks gestation. *New England Journal of Medicine* **329**, 1597–1601.

American Academy of Pediatrics (1987). Guidelines for the determination of death in children. *Pediatrics* **80**, 298–300.

American Academy of Pediatrics Committee on Bioethics (1992). Infants with anencephaly as organ sources: ethical considerations. *Pediatrics* **89**, 1116–1119.

(1995). Informed consent, parental permission, and assent in pediatric practice. *Pediatrics* **95**, 314–317.

American College of Chest Physicians/Society of Critical Care Medicine Consensus Panel (1990). Ethical and moral guidelines for the initiation, continuation, and withdrawal of intensive care. *Chest* **97**, 949–958.

American Medical Association Council on Ethical and Judicial Affairs (1991). Guidelines for the appropriate use of do-not-resuscitate orders. *JAMA* **265**, 1868–1871.

(1993). Report 49: ethical considerations in the allocation of organs and other scarce medical resources among patients. *Code of Medical Ethics Reports* **4** (2), 140–173.

(1995a). The use of anencephalic neonates as organ donors. *JAMA* **273**, 1614–1618.

(1995b). Ethical issues in managed care. *JAMA* **273**, 330–335.

American Thoracic Society Bioethics Task Force (1991). Withholding and withdrawing life-sustaining therapy. *American Review of Respiratory Disease* **144**, 727–731.

Angell, M. (1991). The doctor as double agent. *Kennedy Institute of Ethics Journal* **3**, 279–286.

Annas, G. J. (1994). Asking the courts to set the standard of emergency care: the case of Baby K. *New England Journal of Medicine* **330**, 1542–1545.

(1995). Reframing the debate on health care reform by replacing our metaphors. *New England Journal of Medicine* **332**, 744–747.

(1996). When death is not an end. *New York Times* March 2, 1996.

(2004). Extremely preterm birth and parental authority to refuse treatment – the case of Sidney Miller. *New England Journal of Medicine* **351**, 2118–2123.

Anon. (1997). Japan's parliament approves bill to allow heart, lung, transplants. *San Jose Mercury News* June 18, 1997.

Anspach, R. R. (1993). *Deciding Who Lives: Fateful Choices in the Intensive-Care Nursery.* Berkeley, CA: University of California Press.

Arras, J. (1991). Beyond Cruzan: individual rights, family autonomy and the persistent vegetative state. *Journal of the American Geriatrics Society* **39**, 1018–1024.

Ashwal S., Bale, J. F. Jr., Coulter, D. L., *et al.* (1992). The persistent vegetative state in children: report of the Child Neurology Society Ethics Committee. *Annals of Neurology* **32**, 570–576.

Ashwal, S., Eyman, R. K., and Call, T. L. (1994). Life expectancy of children in a persistent vegetative state. *Pediatric Neurology* **10**, 27–33.

Austin, J. A. (1998). Why patients use alternative medicine: results of a national study. *JAMA* **279**, 1548–1553.

Bailey, L. L., Wood, M., Razzouk. A., Arsdell, G. V., Gundry, S., and the Loma Linda University Pediatric Heart Transplant Group (1989). Heart transplantation during the first 12 years of life. *Archives of Surgery* **124**, 1221–1226.

Bando, K., Turrentine, M. W., Sun, K., *et al.* (1996). Surgical management of hypoplastic left heart syndrome. *Annals of Thoracic Surgery* **62**, 70–77.

Baum, D., Bernstein, D., Starnes, V., *et al.* (1991). Pediatric heart transplantation at Stanford: results of a 15-year experience. *Pediatrics* **88**, 203.

Beath, S. V. (2004). Small bowel transplant. In *Pediatric Gastrointestinal Disease*, 4th edn, ed. W. A. Walker *et al.* Hamilton, Ont: Decker.

Benner, P. (2004). Relational ethics of comfort, touch and solace: endangered arts? *American Journal of Critical Care* **13**, 346–349.

Benner, P. and Wrubel, J. (1989). *The Primacy of Caring.* Menlo Park, CA: Addison-Wesley.

Bernat, J. L., Culver, C. M., and Gert, B. (1981). On the definition and criterion of death. *Annals of Internal Medicine* **94**, 389–394.

(1982). Defining death in theory and practice. *Hastings Center Report* **12**, 5–9.

Bleich, J. D. (1989). The determination of death. *The New York State Task Force on Life and the Law.*

Boucek, M. M., Novick, R. J., Bennett, L. E., Fiol, B., Keck, B. M., and Hosenpud, J. D. (1997). The Registry of the International Society of Heart and Lung Transplantation: first official pediatric report – 1997. *Journal of Heart and Lung Transplantation* **16**, 1189–1206.

Bove, E. L. (1998). Current status of staged reconstruction for hypoplastic left heart syndrome. *Pediatric Cardiology* **19**, 308–315.

Brock, D. W. (1989). Death and dying. In *Medical Ethics: an Introduction*, ed. R. M. Veatch. Boston, MA: Jones and Bartlett.

(1991). The ideal of shared decision making between physicians and patients. *Kennedy Institute of Ethics Journal* **1**, 28–47.

(1995). Justice and the ADA: does prioritizing and rationing health care discriminate against the disabled? *Social Policy and Philosophy* **12**, 159–185.

(2000). Health care, resource prioritization and discrimination against persons with disabilities. In *Americans with Disabilities: Exploring Implications of the Law for Individuals and Institutions*, ed. L. Francis and A. Silvers. New York, NY: Routledge.

Brody, B. (1991). Quality of scholarship in bioethics. *Journal of Medicine and Philosophy* **15**, 161–78.

Brody, H. (1989). Transparency: informed consent in primary care. *Hastings Center Report* **19** (5), 5–9.

Bryk, M. and Siegel, P. T. (1997). My mother caused my illness: the story of a survivor of Munchausen by proxy syndrome. *Pediatrics* **100**, 1–7.

Callahan, D. (1998). Managed care and the goals of medicine. *Journal of the American Geriatrics Society* **46**, 385–388.

Cantor, N. L. (1996). Can healthcare providers obtain judicial intervention against surrogates who demand "medically inappropriate" life support for incompetent patients? *Critical Care Medicine* **24**, 883–887.

Capron, A. M. (1978). Legal definition of death. *Annals of the New York Academy of Sciences* **315**, 349–362.

Childress, J. F. (1982). *Who Should Decide? Paternalism in Health Care.* New York, NY: Oxford University Press.

(1996). Moral norms in practical ethical reflection. In *Christian Ethics: Problems and Prospects*, ed. L. S. Cahill and J. F. Childress. Cleveland, OH: Pilgrim Press.

Churchill, L. R. (1997). "Damaged humanity": The call for a patient-centered medical ethic in the managed care era. *Theoretical Medicine* **18**, 113–126.

Cohen, C. and Benjamin, M. (1991). Alcoholics and liver transplantation. *JAMA* **265**, 1299–1301.

Connelly, R. (2003). Ethical issues in the use of covert video surveillance in the diagnosis of Munchausen syndrome by proxy: the Atlanta study. An ethical challenge for medicine. *HEC Forum* **15**, 21–41.

Cooper, M. C. (1990). Reconceptualizing nursing ethics. *Scholarly Inquiry for Nursing Practice* **4**, 209–221.

(1991). Principle oriented ethics and the ethics of care: a creative tension. *Advances in Nursing Science* **14** (2), 22–31.

Cowart, D. and Burt, R. (1998). Confronting death: who chooses, who controls? *Hastings Center Report* **28** (1), 14–24.

DeBolt, A. J., Stewart, S. M., Kennard, B. D., Petrik, B. D., and Andrews, W. S. (1995). A survey of psychosocial adaptation in long-term survivors of pediatric liver transplants. *Children's Health Care* **24**, 79–96.

Devettere, R. J. (1990). Neocortical death and human death. *Law, Medicine and Hospital Care* **18**, 96–104.

Dicke, W. (1996). Anselm L. Strauss dies at 79: leader in medical sociology. *New York Times* September 16, 1993.

Diekema, D. S. (1995). Unwinding the COBRA: new perspectives on EMTALA. *Pediatric Emergency Care* **11**, 243–248.

Diem, S. J., Lantos, J. D., and Tulsky, J. A. (1996). Cardiopulmonary resuscitation on television: miracles and misinformation. *New England Journal of Medicine* **334**, 1578–1605.

Donn, S. M. (1996). Neonatal resuscitation. In *Risk Management Techniques in Perinatal and Neonatal Practice*, ed. S. M. Donn and C. W. Fisher. Armonk, NY: Futura Press, pp. 391–405.

Dresser, R. and Robertson, J. (1989). Quality of life and non-treatment decisions for incompetent patients: a critique of the orthodox approach. *Law, Medicine and Health Care* **17**, 234–244.

Duff, R. S. (1987). "Close-up" versus "distant" ethics: deciding the care of infants with poor prognosis. *Seminars in Perinatology* **11**, 244–253.

Dunn, P. M. and Levinson, W. (1996). Discussing futility with patients and families. *Journal of General Internal Medicine* **11**, 689–93.

Dworkin, G. (1983a). Paternalism. In *Paternalism*, ed. R. Sartorius. Minneapolis, MN: University of Minnesota Press, pp. 19–34.

   (1983b). Paternalism: some second thoughts. In *Paternalism*, ed. R. Sartorius. Minneapolis, MN: University of Minnesota Press, pp. 105–112.

   (1998). *The Theory and Practice of Autonomy*. Cambridge: Cambridge University Press.

Dworkin, R. B. (1973). Death in context. *Indiana Law Journal* **48**, 623–639.

   (1993). *Life's Dominion*. New York, NY: Knopf.

Eisenberg, D. M., Kessler, R. C., Foster, C., Norlock, F. E., Calkins, D. R., and Delbanco, T. L. (1993). Unconventional medicine in the United States. *New England Journal of Medicine* **328**, 246–252.

Ellsbury, K. E. and Montano, D. E. (1990). Attitudes of Washington state primary care physicians toward capitation-based insurance plans. *Journal of Family Practice* **30**, 89–94.

Ellsbury, K. E., Montano, D. E., and Manders, D. (1987). Primary care physicians' attitudes about gatekeeping. *Journal of Family Practice* **25**, 616–619.

Ellsbury, K. E., Montano, D. E., and Krafft, K. (1990). A survey of the attitudes of physician specialists toward capitation-based health plans with primary care gatekeepers. *Quality Review Bulletin* **16**, 294–300.

Emanuel, E. J. (1995). Medical ethics in the era of managed care: the need for institutional structures instead of principles for individual cases. *Journal of Clinical Ethics* **6**, 335–338.

Emanuel, E. J. and Emanuel L. L. (1992). Four models of the physician–patient relationship. *JAMA* **267**, 2221–2226.

Emanuel, E. J. and Steiner D. (1995). Institutional conflict of interest. *New England Journal of Medicine* **332**, 262–267.

Emanuel, L. L., Barry, M. J., Stoeckle, J. D., Ettelson, L. M., and Emanuel, E. J. (1991). Advance directives for medical care: a case for greater use. *New England Journal of Medicine* **324**, 889–895.

Engelhardt, H. T. J. (1996). *The Foundations of Bioethics*, 2nd edn. New York, NY: Oxford University Press.

Faber-Langedoen, K. (1994). The clinical management of dying patients receiving mechanical ventilation. *Chest* **106**, 880–888.

Faden, R. R., Beauchamp, T. L., and King, N. M. P. (1986). *A History and Theory of Informed Consent*. New York, NY: Oxford University Press.

Fadiman, A. (1997). *The Spirit Catches You and You Fall Down: a Hmong Child, her American Doctors, and the Collision of Two Cultures.* New York, NY: Farrar, Straus and Giroux.

Farrell, M. M. and Levin, D. L. (1993). Brain death in the pediatric patient: historical, sociological, medical, religious, cultural, legal and ethical considerations. *Critical Care Medicine* 21, 1951–1965.

Fletcher, J. C., Lombardo, P. A., Marshall, M. F., and Miller, F. G. (1997). *Introduction to Clinical Ethics*, 2nd edn. Frederick, MD: University Publishing Group.

Foreman, E. N. and Ladd, R. E. (1991). *Ethical Dilemmas in Pediatrics: a Case Study Approach.* Lanham, MD: University Press of America.

Fost, N. C. (1995). Medical futility: commentary. In *Ethics and Perinatology*, ed. A. Goldworth, W, Silverman, D. K. Stevenson, and E. W. D. Young. New York, NY: Oxford University Press, pp. 70–81.

Fost, N. C., Chudwin, D., and Wikler, D. (1980). The limited moral significance of "fetal viability." *Hastings Center Report* 10 (6), 10–13.

Fox, E. and Stocking, C. (1993). Ethics consultants' recommendations for life-prolonging treatment of patients in a persistent vegetative state. *JAMA* 270, 2578–2582.

Frader, J. E. and Caniano, D. A. (1998). Research and innovation in surgery. In *Surgical Ethics*, ed. L. B. McCullough, J. W. Jones, and B. A. Brody. New York, NY: Oxford University Press, pp. 216–241.

Frader, J. E. and Thompson, A. (1994). Ethical issues in the pediatric intensive care unit. *Pediatric Clinics of North America* 41, 1405–1421.

Fried, C. (1975). Rights and health care: beyond equity and efficiency. *New England Journal of Medicine* 293, 241–245.

Friedman, J. A. (1990). Taking the camel by the nose: the anencephalic as a source for pediatric organ transplants. *Columbia Law Review* 90, 917–978.

Fyler, D. C., Rothman, K. J., Buckley, L. P., Cohn, H. E., Hellenbrand, W. E., and Castaneda, A. (1981). The determinants of 5 year survival of infants with critical congenital heart disease. In *Pediatric Cardiovascular Disease*, ed. M. A. Engle. Philadelphia, PA: Davis, pp. 393–405.

Gadow, S. (1983). Existential advocacy: philosophical foundations of nursing. In *Nursing: Images and Ideals*, ed. S. F. Spiker and S. Gadow. New York, NY: Springer, pp. 79–101.

Gaylin, W. (1974). Harvesting the dead. *Harpers (New York)* 249 (1492), 23–28.

Gaynon, P. S., Qu, P. R., Chappell, R. J., *et al.* (1998). Survival after relapse in childhood acute lymphoblastic leukemia: impact of site and time to first relapse – the Children's Cancer Group Experience. *Cancer* 82, 1387–1395.

Gervais, K. G. (1995). Death, definition and determination of perspectives. In *Encyclopedia of Bioethics*, ed. W. T. Reich, rev. edn. New York, NY: Macmillan, pp. 540–549.

Gillick, M. R., Hesse, K., and Mazzapica, N. (1993). Medical technology at the end of life: what would physicians and nurses want for themselves? *Archives of Internal Medicine* 153, 2542–2547.

Grady, D. (1998). Articles question safety of dietary supplements. *New York Times* September 17, 1998.

Grant, D. (1989). Intestinal transplantation: current status. *Transplant Proceedings* 21, 2869–2871.

Gutgesell, H. P. and Massaro, T. A. (1995). Management of hypoplastic left heart syndrome in a consortium of university hospitals. *American Journal of Cardiology* **76**, 809–811.

Hall, M. A. (1994). Rationing health care at the bedside. *New York Law Review* **69**, 693–780.

Halevy, A. and Brody, B. A. (1996). A multi-institution collaborative policy on medical futility. *JAMA* **276**, 571–574.

Hastings Center (1987). *Guidelines on the Termination of Life-Sustaining Treatment and the Care of the Dying*. Bloomington, IN: Indiana University Press.

Hehrlein, F. W., Yamamoto, T., Orime, Y., and Bauer, J. (1998). Hypoplastic left heart syndrome: which is the best operative strategy? *Annals of Thoracic and Cardiovascular Surgery* **4**, 125–132.

Hemenway, D., Killen, A., Cashman, S. B., Parks, C. L., and Bicknell, W. J. (1990). Physicians' responses to financial incentives: evidence from a for-profit ambulatory care center. *New England Journal of Medicine* **322**, 1059–1063.

Hillman, A. L. (1987). Financial incentives for physicians in HMOs: is there a conflict of interest? *New England Journal of Medicine* **317**, 1743–1748.

Hillman, A. L., Pauly, M. V., and Kerstein, J. J. (1989). How do financial incentives affect physicians' clinical decisions and the financial performance of health maintenance organizations? *New England Journal of Medicine* **321**, 86–92.

Horning, S. J., Chao, N. J., Negrin, R. S., *et al.* (1997). High-dose therapy and autologous hematopoietic progenitor cell transplantation for recurrent or refractory Hodgkin's disease: analysis of the Stanford University results and prognostic indices. *Blood* **89**, 801–813.

Howard, L. and Malone, M. (1996). Current status of home parenteral nutrition in the United States. *Transplant Proceedings* **28**, 2691–2695.

Howe, E. G. (1995). Managed care: "new moves," moral uncertainty, and a radical attitude. *Journal of Clinical Ethics* **6**, 290–305.

Huxtable, R. J. (1992). The myth of beneficent nature: the risks of herbal preparations. *Annals of Internal Medicine* **117**, 165–166.

Iannettoni, M. D., Bove, E. L., Mosca, R. S., *et al.* (1994). Improving results with first-stage palliation for hypoplastic left heart syndrome. *Journal of Thoracic and Cardiovascular Surgery* **107**, 934–940.

Institute of Medicine (1997). *Approaching Death: Improving Care at the End of Life*. Washington, DC: National Academy Press.

International Working Party (1996). *Report on the Vegetative State*. London: Royal Hospital for Neuro-disability.

Jecker, N. S. (1990). Integrating medical ethics with normative theory: patient advocacy and social responsibility. *Theoretical Medicine* **11**, 125–139.

(1995). Business ethics and the ethics of managed care. *Trends in Health Care, Law and Ethics* **10**, 51–66.

Jecker, N. S. and Jonsen, A. R. (1997). Managed care: a house of mirrors. *Journal of Clinical Ethics* **8**, 230–241.

Johnson, G. T. (1990). Restoring trust between patient and doctor. *New England Journal of Medicine* **322**, 195–197.

Joint Commission for Accreditation of Healthcare Organizations (1997). *Patient Rights and Organization Ethics: Comprehensive Manual for Hospitals.* Chicago, IL: JCAHO, R 1–32.

Jonsen, A. R. (1986). Blood transfusions and Jehovah's witnesses: the impact of the patient's unusual beliefs in critical care. *Critical Care Clinics* **2**, 91–99.

Kant, I. (1983). The metaphysical principles of virtue (Part II of *The Metaphysics of Morals*), trans. J. W. Ellington. In *Kant's Ethical Philosophy*. Indianapolis, IN: Hackett.

Kassirer, J. P. (1993). Medicine at center stage. *New England Journal of Medicine* **328**, 1268–1269.

Katon, W. and Kleinman, A. (1981). Negotiation and other social science strategies in patient care. In *The Relevance of Social Science for Medicine*, ed. L. Eisenberg and A. Kleinman. Dordrecht: D. Reidel, pp. 253–79.

Katz, J. (1984). *The Silent World of Doctor and Patient.* New York, NY: The Free Press.

Keengwe, I. N., Stansfield, F., Eden, O. B., Nelhans, N. D., Dearlove, O. R., and Sharples, A. (1999). Paediatric oncology and intensive care treatments: changing trends. *Archives of Disease in Childhood* **80**, 553–555.

Kelly, G. (1951). The duty to preserve life. *Theological Studies* **12**, 550.

Kern, J. H., Hayes, C. J., Michler, R. E., Gersony, W. M., and Quaegebeur, J. M. (1997). Survival and risk factor analysis for the Norwood procedure for hypoplastic left heart syndrome. *American Journal of Cardiology* **80**, 170–174.

King, N. M. P. (1992). Transparency in neonatal intensive care. *Hastings Center Report* **22** (3), 18–25.

King, N. M. P. and Cross, A. W. (1989). Children as decision makers: guidelines for pediatricians. *Journal of Pediatrics* **115**, 10–16.

Kocoshis, S. A. (1994). Small bowel transplantation in infants and children. *Gastroenterology Clinics of North America* **23**, 727–742.

(2001). Small intestinal failure in children. *Current Science* **4**, 423–442.

Kon, A. A., Ackerson, L., and Lo, B. (2003). Choices physicians would make if they were the parents of a child with hypoplastic left heart syndrome. *American Journal of Cardiology* **91**, 1506–1509.

Kopelman, L. M., Irons, T. G., and Kopelman, A. E. (1988). Neonatologists judge the "Baby Doe" regulations. *New England Journal of Medicine* **318**, 677–683.

Langnas, A. N. (2004). Advances in small intestine transplantation. *Transplantation* **77**, S75–S78.

Lannoye, P. (1994). *The State of Complementary Medicine.* Draft report. Brussels: European Parliament Committee on the Environment, Public Health and Consumer Protection.

Leikin, S. A. (1989). A proposal concerning decisions to forgo life-sustaining treatment for young people. *Journal of Pediatrics* **115**, 17–22.

Lempinen, E. (1997). State's care of disabled assailed. *San Francisco Chronicle* February 26, 1997.

Lerer, R. J. (1990). For three years, I treated the wrong patient. *Medical Economics* **5**, 54–59.

Lesko, L. M., Dermatis, H. L., Penman, D., and Holland, J. C. (1989). Patients', parents' and oncologists' perceptions of informed consent for bone marrow transplantation. *Medical and Pediatric Oncology* **17**, 181–187.

Lewith, G. T. and Watkins, A. D. (1996). Unconventional therapies in asthma: an overview. *Allergy* **51**, 761–769.

Liever, L. (ed.) (1989). *Dax's Case: Essays in Medical Ethics and Human Meaning.* Dallas, TX: Southern Methodist University Press.

Lillehei, R. G., Goott, B., and Miller, F. A. (1959). The physiological response of the small bowel of the dog to ischemia including prolonged *in vitro* preservation of the bowel with successful replacement and survival. *Annals of Surgery* **150**, 543–560.

Lloyd, G. E. R. (ed.) (1978). *Hippocratic Writings.* New York, NY: Penguin Classics.

Luce, J. M. (1995). Physicians do not have a responsibility to provide futile or unreasonable care if a patient or family insists. *Critical Care Medicine* **23**, 760–766.

  (1997a). Making decisions about the forgoing of life-sustaining therapy. *American Journal of Respiratory Critical Care Medicine* **156**, 1715–1718.

  (1997b). Withholding and withdrawal of life support: ethical, legal, and clinical aspects. *New Horizons* **5**, 30–37.

Ludwig, S. (1995). The role of the physician. In *Munchausen Syndrome by Proxy: Issues in Diagnosis and Treatment*, ed. A. V. Levin and M. S. Sheridan. New York, NY: Lexington Books, pp. 287–294.

Lundberg, G. D. (1995). The failure of organized health system reform – now what? *Caveat aeger –* Let the patient beware. *JAMA* **273**, 1539–1541.

Lynch, B. J., Glauser, T. A., Canter, C., and Spray, T. (1994). Neurologic complications of pediatric heart transplantation. *Archives of Pediatrics and Adolescent Medicine* **148**, 973–979.

MacIntyre, A. (1998). *Dependent Rational Animals: Why Human Beings Need the Virtues.* Chicago, IL: Open Court.

Mallory, G. B. and Stillwell, P. C. (1991). The ventilator-dependent child: issues in diagnosis and management. *Archives of Physical Medicine and Rehabilitation* **72**, 43–55.

Malloy, T. R., Wigton, R. S., Meeske, J., and Tape, T. G. (1992). The influence of treatment descriptions on advance medical directive decisions. *Journal of the American Geriatrics Society* **40**, 1255–1260.

Marshall, P. A. (1992). Anthropology and bioethics. *Medical Anthropology Quarterly* **6**, 49–73.

Martin, J. A. and Bjerknes, L. K. (1996). The legal and ethical implications of gag clauses in physician contracts. *American Journal of Law and Medicine* **12**, 433–476.

May, W. F. (1992). The beleaguered rulers: the public obligation of the professional. *Kennedy Institute of Ethics Journal* **2**, 25–41.

McClure, R. J., Davis, P. M., Meadow, R., and Sibert, J. R. (1996). Epidemiology of Munchausen syndrome by proxy, non-accidental poisoning, and non-accidental suffocation. *Archives of Diseases in Childhood* **75**, 57–61.

McCullough, L. B. and Chervenak, F. A. (1994). *Ethics in Obstetrics and Gynecology.* New York, NY: Oxford University Press.

Meadow, R. (1977). Munchausen syndrome by proxy: the hinterland of child abuse. *Lancet* **2**, 343–345.

Medical Task Force on Anencephaly (1990). The infant with anencephaly. *New England Journal of Medicine* **322**, 669–674.

Mejia, R. E. and Pollack, M. M. (1995). Variability in brain death determination practices in children. *JAMA* **274**, 550–553.

Melnick, M. and Myrianthopoulos, N. C. (1987). Studies in neural tube defects II. *American Journal of Medical Genetics* **26**, 797–810.

Merrick, J. C. (1995). Critically ill newborns and the law: the American experience. *Journal of Legal Medicine* **16**, 189–209.

Michaels, M. G., Frader, J., and Armitage, J. (1993). Ethical considerations in listing fetuses as candidates for neonatal heart transplantation. *JAMA* **269**, 401–403.

Micozzi, M. S. (1996). *Fundamentals of Complementary and Alternative Medicine*. New York, NY: Churchill Livingstone.

Miller, F. G. and Fins, J. J. (1996). Sounding board: a proposal to restructure hospital care for dying patients. *New England Journal of Medicine* **334**, 1740–1742.

Miller, G., Tesman, J. R., Ramer, J. C., Baylen, B. G., and Myers, J. L. (1996). Outcome after open-heart surgery in infants and children. *Journal of Child Neurology* **11**, 49–53.

Miller, R. B. (1996a). Love and death in a pediatric intensive care unit. *Annual of the Society of Christian Ethics* **16**, 21–39.

(1996b). *Casuistry and Modern Ethics: a Poetics of Practical Reasoning*. Chicago, IL: University of Chicago Press, 1996.

(2003). *Children, Ethics and Modern Medicine*. Bloomington, IN: Indiana University Press.

Milstein, A. (1997). Managing utilization management. *Health Affairs* **16**, 87–90.

Mitchell, I. (1995). Research in Munchausen syndrome by proxy. In *Munchausen Syndrome by Proxy: Issues in Diagnosis and Treatment*, ed. A. V. Levin and M. S. Sheridan. New York, NY: Lexington Books, pp. 423–431.

Morreim, E. H. (1991). Economic disclosure and economic advocacy: new duties in the medical standard of care. *Journal of Legal Medicine* **12**, 275–329.

(1994). Profoundly diminished life: the casualties of coercion. *Hastings Center Report* **24** (1), 33–42.

(1995). *Balancing Act: the New Medical Ethics of Medicine's New Economics*. Washington, DC: Georgetown University Press.

(1997). To tell the truth: disclosing the incentives and limits of managed care. *American Journal of Managed Care* **3**, 35–43.

Morrow, W. R., Naftel, D., Chinnock, R., *et al.* (1997). Outcome of listing for heart transplantation in infants younger than six months: predictors of death and interval to transplantation. *Journal of Heart and Lung Transplantation* **16**, 1255–1266.

Moscowitz, E. H. and Nelson, J. L. (1995). The best laid plans. *Hastings Center Report*. Special supplement, November–December, S3–S6.

Moss, A. H. and Siegler, M. (1991). Should alcoholics compete equally for liver transplantation? *JAMA* **265**, 1295–1298.

Multi-Society Task Force on PVS (1994). Medical aspects of the persistent vegetative state. *New England Journal of Medicine* **330**, 1499–1508, 1572–1579.

Murray, T. H. (1996). *The Worth of a Child*. Berkeley, CA: University of California Press.

Murphy, D. J. and Barbour, E. (1994). GUIDe: a community effort to define futile and inappropriate care. *New Horizons* **2**, 326–331.

Natowicz, M., Chatten, J., Clancy, R., *et al.* (1988). Genetic disorders and major extracardiac anomalies associated with the hypoplastic left heart syndrome. *Pediatrics* **82**, 698–706.

Nelson, H. L. and Nelson, J. L. (1995). *The Patient in the Family: an Ethics of Medicine and Families.* New York, NY: Routledge.

Nelson, L. J., Rushton, C. H., Cranford, R. E., Nelson, R. M., Glover, J. J., and Truog, R. D. (1995). Forgoing medically provided nutrition and hydration in pediatric patients. *Journal of Law, Medicine and Ethics* 23, 33–46.

Nichols, D. G., Walker, L. K., Wingard, J. R., *et al.* (1994). Predictors of acute respiratory failure after bone marrow transplantation in children. *Critical Care Medicine* 22, 1485–1491.

Nitschke, R., Humphrey, G. B., Sexauer, C. L., *et al.* (1982). Therapeutic choices made by patients with end-stage cancer. *Journal of Pediatrics* 101, 471–476.

Nixon, J. and Pearn, J. (1977). Emotional sequelae of parents and sibs following the drowning or near-drowning of a child. *Australian and New Zealand Journal of Psychiatry* 11, 265–268.

Norwood, W. I., Jacobs, M. L., and Murphy, J. D. (1992). Fontan procedure for hypoplastic left heart syndrome. *Annals of Thoracic Surgery* 54, 1025–1030.

OPTN (2003). *Organ Procurement and Transplantation Network/Scientific Registry of Transplantation Recipients Annual Report.* www.optn.org/data/Annualreport.asp [visited February 14, 2005].

Orentlicher, D. (1995). Physician advocacy for patients under managed care. *Journal of Clinical Ethics* 6, 311–314.

  (1996a). Destructuring disability: rationing of health care and discrimination. *Harvard Civil Rights and Civil Liberties Law Review* 31 (1).

  (1996b). Paying physicians more to do less: financial incentives to limit care. *University of Richmond Law Review* 30, 155–197.

  (2000). Utility, equality and health care needs of persons with disabilities: interpreting the ADA's requirement of reasonable accommodation. In *Americans with Disabilities*, ed. L. Francis and A. Silvers. New York, NY: Routledge, pp. 236–243.

Pachter, L. M. (1994). Culture and clinical care: folk illness beliefs and behaviors and their implications for health care delivery. *JAMA* 271, 690–694.

Pahl, E., Fricker, F. J., Armitage, J., *et al.* (1989). Coronary arteriosclerosis in pediatric heart transplant survivors: limitation of long-term survival. *Journal of Pediatrics* 116, 177–183.

Pallis, C. (1982). ABC of brain stem death: reappraising death. *British Medical Journal* 285, 1409–1412.

Pearson, L. (1997). Family-centered care and the anticipated death of a newborn. *Pediatric Nursing* 23, 178–182.

Pellegrino, E. D. (1986). Rationing health care: the ethics of medical gatekeeping. *Journal of Contemporary Health Law and Policy* 2, 23–45.

  (1994). Words can hurt you: some reflections on the metaphors of managed care. *Journal of the American Board of Family Practice* 7, 505–510.

  (1995a). Guarding the integrity of medical ethics: some lessons from Soviet Russia. *JAMA* 273, 1622–1623.

  (1995b). Interests, obligations, and justice: some notes toward an ethic of managed care. *Journal of Clinical Ethics* 6, 312–317.

Pellegrino, E. D. and Thomasma, D. C. (1988). *For the Patient's Good: Toward the Restoration of Beneficence in Health Care*. New York, NY: Oxford University Press.

(1994). *The Virtues in Medical Practice*. New York, NY: Oxford University Press.

Penticuff, J. (1997). Nursing perspectives in bioethics. In *Japanese and Western Bioethics: Studies in Moral Diversity*, ed. K. Hoshino. Boston, MA: Kluwer, pp. 49–60.

Piecuch, R. E., Leonard, C. H., Cooper, B. A., Kilpatrick, S. J., Schlueter, M. A., and Sola, A. (1997). Outcome of infants born at 24–26 weeks' gestation. II. Neurodevelopmental outcome. *Obstetrics and Gynecology* **90**, 809–814.

Pillans, P. I. (1995). Toxicity of herbal products. *New Zealand Medical Journal* **108**, 469–471.

Pisetsky, D. S. (1998). Doing everything. *Annals of Internal Medicine* **128**, 869–870.

Prendergast, T. J. (1995). Futility and the common cold: how requests for antibiotics can illuminate care at the end of life. *Chest* **107**, 836–844.

Prendergast, T. J. and Luce, J. M. (1997). Increasing incidence of withholding and withdrawal of life support from the critically ill. *American Journal of Respiratory Care Medicine* **155**, 15–20.

Present, P. (1987). *Child Drowning Study: a Report on the Epidemiology of Drownings in Residential Pools to Children Under Age Five*. Washington, DC: Directorate for Epidemiology, US Consumer Product Safety Commission.

President's Commission for the Study of Ethical Problems in Medicine and Biomedical and Behavioral Research (1982). *Making Health Care Decisions: the Ethical and Legal Implications of Informed Consent in the Patient–Practitioner Relationship*. Washington, DC: Government Printing Office.

(1983). *Deciding to Forego Life-Sustaining Treatment: a Report on Ethical, Medical, and Legal Issues in Treatment Decisions*. Washington DC: Government Printing Office.

Purtillo, R. B. (1995). Managed care: ethical issues for the rehabilitation of patients. *Trends in Health Care, Law, and Ethics* **10**, 105–108, 118.

Quill, T. (1991). Death and dignity: a case of individualized decision making. *New England Journal of Medicine* **324**, 691–694.

Ramsey, P. (1970). *The Patient as Person*. New Haven, CT: Yale University Press.

Rappaport, L. A., Bellinger, D., and Wypij, D. (1996). Developmental findings at one year. In *Brain Injury and Pediatric Cardiac Surgery*, ed. R. A. Jonas, J. W. Newburger, and J. J. Volpe. Boston, MA: Butterworth–Heinemann, pp. 341–351.

Razzouk, A., Chinnock, R. E., Gundry, S. R., *et al.* (1996). Transplantation as a primary treatment for hypoplastic left heart syndrome: intermediate-term results. *Annals of Thoracic Surgery* **62**, 1–8.

Reilly, R. B., Teasdale, T. A., and McCullough, L. B. (1994). Projecting patients' preferences from living wills: an invalid strategy for management of dementia with life-threatening illness. *Journal of the American Geriatric Society* **42**, 997–1003.

Reiser, S. J. (1994). The ethical life of health care organizations. *Hastings Center Report* **24** (6), 28–35.

Relman, A. S. (1992). What market values are doing to medicine. *Atlantic Monthly* **269** (3), 99–106.

Rhodes, R. and Holzman, I. (2004). The not unreasonable standard in the assessment of surrogates and surrogate decisions. *Theoretical Medicine and Bioethics* **25**, 367–385.

Rhodes, R., Miller, C., and Schwartz, M. (1992). Transplant recipient selection: peacetime vs. wartime triage. *Cambridge Quarterly of Healthcare Ethics* **4**, 327–331.

Richardson, H. S. (1990). Specifying norms as a way to resolve concrete ethical problems. *Philosophy and Public Affairs* **19**, 279–310.

Risser, A. L. and Mazur, L. J. (1995). Use of folk remedies in a hispanic population. *Archives of Pediatric and Adolescent Medicine* **149**, 978–981.

Robertson, J. A. (1975). Involuntary euthanasia of defective newborns: a legal analysis. *Stanford Law Review* **27**, 217.

Robertson, J. A. and Fost, N. (1976). Passive euthanasia of defective newborn infants: legal considerations. *Journal of Pediatrics* **88**, 883–889.

Rodwin, M. A. (1995). Conflicts in managed care. *New England Journal of Medicine* **332**, 604–607.

Rogers, B. T., Msall, M. E., Buck, G. M., *et al.* (1995). Neurodevelopmental outcome of infants with hypoplastic left heart syndrome. *Journal of Pediatrics* **126**, 496–498.

Rosenberg, D. A. (1987). Web of deceit: a literature review of Munchausen syndrome by proxy. *Child Abuse and Neglect* **11**, 547–563.

Ross, L. F. (1998). *Children, Families and Health Care Decision Making.* Oxford: Oxford University Press.

Roulet, M., Laurini, R., Rivier, L., and Calame, A. (1988). Hepatic veno-occlusive disease in newborn infant of a woman drinking herbal tea. *Journal of Pediatrics* **112**, 433–436.

Schneider, C. E. (1998). *The Practice of Autonomy: Patients, Doctors, and Medical Decisions.* New York, NY: Oxford University Press.

Shaw, A. (1977). Defining the quality of life: a formula without numbers. *Hastings Center Report* **7** (5), 11.

Shillington, P. (1995). John's will. *Miami Herald* December 9, 1995.

Siegler, M. (1979). Clinical ethics and clinical medicine. *Archives of Internal Medicine* **139**, 914–915.

Silverman, W. A. (1998). *Where's the Evidence? Debates in Modern Medicine.* Oxford: Oxford University Press.

Silvers, A., Wasserman, D., and Mahowald, M. (1998). *Disability, Difference, Discrimination: Perspectives on Justice in Bioethics and Public Policy.* Lanham, MD: Rowman and Littlefield.

Sinclair, J. C. and Torrance, G. W. (1995). The use of epidemiological data for prognostication and decision making. In *Ethics and Perinatology*, ed. A. Goldworth, W. Silverman, D. K. Stevenson, and E. W. D. Young. New York, NY: Oxford University Press, pp. 120–145.

Slater, J. A. (1994). Psychiatric aspects of organ transplantation in children and adolescents. *Child and Adolescent Psychiatric Clinics of North America* **3**, 557–598.

Society of Critical Care Medicine Task Force on Ethics (1990). Consensus report on the ethics of foregoing life-sustaining treatments in the critically ill. *Critical Care Medicine* **18**, 1435–1439.

Solomon, M. Z., O'Donnell, L., Jennings, B., *et al.* (1993). Decisions near the end of life: professional views on life-sustaining treatments. *American Journal of Public Health* **83**, 14–23.

Southall, D. P., Plunkett, M. C. B., Banks, M. W., *et al.* (1997). Covert video recordings of life threatening child abuse: lessons for child protection. *Pediatrics* **100**, 735–760.

Spencer, E. M., Mills, A. E., Rorty, M. V., and Werhane, P. H. (2000). *Organization Ethics in Health Care.* New York, NY: Oxford University Press.

Sprung, C. L. and Eidelman, L. A. (1996). Judicial intervention in medical decision-making: a failure of the medical system? *Critical Care Medicine* **24**, 730–732.

Sprung, C. E., Eidelman, L. A., and Steinberg, A. (1995). Is the physician's duty to the individual patient or to society? *Critical Care Medicine* **23**, 618–620.

Stahlman, M. (1995). Withholding and withdrawing therapy and actively hastening death I. In *Ethics and Perinatology*, ed. A. Goldworth, W. Silverman, D. K. Stevenson, and E. W. D. Young. New York, NY: Oxford University Press, pp. 163–171.

Stefanovic, V. and Polenakovic, M. H. (1991). Balkan nephropathy: kidney disease beyond the Balkans. *American Journal of Nephrology* **11**, 1–11.

Stone, D. A. (1997). The doctor as businessman: the changing politics of a cultural icon. *Journal of Health Politics, Policy and Law* **22**, 533–556.

Sullivan, W. M. (1995). *Work and Integrity: the Crisis and Promise of Professionalism in America.* New York, NY: Basic Books.

Susman, E. J., Dorn, L. D., and Fletcher, J. C. (1987). Reasoning about illness in ill and healthy children and adolescents: cognitive and emotional developmental aspects. *Journal of Developmental and Behavioral Pediatrics* **8**, 266–273.

  (1992). Participation in biomedical research: the consent process as viewed by children, adolescents, young adults and physicians. *Journal of Pediatrics* **121**, 547–552.

Taylor, C. (1992). *Multiculturalism and "the Politics of Recognition."* Princeton, NJ: Princeton University Press.

  (1995). To follow a rule. In *Philosophical Arguments*. Cambridge, MA: Harvard University Press.

Thomasma, D. C. (1995). The ethics of managed care and cost control. *Trends in Health Care, Law and Ethics* **10**, 33–36, 44.

Todres, I. D. (1992). Ethical dilemmas in pediatric critical care. *Critical Care Clinics* **8**, 219–227.

Tomaske, M., Bosk, A., Eyrich, M., Bader, P., and Niethammer, D. (2003). Risks of mortality in children admitted to the paediatric intensive care unit after haematopoietic stem cell transplantation. *British Journal of Haematology* **121**, 886–891.

Tomlinson, T. and Czlonka, D. (1995). Futility and hospital policy. *Hastings Center Report* **25** (3), 28–35.

Tong, R. (1998). The ethics of care: a feminist virtue ethics of care for healthcare practitioners. *Journal of Medicine and Philosophy* **23**, 131–152.

Trent, J. (1994). *Inventing the Feeble Mind: a History of Mental Retardation in the United States.* Berkeley, CA: University of California Press.

Tresch, D. D., Sims, F. H., Duthie, E. H., and Goldstein, M. D. (1991). Patients in a persistent vegetative state: attitudes and reactions of family members. *Journal of the American Geriatric Society* **39**, 17–21.

Tronto, J. (1999). Care ethics: moving forward. *Hypatia* **14**, 112–119.

Truog, R. D. (1997). Is it time to abandon brain death? *Hastings Center Report* **27** (1), 29–37.

Truog, R. D. and Fletcher, J. C. (1990). Brain death and the anencephalic newborn. *Bioethics* **4**, 200–215.

Truog, R. D., Brett, A. S., and Frader, J. (1992). The problem with futility. *New England Journal of Medicine* **326**, 1560–1564.

Tzakis, A. G., Nery, J. R., Weppler, D., *et al.* (1998). Mycophenolate mofetil in combination with FK506 and steroids for intestinal transplantation. *American Society for Parenteral and Enteral Nutrition*, 22nd Congress Program Book, pp. 336–342.

United Network for Organ Sharing (UNOS) (1992). Minutes: Ethics Committee. Policy statement from the United Network of Organ Sharing Ethics Committee meeting on January 27, 1992.

Vanderhoof, J. A. (1996). Short bowel syndrome in children and small intestinal transplantation. *Pediatric Clinics of North America* **43**, 533–550.

Vanderpool, H. Y. (1995). Death and dying: euthanasia and sustaining life. In *Encyclopedia of Bioethics*, ed. W. T. Reich, rev. edn. New York, NY: Macmillan, pp. 554–563.

Van DeVeer, D. (1980). Autonomy respecting paternalism. *Social Theory and Practice* **6**, 187–207.

Veatch, R. M. (1986). Defining death anew: technical and ethical problems. In *Ethical Issues in Death and Dying*, 2nd edn., ed. R. F. Weir. New York, NY: Columbia University Press, pp. 59–79.

(1989). Allocating organs by utilitarianism is seen as favoring whites over blacks. *Kennedy Institute of Ethics Newsletter* **3** (3), 1–3.

Walters, J., Ashwal, S., and Masek, T. (1997). Anencephaly: where do we now stand? *Seminars in Neurology* **17**, 249–255.

Watson, J. (1988). *Nursing: Human Science and Human Care*. Boston, MA: Jones and Bartlett.

Weir, R. F. (1984). *Selective Nontreatment of Handicapped Newborns: Moral Dilemmas in Neonatal Medicine*. New York, NY: Oxford University Press.

Weir, R. F. (1995). Withholding and withdrawing therapy and actively hastening death II. In *Ethics and Perinatology*, ed. A. Goldworth, W. Silverman, D. K. Stevenson, and E. W. D. Young. New York, NY: Oxford University Press, pp. 172–183.

Whitney, S. N., McGuire, A. L., and McCullough, L. B. (2004). A typology of shared decision making, informed consent, and simple consent. *Annals of Internal Medicine* **140**, 54–59.

Wilde, J. A. and Pedron, A. T. (1993). Privacy rights in Munchausen syndrome. *Contemporary Pediatrics* (November 1993), 86.

Winkenwerder, W. and Ball, J. R. (1988). Transformation of American health care: the role of the medical profession. *New England Journal of Medicine* **318**, 317–319.

Wintemute, G. J. (1990). Childhood drowning and near-drowning in the United States. *American Journal of Diseases of Children* **144**, 663–669.

Woolhandler, S. and Himmelstein, D. U. (1995). Extreme risk: the new corporate proposition for physicians. *New England Journal of Medicine* **333**, 1706–1708.

Yarmolinsky, A. (1995). Supporting the patient. *New England Journal of Medicine* **332**, 602–603.

Zamula, W. W. (1987). *Social Costs of Drownings and Near-Drownings from Submersion Accidents Occurring to Children Under Five in Residential Swimming Pools*. Washington, DC: Directorate for Economic Analysis, US Consumer Product Safety Commission.

Zitelli, B. J., Seltman, M. F., and Shannon, R. M. (1987). Munchausen's syndrome by proxy and its professional participants. *American Journal of Diseases of Children* **141**, 1099–1102.

Zoloth-Dorfman, L. and Rubin, S. (1995). The patient as commodity: managed care and the question of ethics. *Journal of Clinical Ethics* **6**, 339–357.

Index